Hospital Volume, Physician Volume, and Patient Outcomes

Harold S. Luft
Deborah W. Garnick
David H. Mark
Stephen J. McPhee

Hospital Volume, Physician Volume, and Patient Outcomes

Assessing the Evidence

Health Administration Press Perspectives
Ann Arbor, Michigan 1990

95   94   93   92   91   90   5   4   3   2   1

Library of Congress Cataloging-in-Publication Data

Hospital volume, physician volume, and patient outcomes : assessing
    the evidence / Harold S. Luft ... [et al.].
    p.   cm.
    Includes bibliographical references.
    ISBN 0-910701-46-6
    1. Hospital care—Evaluation.   2. Hospitals—Utilization.
I. Luft, Harold S.
    [DNLM: 1. Health Services Research—United States.   2. Outcome
and Process Assessment (Health Care)   3. Quality Assurance, Health Care—
United States.   W 84 AA1 H79]
RA972.H685   1990   362.1'1—dc20
DNLM/DLC for Library of Congress   90-4003 CIP

The editors are grateful to the authors and publishers for their contributions to this book. Because of the variety of sources, references were not changed to a consistent style, but follow the citation style of the book or journal in which they first appeared.

NWSt
IADJ4688

Health Administration Press
A division of the Foundation of the
    American College of Healthcare Executives
1021 East Huron Street
Ann Arbor, Michigan 48104-9990
(313) 764-1380

Contents

Acknowledgments

A number of people have helped to make this volume possible. First, without the authors of the papers reviewed in this book we would not have had so rich a body of research to review. The impetus for our work came from Jane Sisk of the U.S. Congress Office of Technology Assessment (OTA), who commissioned us to do a review of research on the relationship between hospital volume and patient outcomes as a chapter of the publication *The Quality of Medical Care: Information for Consumers*. Her encouragement and the work of her staff, especially Pauline Erenhaft, helped us to focus our analysis. She assembled a set of reviewers, including Robert DuBois, Ann Barry Flood, Jinnet Fowles, Joyce Kelly, Leslie Roos, Stephen Shortell, Frank Sloan, and Ronald Williams. They, along with other anonymous reviewers of our chapter for OTA and the book manuscript, have contributed substantially to the quality of this book. Any errors remain our own. The National Center for Health Services Research and the Office of the Inspector General, Department of Health and Human Services, provided funding for the authors' own research on this topic. The Institute for Health Policy Studies, University of California, San Francisco, provided institutional support. The Henry J. Kaiser Family Foundation provided support for Hal Luft as a Fellow at the Center for Advanced Study in the Behavioral Sciences.

Jan Tetreault was instrumental in conducting the automated literature search, organizing our review of the literature, and editing and preparing early drafts. Lucy Marton, Corinne Miller, Virginia Heaton, Leslie Lindzey, and Deanna Knickerboker provided key administrative support throughout the project and prepared the final manuscript. Kathleen Much edited the drafts of our book chapters and Lynn Gale provided statistical consulting. Lincoln Moses, Lissy Jarvik, and Robert Rosenthal provided helpful comments on Chapter 4. Without the efforts and support of all of these people, we could not have written this book.

Part I
An Overview of the Literature

Chapter 1

Introduction and Background

The idea that volume and outcome in medical care might be related is not a new one. Medical training involves a substantial amount of "learning by doing," so it is natural to think that, with greater experience, one becomes more skilled. Whether this same relationship applies at the hospital level, however, is a different question. Since the 1970s, a growing body of research has addressed the empirical relationship between the number of patients with a specific diagnosis or surgical procedure and their outcomes after treatment by a particular physician or in a particular hospital. This has led to recommended minimum volumes for certain types of services, such as open-heart surgery. In addition to such regulatory approaches based on volumes, health insurers and even the Medicare program are considering selective contracts with certain providers using volume as one of the criteria.

Despite the growing acceptance in the policy community of the relationship between volume and outcome, a careful review of the available data suggests that the evidence of a relationship is quite strong for some types of patients and quite weak for others. Thus one must be careful about generalizing such findings. It is also clear that there are many unanswered questions about the observed relationship. For example, is the underlying process really one of accumulated experience, or do outcomes depend on current volume levels? Will a team averaging 50 procedures a year for five years have better or worse outcomes than a new group with 100 procedures in their first year? To what extent is it physician volume rather than hospital volume that matters, and how do the operating room staff, postoperative nursing staff, medical consultants, other staff, and equipment contribute to the "hospital effect"? Finally, is the implicit causal relationship from outcome to volume, rather than from volume to outcome? That is, might it be the case that some professionals perform better than others and that, because of their high quality, they get more referrals and, therefore, higher volumes?

This book provides a critical overview of the research on the volume-outcome relationship. Unlike the excellent study by Flood and Scott (1987), the book does not report detailed findings from particular data. Instead, we offer an examination of peer-reviewed literature and a discussion of both consistent and inconsistent results across studies and procedures and diagnoses. By examining various studies with widely differing data, settings, and methodological approaches, one is better able to determine which conclusions are well supported by the empirical evidence and which conclusions are based on only a few findings or are frequently contradicted.

In addition to exploring the evidence behind the volume-outcome relationship, this book illustrates the role of research methods in shaping our understanding of an empirical relationship. It does not focus on statistics or quantitative techniques, but instead offers an example of how to interpret and digest empirical research. Readers may want to approach the book with the dual focus in mind. The remainder of this chapter describes the background of the study and the analytic approach. Readers who are interested primarily in the evidence on the volume-outcome relationship might then focus on Chapter 2: Theoretical and Methodological Issues in the Volume-Outcome Relationship; Chapter 3: Description of Research Studies; Chapter 5: Summary of Research Findings; Chapter 6: Diagnosis- and Procedure-Specific Research Results; and Chapter 7: Future Research and Policy Options. Twelve of the 25 published studies are reprinted in Chapters 8–19 for more careful review. Readers interested primarily in methodological questions might focus on Chapters 2 and 3, and then give careful attention to Chapter 4: Does Method Matter? The Influence of Method on Findings. The introductions to Chapters 8–19 provide a guide to the literature, focusing on important methodological issues and contrasting the approaches and findings of one study with those in other studies.

Although research is meant to be scientifically objective, there is always the potential for subtle and not-so-subtle biases to influence the choice of questions, study design, and interpretation of findings. We are particularly concerned about this problem for two reasons. First, this book is largely a re-analysis and interpretation of published material. In some instances, we have even reinterpreted data. Readers might question whether we are truly unbiased or whether we are putting a certain "spin" on the evidence to make it fit an underlying hypothesis or point of view. Second, since the authors of this book have also written 8 of the 25 studies reviewed herein, readers might be concerned that we have tried to defend our own research. While we have attempted to be impartial, the most convincing evidence of that will be the reader's own interpretations of the evidence. In order to address this concern, we have included substantial detail on all the studies and reprints of nearly half the literature. (Papers were chosen for inclusion not on the basis of their findings but because they demonstrate certain methodological approaches.)

BACKGROUND

While in Boston during a sabbatical, John Bunker, a Stanford University anesthesiologist and health services researcher, noticed a newspaper story about a small suburban hospital in which the mortality rate after open-heart surgery was several times that of the high-volume Boston teaching hospitals. Upon returning to Stanford, he discussed this with his colleagues, Alain Enthoven and Harold Luft. Enthoven knew of studies in the aircraft industry that showed falling costs with accumulating experience and it seemed plausible that the same phenomenon could occur in surgical care. With support from the Henry J. Kaiser Family Foundation, the three colleagues designed a research study using discharge abstract data from a national sample of hospitals. (Interestingly, the foundation has also helped this work come full circle through Luft's Fellowship at the Center for Advanced Study in the Behavioral Sciences.) A paper in the *New England Journal of Medicine* in 1979 was the first to examine the volume-outcome relation across a series of surgical procedures.

After his move to the Institute for Health Policy Studies at the University of California, San Francisco, Luft's continued interest in the volume-outcome relationship led to a series of studies using both national and California state discharge abstract data. Each study led to further questions, particularly about the role of selective referrals to better quality physicians and hospitals. After over a decade of research, we have learned a great deal about the volume-outcome relationship, but there is still more to learn.

In the middle of 1987, the Office of Technology Assessment asked the authors of this book to undertake a review of the literature on the relationship between volume and outcome. This was to be part of their report in response to congressional interest in "whether valid information on hospital and physician quality could be developed and distributed to the public to assist their choice of health care providers" (U.S. Congress 1988). Since we had already written extensively on the topic, we worked with the OTA staff to develop a set of protocols to identify and evaluate studies in an impartial fashion. This led to an extensive paper, and a brief version was published as Chapter 8 of the OTA report. Some of the tables in this book are based on those in the original report, but they include minor revisions and corrections.

Analytic Approach

Our approach falls somewhere between that of a classic literature review and that of a meta-analysis. The former typically reviews a body of literature study by study, with careful consideration of the methods, problems, and results of each.

The reviewer often weaves together findings from various sources in order to present a comprehensive discussion of the findings. The weighting of conflicting evidence is often implicit, although a good reviewer will explain why some findings are less believable than others.

As the number of studies increases, one may ask whether it is possible to combine results of many studies in some formal way to develop more precise estimates of the true effects. The meta-analysis approach developed by Glass (1976) and expanded by Rosenthal (1984), Light and Pillemer (1984), and others, is designed to allow such combining of results across studies. In the classic meta-analysis there are numerous studies of an intervention, such as a new teaching technique, and a standardized set of outcome measures, such as achievement test scores. If the experiments were well executed and reported, the data are often available in the published reports to allow one to combine the results across studies, thereby expanding the sample size and increasing the precision of the estimates.

If the available studies are not all well executed, or if they differ markedly in their approaches, populations, and methods, then it is impossible to directly combine findings. Our review of the studies of the relationship between volume and outcome falls between a classic literature review and a meta-analysis. The evidence cuts across a large number of surgical procedures and a small number of medical diagnoses. The methods used vary markedly, from rather simple comparisons of outcomes across volume groups to complex simultaneous-equation models testing several causal relationships. Sample sizes, outcome measures, and the representation of volume often vary across studies. Sufficient data are almost never presented in an article to transform the findings to test for their consistency with those of other articles. Thus, a formal meta-analysis is quite impossible. This does not mean, however, that one must rely on the more impressionistic literature review approach.

There is an important middle ground between literature reviews and formal meta-analyses, although it is sometimes placed under the heading of meta-analysis. For example, Luft (1978) found that some studies showed health maintenance organization (HMO) enrollees received more preventive services than comparison groups, but that other studies showed they received the same or less. However, simply classifying the studies according to whether the "comparison group" had coverage for preventive services explained the inconsistent findings.

The following analysis is also based on this middle approach. We treat the findings presented in the various studies as data points for further analysis, much as one would do in a meta-analysis. The differences in approaches across studies, however, make it impossible to combine findings in a very sophisticated manner. Instead, we merely ask: What is the implicit shape of the curve relating outcome to volume as presented by the authors of the study? For example, does it indicate a continuously falling mortality rate, does it flatten out at a certain point, or does it begin to rise again above a certain volume level? Once all the findings are categorized, one can examine them for patterns with respect to certain other variables, such as medical diagnoses as opposed to surgical procedures, physician volume as opposed to hospital volume, and consistency among studies of a given procedure or diagnosis.

Consistency of findings across studies is quite a weak criterion for accepting an interpretation. It ignores differences in magnitudes, and, perhaps more important, it risks succumbing to the "file drawer phenomenon," in which studies with negative findings are either rejected by journals or abandoned by researchers (Rosenthal 1979). In the long run, however, many of the negative studies eventually appear, so the bias may be less important than Rosenthal once believed (Rosenthal and Rubin 1988). Although one cannot be sure of the bias in volume-outcome studies, it may be helpful that the published reports often include results for a large number of diagnoses and procedures. If this is generally so, then negative results are more likely to be published for two reasons: (1) they come "bundled" with positive results, and (2) a series of negative results is much more "interesting" than an isolated negative finding.

Chapter 4 looks beyond the simple measures of consistency in terms of the shape of the curve, exploring the implications of the different methods. Since reworking the data used in the various studies would have been an enormous undertaking, we chose a far simpler approach. Two sets of patient data were used, one for patients undergoing coronary artery bypass graft surgery—a complex procedure undertaken at approximately one hospital in five—and one for patients undergoing cholecystectomy—a far more commonly available procedure. We applied the various methods used in the 25 studies to determine if different findings would have been reached. While in most cases results are consistent across methods, quite different findings would have been reported in a few notable instances.

Selection of Articles

In selecting articles for review, we began with studies we had examined during the course of our previous research on the volume-outcome relationship, took pertinent references from the bibliographies of these studies, and perused recent issues of several journals. We also searched the medical and health administration sections of the data base of the National Library of Medicine, using subject headings such as "outcome and process assessment (health care)" and "patient outcome assessment." We also perused recent issues of journals that appeared often in our search. Finally, we wrote asking persons who have published pertinent research[1] to review our preliminary list.[2]

We then established a set of study inclusion criteria. Studies were included if they examined a sufficient number of hospitals (more than 20) and cases to offer a reasonable likelihood of statistically valid volume-outcome results *or* if the study purported to examine the volume-outcome relationship. Thus some studies that focus primarily on questions other than the volume-outcome relationship have been included, since they may shed light on our topic. Others that may be unable to shed much light because of their small samples have been included nonetheless, because some may interpret them as rejecting the hypothesis of a relationship.

Examination of Selected Articles

During our literature search we read abstracts of approximately 100 papers, thoroughly reviewed 50 of these, and identified 25 papers that presented reportable findings on the volume-outcome relationship. The excluded papers generally failed to have empirical findings (e.g., editorials or policy statements) or presented evidence on only a single setting or a handful of settings. Each of the four authors of this book reviewed at least a quarter of the articles and completed two review forms for each article.

On the first form, the reviewer wrote a brief abstract (see Chapter 3) and provided the following information about each paper: authors, title, authors' institutional affiliations, and publication reference; procedures or diagnoses; volume measure; outcome measure; study period; provider characteristics (including type, number, and setting); patient characteristics controlled for; hospital, provider, or other control variables; unit of analysis; specification of dependent variable and volume variable; statistical method; results and comments.

An article could provide information on one or more diagnoses or procedures. For each medical diagnosis or surgical procedure in each paper, the reviewer provided the following information on the second form: authors, title, procedure or diagnosis (ICD-9-CM code), specification of volume (including mean and range), specification of outcome (including mean and range), number of providers or patients, procedure or diagnosis characteristics unique to this study, results, and shape of volume-outcome curve.

About two-thirds of the studies were reviewed by two readers. Since the interpretations of both reviewers were essentially the same, only one reader was used for the remaining studies. The studies and the forms were then redistributed among the researchers by procedure or diagnosis. Thus the "unit of observation" is the "study finding," or the results for a particular procedure or diagnosis within a given study. The reviewers compared the results for each procedure or diagnosis across studies, summarized them, and presented them graphically (see Tables 5.2 and 5.3). The summaries were reviewed by all four authors to clarify interpretations and reach a consensus. Once the definitions were clarified, the assignment of findings was consistent across reviewers. As we worked through the analysis, further questions about data, methods, and findings were resolved by referring back to the original published papers.

NOTES

1. These included Robert DuBois, Ann Flood, Jinnet Fowles, Joyce Kelly, Leslie Roos, Stephen Shortell, Frank Sloan, and Ronald Williams.
2. Although we were informed of two studies being carried out as master's and doctoral projects, we chose to limit our review to works already published or in press.

Chapter 2

Theoretical and Methodological Issues in the Volume-Outcome Relationship

Before considering the available evidence on the volume-outcome relationship, it is important to address a series of theoretical, methodological, and data questions. A consideration of these questions helps not only to place individual studies in context but also in understanding why findings may vary across studies. The theoretical issues include the nature of the causal linkages, the significance of physician volume, and the pattern of effects over time. Methodological issues include the types of outcome measures and the ways in which volume is specified. Many issues affect the selection of statistical methods. These include approaches to the adjustment for differences in severity of illness among patients, the choice of the hospital or the patient as the unit of observation, the type and exact source of data, and the selection of procedures and diagnoses for study. Finally, we consider the validity and reliability of the data and how they affect the procedures and diagnoses chosen for analysis.

In a review of the literature one is often tempted to compare all studies to the "state of the art," but that is neither fair nor appropriate. Many of the studies used state-of-the-art approaches when they were undertaken. Some researchers might have preferred to use different approaches but were constrained by the availability of data. Others may have chosen simple techniques in order to reach a policy-oriented audience, rather than attempting to explain more complex methods. These issues will be highlighted in Chapters 8 to 19. The more important issue of whether the different methods affect the "bottom line" results will be discussed in Chapter 4. The remainder of this chapter will outline some of the factors that need to be considered in exploring the different approaches.

WHAT ARE THE CAUSAL LINKAGES?

The volume-outcome curve depicted in Figure 2.1 merely represents an association. Although one may be tempted to interpret it as representing a causal relationship, several problems arise; some of these are standard problems in exploring any empirical data for causal relationships. For example, it is not legitimate to say that "as volume increases, mortality falls" and take this to mean that increasing volume in a hospital will improve outcomes, or that reducing volume will worsen outcomes. Since the data are almost always taken from a cross-section of hospitals observed at a specific time, rather than the history of mortality at a given hospital as its volume rises or falls, one cannot legitimately conclude anything about the effect of *changes* in volumes on outcomes.

In addition, some unmeasured factors may account for the observed relationship. For example, suppose that having a teaching program is the true cause of better outcomes. Since teaching hospitals tend to have high volumes, there would appear to be a correlation between volume and outcome. In fact, volume has no effect on outcome in this case, other than through its association with teaching status. A second type of error would occur if some hospitals achieve

Figure 2.1:   Hypothesized Relationship between Volume and Outcome

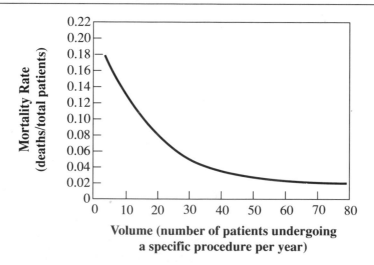

**Volume (number of patients undergoing
a specific procedure per year)**

high volumes by using broad indications for surgery. If this is the case, hospitals that admit large numbers of healthy patients for procedures will be more likely to have good outcomes. These errors in interpretation are fairly obvious.

A third type of error in causal interpretation is more subtle and contentious. Although it is usually assumed that volume affects outcome, the causality may work in the opposite direction, so that the curve should be flipped over, indicating that low mortality rates attract high volumes. Some researchers have contrasted two different explanations of the volume-outcome relationship, a "practice makes perfect" hypothesis and a "selective referral" hypothesis.

The Practice-Makes-Perfect Hypothesis

The discussion of the effects of volume on outcome often becomes confusing because two different causal models underlie what is often estimated as the effect of volume on outcome. The first is appropriately labelled the "experience," "learning," or practice-makes-perfect effect and refers to the experience accumulated over time by doing a procedure or treating a certain type of patient. This explanation rests on the general notion that increased experience results in more finely developed skills and, therefore, in better outcomes. Evidence from various industries shows that production costs per unit fall as a firm accumulates experience (Asher 1956). The second causal model focuses on what is really a scale effect—that is, hospitals or physicians with high volumes at a particular point in time achieve better outcomes. Although accumulated experience is related to volume per unit of time, the two are not identical. Clearly, a surgeon with a high operative load develops experience much faster than one with a low volume, but cumulative experience among physicians can vary widely at given yearly volume levels. Therefore, one might expect age to be a crucial variable in analyses with physician-specific data.

The direct analogy between the manufacturer's "learning curve" described by Asher and the development of a particular medical care skill is probably most valid during the training of a physician. Although each person has an individual learning curve, the flat portion of the curve, where increases in volume are associated with little change in outcomes, is probably attained during the training period. There may also be an organizational learning curve, so that as experience is gained with certain types of patients, standard protocols are developed that make it easier to treat subsequent patients. Thus experience accumulated over many years is not a likely explanation for the observed relationship.

Another feature of the scale effect is the deterioration of skills with lack of practice. In a comparison of two equally trained surgeons, the one who consistently performs many of the procedures in question will maintain—or continue to improve—his or her skills, and the one who performs few such procedures will become progressively less proficient. Similarly, nurses and other staff members who are more familiar with certain types of patients may become or remain more proficient in working with them. Higher volumes may make it possible for hospitals to purchase specialized equipment for such patients (Flood, Scott, and Ewy 1984a). High volumes may also allow the hiring of several people, such as heart pump technicians, to handle a high number of open-heart surgery patients. With several highly skilled people for each position on the team, such hospitals may be far better equipped to handle emergency procedures. Thus one can describe this type of volume effect as an economy of scale with respect to both skills and equipment, if "production cost" is expanded to include the adverse consequences of poor outcomes.

Given the available data, it has been almost impossible to distinguish the learning effect from the scale effect. To do so, one would have to measure both current volume and the accumulated experience of the relevant professionals and organizations. The problem is more complex than in manufacturing studies, in which each worker is assumed to have a negligible individual effect on the efficiency of producing a complex output such as a Boeing 747. In such cases, one need only compare production costs over time as the assembly line works at varying speeds. The assumption is that most of the individual learning is incorporated in the organizational process.

In the case of a surgical procedure, there certainly may be some important organizational learning, as the operating room team, for example, becomes used to the "style" of a new surgeon. This style may be quite similar for all of this surgeon's operations, not just the particular one under study. Accumulated experience with that procedure, however, may affect the surgeon's ability to handle certain complicating factors, and volume may have a separate effect in making such experiences more common. It must be easier to deal with the "one in a hundred" complications if these occur once a month than if they occur once every few years. In the absence of detailed data allowing the separate estimation of accumulated experience and contemporaneous volume or scale effects, and for ease of discussion, we will follow the bulk of the literature and refer to the effect of volume on outcome to include both scale and experience effects.

The Selective-Referral Hypothesis

The selective-referral hypothesis holds that the observed inverse relationship between volume and outcome arises from the attraction of more patients to physicians and hospitals with better outcomes. The notion that patients in some instances may look for hospitals or physicians with better procedure-specific adjusted mortality rates seems implausible to those who claim that the variation in mortality by disease or procedure is too small to influence patient choice (Flood, Scott and Ewy 1984a). If complications are correlated with mortality, however, variations in outcomes may be large enough to be noticed by patients' primary physicians, who choose specialists for referral. Although it is difficult to identify an individual hospital or physician as having significant death rates that are worse than average (Luft and Hunt 1986), referral patterns may be based on a simpler set of decision rules that are designed to avoid the worst outcomes, rather than search for the best. For example, suppose primary physicians select specialists within the appropriate field at random, but switch referrals after even one "bad outcome," such as a death or complication. Patients in this system are eventually directed away from providers whose outcomes are worse than average, and specialists with better outcomes will end up with higher volumes. If physicians share their referral decisions with one another, this process will lead even more quickly to selective referrals to the better providers, but some patients will still be sent to providers with average or below-average quality.

Even if the majority of patients go to the nearest hospital or otherwise make decisions independent of perceived outcomes, a minority seeking or referred to the "best provider in town" (or referred away from poor-quality providers) will result in a selective-referral pattern for specific diagnoses and procedures. All this means is that hospitals with better outcomes will have higher volumes and poor-outcome hospitals will have lower volumes than one would expect in the absence of outcome-sensitive referrals. It is important to note that the selective-referral effect need not be very large, nor does its presence rule out the possibility that outcomes are influenced by volume or scale. The question, therefore, is whether *some* patients are influenced in their choice of physicians and hospitals by relative performance, not whether *all* patients are so influenced.

The principal empirical objection to the selective-referral hypothesis is that some studies show little relationship between outcomes and hospital characteristics traditionally considered to be markers of good performance, such as teaching status or board certification of physicians (Flood, Scott, and Ewy 1984b; Luft 1980). But these measures are rather blunt indicators of special expertise. It is not uncommon for a teaching hospital to be outstanding in the treatment of one diagnosis or procedure—for example, cardiovascular surgery—but not to be particularly distinguished in another, such as neurosurgery.

If externally measurable variables, such as board certification or medical school affiliation, are insensitive to differences in outcomes that may influence referrals, then higher-than-expected volume for a specific procedure or diagnosis may, in fact, be the best single indicator of exceptionally good outcomes. If so, at least part of the causal linkage is from outcomes to volumes. As an analogy, consider the situation of a new visitor to a city. The hotel's restaurant guide provides a description of the local options, including the type of food, the price range, and where the chef trained. This information may be of some guidance in finding the best restaurant, but our visitor is likely to continue to be uncertain. A better indication of relative quality might be the crowd at each establishment. Our visitor would probably be wise to avoid places that are nearly empty, and, if there is no hurry, a long line would be not only a measure of popularity but perhaps the best single indicator of good food within a given price range. One would not, however, argue that the food is good simply because the lines are long (or the chef has enough practice). Of course, the restaurant example raises many other issues—one is more likely to be impressed by an establishment filled with locals than one full of out-of-towners, or by a busy place in an out-of-the-way location. The availability of local alternatives is an obvious factor to take into account. Just as one might place more credence in crowds as an indicator of quality for fine restaurants than for fast-food establishments, the importance of selective referral may vary across procedures and diagnoses.

Although different models sometimes have the same empirical implications, the appropriate causal model is often necessary for the interpretation of various statistical methods. Unfortunately, it is often difficult, or even impossible, to test alternative causal models with the data at hand. The more sophisticated techniques designed to test simultaneous paths of causation assume a well-specified and well-estimated model. Unfortunately, the attempts to estimate such models have not been fully convincing, even to their authors (Luft 1980; Luft, Hunt, and Maerki 1987). For some purposes, however, the exact chain of causation may not be the paramount issue. But we must be alert to the fact that most studies are appropriately interpreted as testing the existence of a relation between volume and outcome, not its direction. Unfortunately, none of the studies in the volume-outcome literature explores in detail the complex referral relationships among patients, primary care physicians, and specialists. All the available evidence is indirect and, therefore, less than fully convincing. Our view is that the case concerning causation is far from settled.

Unfortunately, the two causal models have substantially different policy implications. If the observed patterns reflect only the "volume affects outcome" phenomenon, then any effort to concentrate patients in selected hospitals will improve outcomes. Thus Medicaid programs or preferred provider organizations that obtain low prices from hospitals in return for more patients would be justified on grounds of both economy and quality (Iglehart 1984; Trauner 1983). Moreover, one could make this argument without assessing the quality of the contractors, since one could assume that increasing volume would improve quality. On the other hand, if the observed patterns are entirely due to intelligent selective referrals, where patients are channeled to the best providers, then contracting on the basis of price will not necessarily result in beneficial patient care outcomes. Since regionalization alone would not, under this model, improve outcomes, selective contracting could markedly worsen patient care.

DO HOSPITAL AND PHYSICIAN VOLUME
INFLUENCE OUTCOMES?

Although most of the published research relates to hospital volume, a small but growing body of literature focuses on the relative importance of physician volume in contrast, or in addition, to hospital volume. The uncertainty in this area reflects our limited understanding of the reasons underlying the observed relation between volume and outcome. For example, is the observed association for patients undergoing a surgical procedure related to the volume or experience of the surgeon, anesthesiologist, operating room staff, postoperative recovery room staff, or other staff in the hospital? Are problems in surgical techniques or problems with postoperative monitoring causing poor outcomes? Answers to these questions would require extensive chart reviews from many hospitals across many procedures and diagnoses because, until recently, detailed data on physicians have not been available on hospital discharge data sets.

The 20 states with publicly mandated hospital discharge data systems that include physician information vary with respect to (1) the use of a physician identifier that can be linked across hospitals, (2) the number of years of data, (3) the public availability of these data to research, and (4) the number of physicians listed (Hughes and Lee 1990). Arizona, Connecticut, Minnesota, Maryland, Nevada, New Jersey, New York, North Carolina, Pennsylvania, South Carolina, Tennessee, and Washington collect physician data using a physician license number or statewide number (rather than a hospital-specific identification number) and make these data publicly available (generally after a review process and in an encrypted format).

Even if physician volume is most important, hospital volume is also likely to be important. For example, a hospital with several high-volume and several low-volume surgeons may develop monitoring methods and standard procedures for the nursing and other staff that catch potential errors and problems and institute corrective actions. Thus a low-volume surgeon may be "protected" by the organizational safeguards in a high-volume hospital. The generally high correlation between hospital and physician volume must also be investigated in order to produce valid empirical estimates.

WHAT ARE THE EFFECTS OVER TIME?

To understand the underlying causal relationships, we must add some time dimension. If we consider the practice-makes-perfect hypothesis, the fact that a beginning surgeon will eventually perform 200 procedures during the year should not affect the outcomes of the first patients he or she operates on in that year. Thus, with a new surgeon, one immediately faces a confounding of the learning and scale effects. If one has no reason to believe that a physician is a new practitioner or that a hospital has introduced a new procedure, one assumes that a physician or hospital with a volume of 200 procedures in any one year probably has had about that many procedures in prior years. We assume implicitly that all volumes have reached some steady-state level. In reality, new physicians enter practice, new procedures are developed, hospitals offer new services, and past volume levels may differ from current (and future) ones. Thus, if outcomes truly improve as volume increases—for example, from 100 to 200 patients per year—how long does it take the outcomes to improve if the higher volume is suddenly achieved? Again, changes in outcomes may be separate from an experience effect. For example, it is likely that accumulated experience matters little after 100 or so procedures, but volume effects may continue to be important. Does a sudden increase in volume, perhaps because a neighboring hospital closed a specialized unit, immediately improve outcomes, or might they even worsen for a period?

Timing is also important for considering the selective-referral hypothesis. If outcomes or reputations influence referrals, what is the time lag involved? Do referring physicians ignore an occasional higher-than-expected mortality rate and notice only those results that are consistently better or worse than average? Or can even small changes in outcomes cause shifts in referral patterns? Furthermore, is it possible to reverse a trend of falling referrals by improving outcomes? These questions have not been explored in any empirical studies to date.

WHAT OUTCOME MEASURES ARE USED?

Four measures of patient outcome were used in the research we reviewed: (1) in-hospital mortality, (2) mortality within a fixed period of time, (3) complications or health status measures, and (4) long hospital stays as a proxy for complications.

Mortality is a clearly defined outcome, although the causes of any particular death may be difficult to determine. Therefore, researchers have generally focused on total mortality for a group of patients, perhaps after adjustment for case mix, rather than what might be called "avoidable" deaths. The latter may be determined by careful review of each patient's treatment by experienced physicians to determine whether greater skill or avoidance of errors might have led to a better outcome (DuBois, Brook, and Rogers 1987). Although the classification of a death as avoidable or preventable is somewhat arbitrary, it provides a more sensitive measure of poor or exceptionally good quality by eliminating the large number of unavoidable deaths. Careful case-mix adjustment for patient severity attempts to do the same things statistically (see below).

Information on deaths occurring during the hospital stay is routinely available from hospital discharge abstracts. Except for patients who are irreversibly ill and in pain, in-hospital mortality is indubitably an adverse outcome. (One almost never sees studies of this type focusing on patients with advanced cancer, for instance.) Nevertheless, using mortality as an outcome measure carries some important limitations. For some procedures and diagnoses, mortality is so rare an event that it is difficult to determine whether an occasional death indicates a pattern of poor quality or mere chance.

Important biases also may be introduced, since hospital-controlled discharge policies can affect inpatient mortality rates. For instance, hospitals will exhibit lower mortality rates if patients with severe complications are transferred to other regional tertiary hospitals or terminal patients to hospices. Furthermore, in hospitals with longer average stays there is a greater chance of observing a death. For example, suppose that Hospital A typically keeps patients for ten days after a certain surgical procedure, but Hospital B works to get patients on their feet quickly and discharges them after a week. Even if the same fraction of patients from each hospital experiences a fatal heart attack on the eighth to tenth day after surgery, these deaths will be counted in the in-hospital mortality rate of only Hospital A.

Because of these biases, some researchers calculate mortality rates with respect to a fixed window, such as 30 days after admission or operation (U.S. DIIIIS 1988). Linkage of several data sources to determine postdischarge mortality is possible with Medicare patients, for whom an ongoing enrollment file allows the determination of postdischarge deaths. For other patients, follow-up is far more complicated because most U.S. insurance systems cannot determine whether the lack of current enrollment is due to death or a change of coverage. Even with linked data, problems arise in the use of postdischarge mortality data. If the window is too short, some patients will be counted as being alive even though they subsequently die without ever leaving the hospital. The use of respirators and other life-support systems makes this concern more than just hypothetical. On the other hand, the longer the window of observation extends after discharge, the greater the likelihood that an individual patient died of causes unrelated to the hospital care. There are also questions of whether to begin counting from the day of admission or the day of surgery, how to handle patients still in the hospital at the end of the observation period, and which hospital should be "credited" with a death when a patient is transferred to or readmitted from another facility within the observation period.

Complications and other measures of health status are less objectively measured than mortality. In some instances, a clearly identified procedure, such as a reoperation, indicates a poor outcome (Roos, et al. 1986). (Not all such procedures are indicative of poor outcomes, but unusually high rates are.) Other measures, such as wound infections, have been used (Farber, Kaiser, and Wenzel 1981), but they are not reliably coded from hospital to hospital. Patient assessments of health status or functional status can be measured through interviews or questionnaires (Flood and Scott 1987), but such primary data collection is far more expensive than strategies relying on routinely collected data. Because of the cost of primary data collection, such studies include a relatively small number of hospitals, and it may be difficult to generalize their results. It is also possible to measure complications during only the initial hospital stay or over a longer period of time. Each approach, of course, has implications analogous to those raised with respect to in-hospital mortality versus fixed window mortality.

Luft and his colleagues propose that the proportion of patients who stay a very long time in the hospital is a proxy for complication rates (Showstack et al. 1987; Hughes, Hunt, and Luft 1987; Hughes et al. 1988). Although it is an indirect measure of outcome, they argue that if one chooses a length of stay exceeded by only 10 percent of all patients with a given diagnosis or procedure, then a hospital with far more than 10 percent of its patients staying that long or longer may be experiencing poor outcomes. Although this notion is plausible, it has not yet been validated. To do so would require medical record reviews to determine whether those patients with very long stays truly have complications resulting from ineffective care, or stay longer for other reasons, such as a scarcity of nursing home beds. In Chapter 4, however, we explore the implications of using some of the alternative measures of outcomes.

HOW IS VOLUME SPECIFIED?

Volume is typically measured per year, although some studies use other periods, such as an annual average based on a two-year period or, in one case, up to 7½ years (Pilcher et al. 1980).

Once the period of time for the volume measure is determined, it can be expressed in various forms:

- Categorical variables (e.g., low- and high-volume groups, or a four- or five-category classification)

- A continuous variable (e.g., a count of patients, which allows for a linear relation)

- A quadratic formulation (e.g., volume and volume-squared, which allow for linear, U-shaped or inverted U-shaped curves)

- Log of volume (which allows for a stronger effect at low volumes and progressively weaker effects at higher volumes—a "rounded L" effect)

- A combination of measures (e.g., the proportion of patients in a hospital [a continuous measure] treated by surgeons with low volumes [a dichotomous variable])(Hughes, Hunt, and Luft 1987)

The method of specifying volume may seem to be esoteric, but it leads to important policy implications. For example, testing a simple continuous variable may show that as volume increases, outcomes improve. But using only a continuous variable (without a quadratic term or a log transformation) may mask the fact that outcomes are dramatically worse only below a particular volume level. Thus one may be led to the interpretation that outcomes improve with volume rather than that outcomes are very bad in hospitals with volumes below x, and that there is little relationship between volume and outcome above that point.

Unfortunately, few studies explicitly compare various indicators of volume. The categorical approach is the most robust, if enough categories are used, in that it allows one to represent the widest range of relationships. However, the volume cutoffs must be determined in advance and they must be procedure specific. For example, a hospital with 50 total hip replacements is a high-volume facility, but one with 200 cardiac catheterizations is a low-volume center. A quadratic formulation is easier to use and allows the calculation of the volume at which poor outcomes are minimized (Maerki, Luft, and Hunt 1986; Sloan, Perrin, and Valvona 1986). It is difficult, however, to distinguish a U-shaped curve from a rounded-L shape if there are few very high volume observations. For some analyses, such as simultaneous-equation models, in which volume is also a dependent variable, one must specify a single variable, such as volume or log volume (Hughes, Hunt, and Luft 1987; Luft, Hunt, and Maerki 1987).

Our categorization of findings recognizes the difficulties in distinguishing the results of the various expressions of volume. We lump together many of the functional forms simply because the data are not available to distinguish them. For example, if only an inverse log form was tested, we cannot determine if a U might provide a better fit. Furthermore, the wide range of sophistication in approaches makes comparisons even more difficult. One cannot look for answers to sophisticated questions, such as the importance of volume as a function of outcome relative to outcome as a function of volume, in studies that do not investigate them. On the other hand, complex models sometimes obscure the answer to simple questions. For example, we usually ask whether there is an observed relationship between volume and outcome. In some of the simultaneous-equation studies, simple correlations were found for some procedures (Luft, Hunt, and Maerki 1987), but in the two-equation model, the coefficient for the influence of outcomes on volume was significant but the coefficient of volume on outcome was not. If one only focused on the classic equation showing outcome as a function of volume, one would have to report the absence of an effect.

WHAT STATISTICAL METHODS ARE USED?

In the studies we reviewed, statistical methods range from simple comparisons of high- and low-volume groups to fairly sophisticated causal models. In some instances, the results for various volume levels are presented for qualitative observation without tests of statistical significance (Luft, Bunker, and Enthoven 1979). Regression models are commonly used because they can include a large number of patient and hospital variables as explanatory factors (Shortell and LoGerfo 1981; Showstack et al. 1987; Sloan, Perrin, and Valvona 1986; Williams 1979). In some cases, logistic models are used to account explicitly for the yes-or-no nature of patient mortality (Kelly and Hellinger 1986; Riley and Lubitz 1985; Roos et al. 1986). Three papers use simultaneous-equation models to estimate both the influence of volume on outcomes and the influence of outcomes on volume (Hughes, Hunt, and Luft 1987; Luft 1980; Luft, Hunt, and Maerki 1987).

HOW DO RESEARCHERS ACCOUNT FOR DIFFERENCES IN PATIENT SEVERITY OF ILLNESS?

One serious problem in analysis of the volume-outcome relationship is the potential confounding effect of differences in patient severity of illness. Every patient is different and individual factors strongly influence outcomes. Even if these patient differences are random, the estimation of a volume-outcome relationship will be more difficult because of the "noise" created by these random effects. For example, Figure 2.2 plots the inpatient mortality rates for patients undergoing coronary artery bypass graft surgery in 78 California hospitals in 1983. Although there appears to be a general downward-sloping pattern with respect to volume, there is substantial variation among hospitals at given volume levels, which may be due to patient factors. From the analyst's perspective, the problem is that clinicians are aware of the importance of patient-specific factors in determining outcomes. In the absence of convincing evidence that patient factors do *not* account for differences in hospital-level results, the potential for alternative explanations is always present.

The crucial question is whether more (or less) severely ill patients are consistently being treated in high-volume hospitals. (If selective referrals occur for any reason, one could no longer support the *assumption* of random differences in severity across hospitals.) If so, selective referral could, in theory, produce an observed association between outcome and volume due entirely to patient case mix. For example, hospitals with less stringent requirements for admission could boost their volumes and improve their outcomes by having a high proportion of healthier patients. Whether this is the case, of course, is an empirical question.

Determining whether the volume-outcome relationship is the result of case mix would be possible if large numbers of patients were randomly assigned or referred to institutions with varying volume levels. Such random assignment, with sufficiently large numbers of patients, would reduce to insignificance the likelihood that patient factors accounted for the observed differences in outcomes. One would then have a "gold standard" test of whether high volume leads to better outcomes. It would say little about the impact of severity differences or selective referral in the nonexperimental situation. Manning, Liebowitz, and Goldberg (1984) report on an analogous problem with respect to health maintenance organizations. Such an experiment is obviously impractical; it would not only be enormously expensive, but also ethically impossible. Thus one is left with attempts to control for case-mix differences through various statistical means. Unfortunately, such approaches are never entirely convincing to the skeptical reader. One must decide, however, whether the likely problems can fully explain the reported results. That is, if the findings are still contrary to one's expectations, can plausible biases due to unexplained variables account for the observed results?

There are two general approaches to dealing with differences in patient case mix among hospitals. The first is to specify the procedure or diagnosis for study as carefully and narrowly as possible. In this approach, very specific and detailed patient selection criteria result in a reasonably homogeneous group of patients. For example, patients undergoing simultaneous coronary artery bypass graft (CABG) surgery and heart valve replacement surgery have mortality rates about three times as high as those undergoing CABG surgery alone. Some hospitals may specialize in uncomplicated CABG surgery; others may have a large share of patients who also require valve replacement surgery. Comparing their outcomes and volumes may be biased, unless one selects patients with CABG surgery alone.

The second approach, which can be combined with the first, is to include variables in the analysis that may capture risk differences among the patients included in the study. In theory, each of these additional variables could be used to stratify further the study population of patients, but one is limited in this endeavor by an ever-shrinking sample size. Therefore, in many studies, patient selection criteria are combined with statistical controls. The patient's age, race, and gender are classic variables of this type. Transfer from another hospital is often a powerful indicator of a patient at higher risk of a poor outcome (Luft 1980). Counts of the number of secondary diagnoses or procedures or the presence of specific diagnoses or procedures also are used (Luft, Bunker, and Enthoven 1979; Showstack et al. 1987; Sloan, Perrin, and Valvona 1986). In some instances, diagnostic information is combined to form a disease "stage" indicating the severity of the principal diagnosis (Kelly and Hellinger 1986; Kelly 1988). Ideally, one would like to include physiological measures of severity and patient status captured on admission or before surgery. In most cases, however, the cost of collecting such data has forced researchers to rely on far less desirable, but routinely collected data. A recent study by Roos, Roos, and Sharp (1987) suggests that some administrative data, such as insurance claims, may be as useful a predictor of poor outcomes as the more precise clinical indicators available in the chart. While the data have been used for analyses of Canadian patients, the Medicare claims data now available in the United States have not yet been used for research on the volume-outcome relationship.

The problem of case-mix differences has been highlighted in recent attempts to use mortality data to evaluate individual hospital performance (Blumberg 1986). Not surprisingly, many hospitals that were identified by the U.S. Department of Health and Human Services (DHHS) as having poor outcomes (based on data collected in 1986) claimed that a sicker-than-average case mix caused their poor rating (U.S. DHHS 1987). DuBois, Brook, and Rogers (1987) showed that there is indeed a sicker case mix in hospitals identified as outliers. Subsequent data releases included better adjustments for case mix (U.S. DHHS 1988), but one can never be sure that all of the patient characteristics that are important have been taken into account. To some extent, this problem of inade-

Figure 2.2:   Inpatient Mortality Rates by Volume of Patients Undergoing
Coronary Artery Bypass Graft Surgery in California, 1983

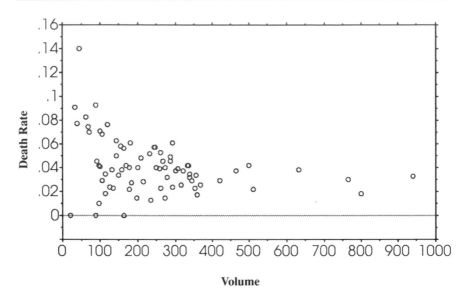

Figure 2.3:   Ratio of Actual to Expected Mortality Rates by Volume of Patients
Undergoing Coronary Artery Bypass Graft Surgery in California, 1983

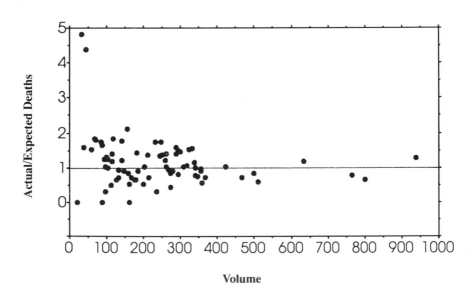

quate case-mix adjustment is less troublesome if the focus is on *patterns of outcomes*—say, with respect to volume—rather than on *individual hospitals*. If a specific hospital is identified as having a mortality rate that is significantly above average, the hospital administration is likely to respond that unmeasured differences in case mix account for the observed results. In fact, careful examination of the medical records may reveal that a few patients who enter the hospital with severe problems account for the elevated mortality rate. However, in order for an analytical study of the volume-outcome relationship to be seriously compromised by case mix, there must be unmeasured differences in case severity across hospitals, and they must be correlated with volume. Random errors merely reduce one's ability to detect a true relationship. Only if the omitted variables, such as severity, are correlated with the explanatory factors, such as volume, will the estimated relationship be biased.

One can sometimes test the plausibility of the "inadequately measured variable" argument by examining relationships with the available data. For example, age, gender, and the presence of certain comorbidities are known risk factors. If these data suggest that high-volume hospitals have a sicker case mix, then it is more difficult to accept the argument that unmeasured severity factors work in the opposite direction, after statistically accounting for age, gender, and comorbidities. That is, one would have to argue that high-volume hospitals have a disproportionate share of people in the measured high-risk categories, but that the patients *within* these categories are healthier than average. On the other hand, if high-volume hospitals had healthier-than-average case mixes, it would be easier to believe the argument that unmeasured factors indicating even less severity could explain the better results observed in those hospitals.

The role of case-mix adjustments can be seen in the following example. In Figure 2.2, the mortality rates vary substantially for individual hospitals at approximately the same volume levels. These data are for CABG patients, chosen as a reasonably homogeneous group, but the data are otherwise unadjusted for case mix. The data include patients undergoing only CABG surgery; all patients with heart valve operations are excluded from the outcome data. In the paper from which these data were drawn, a number of variables were included in the regression analysis to control for case mix. These variables include whether the operation was performed on the first or second day after admission (suggesting a scheduled procedure), age, gender, ethnic group, presence of acute myocardial infarction, congestive heart failure, or angina, and a coronary angiography during the same hospitalization (Showstack et al. 1987). Given these variables, one can compute a probability of death for each patient and, by aggregating the records for all patients in a hospital, the expected mortality rate for each hospital.

Figure 2.3 presents the ratio of actual to expected death rates for the same hospitals that are depicted in Figure 2.2. The same basic relationship between volume and outcome is apparent after we control for case mix. This is not to say that the case-mix variables are useless; at the level of individual patient predictions, they increase the explanatory power of the regression from 0.0009 using volume categories alone to 0.03 (neither figure is very high, but the 0.03 value is reasonable for patient-level analyses) (Flood, Scott, and Ewy 1984a). Case mix matters for individual patients and hospitals, but at least in this data set, case-mix variables are not correlated with volume, so the estimated coefficients for the volume effects are almost identical with and without the case-mix variables (see Chapter 4). Without detailed analyses of other data sets, it is impossible to determine whether the volume-outcome results for other procedures and diagnoses are similarly insensitive to patient risk factors.

HOSPITAL OR PATIENT AS THE UNIT OF ANALYSIS?

Since the underlying data refer to individual patient outcomes, some researchers use the patient as the unit of observation in a regression model to "predict" the patient's outcome (Farber, Kaiser, and Wenzel 1981; Kelly and Hellinger 1986; Roos et al. 1986; Showstack et al. 1987). They include as many patient risk factors as possible, along with variables indicating the number of patients with the procedure or diagnosis in the hospital per year. Regressions using the patient as the unit of analysis typically explain only a small part of the variation (e.g., low R^2), indicating a limited ability to predict whether an individual patient will live or die, even though many of the variables, such as volume, may be highly significant.

Other researchers argue that, since the focus of volume-outcome studies is on the performance of hospitals at different volume levels, the correct measure of degrees of freedom is the number of hospitals, not the number of patients (Whiting-O'Keefe, Henke, and Simborg 1984). (If one is focusing on physician volume, then the analogous approach would be to use the aggregation of a physician's patients as the unit of observation.) These researchers estimate regression models using the hospital as the unit of analysis. They include the proportion of patients with each risk factor to predict a composite expected poor outcome rate based on case mix in the hospital (Luft, Hunt, and Maerki 1987; Shortell and LoGerfo 1981; Sloan, Perrin, and Valvona 1986). In some cases, they even estimate a patient-based outcome equation and then use it to calculate a probability of dying for each patient. These probabilities are aggregated for all patients in the hospital to get an expected death rate (Flood, Scott, and Ewy 1984a).

One should not be misled by the high levels of significance for coefficients or the low R^2s in patient-level analyses, as there is a reasonable middle ground. For example, one could use patient-level analyses but rely upon the number of hospitals for the degrees of freedom when examining volume measures (Flood, Scott, and Ewy 1984a). In practice, the choice of approach is often governed by data availability and cost. Some data have not been available at the patient level, so researchers have had to make do with hospital-level statistics. The computational costs and data logistics are certainly simpler if one needs to deal only with hundreds or a few thousand hospital observations, rather than with hundreds of thousands of patient records. There are, however, some situations in which the hospital is more clearly the appropriate unit of analysis. For example, it would be hard to imagine using patients as the unit of observation for studies of hospital mortality rates over time (Sloan, Perrin, and Valvona 1986) or the effect of outcomes on volume (Luft, Hunt, and Maerki 1987).

WHAT DATA ARE USED AND HOW RELIABLE ARE THEY?

Three principal types of data have been used to examine patient outcomes:

- Data drawn from medical records or prospectively collected as part of the research project (Farber, Kaiser, and Wenzel 1981; Flood et al. 1979)

- Data from routinely collected case abstracts provided by the hospitals for all patients (Flood, Scott, and Ewy 1984a; Kelly and Hellinger 1986; Luft, Bunker, and Enthoven 1979; Showstack et al. 1987)

- Insurance claims data to track patients in and out of the hospital (Riley and Lubitz 1985; Roos, Roos, and Sharp 1987; Wennberg et al. 1987)

The most detailed measures of patient risk factors are found in prospectively collected data. Such data also provide measures of outcomes beyond mortality, such as postoperative wound infection rates or evaluation of patient health status at a given time. These data may provide information concerning what went wrong in identifying causal factors underlying poor outcomes. The principal drawback is that such data are costly and, therefore, that studies using them tend to be restricted to a very small number of hospitals.

Routinely collected case abstract data provide breadth but not much depth. For example, many states, including Maryland, California, and New York, collect such data from all hospitals and make them available to researchers for a nominal sum. The Commission on Professional and Hospital Activities (CPHA) has similar data from up to 1,700 hospitals across the country, but hospital identifiers are not available to researchers. Discharge abstract data are also available for Medicare patients from the Office of Statistics and Data Management of the Health Care Financing Administration (HCFA).

There are several limitations to case abstract data. One potential problem is that the diagnosis data pertain to discharge status rather than admission. Relatively little information is provided on test results, such as biopsies, that provide information on the severity of illness. (The data from the CPHA include some information on blood pressure, hemoglobin, and other tests. New data systems with severity measures, such as MedisGroups and the Computerized Severity

Index, also include far more detailed data. These sources have not, however, been used for volume-outcome research.)

In addition, this routinely collected information depends on the accuracy of the hospital's medical records abstractors in the coding of diagnoses and procedures from charts. Hospitals that code diagnoses in more detail may appear to have a sicker case mix. The Medicare Provider Analysis and Review (MEDPAR) files from HCFA allow for a principal diagnosis and up to four additional diagnoses, a limitation that may introduce bias. Some investigators have suggested that, because of this limit, acute problems may take precedence over chronic illnesses on the medical chart's diagnosis list in patients with several acute medical problems (Jencks, Williams, and Kay 1988). Several studies of the accuracy of hospital abstracting suggest a high error rate (Institute of Medicine 1980). Since the introduction of Medicare's prospective payment system (PPS) in 1983, the reliability and consistency, if not the validity, of case abstract coding among hospitals have most likely improved because hospital payment based on case mix has given medical record abstracting much more importance (Hsia et al. 1988). Errors not associated with volume will have little effect on the relationships we are exploring, although such errors will make it more difficult to detect a volume-outcome relationship.

Claims data also have the advantage of breadth, with Medicare claims data available from almost all U.S. hospitals. Unfortunately, claims data, particularly non-Medicare insurance data, often include even less information concerning diagnoses than routinely collected case abstract data. With some manipulation, claims data can be used to provide information on postdischarge patient status. In "universal" systems, such as the one used in Manitoba, Canada, and Medicare in the United States, eligibility files can be used to determine postdischarge deaths (Roos and Roos 1983). Repeated admissions or outpatient visits for selected procedures can also be used as measures of postdischarge complications. Unfortunately, coding problems for claims data may be even worse than for hospital discharge abstracts. This is particularly true for medical diagnoses; surgical procedures are generally well coded (Chassin et al. 1987).

WHICH DIAGNOSES AND PROCEDURES
HAVE BEEN STUDIED?

Table 2.1 presents a summary listing of the 15 procedures and diagnoses investigated in the 25 major studies we reviewed. In general, we chose procedures and diagnoses that have been the subject of several different studies of the volume-outcome relationship, preferably by different researchers. Thus a few studies include data on selected procedures not shown in Table 2.1. This approach was used to explore the underlying generalizability of the research.

The studies are grouped in the left-hand column by research team and the publication date of the first article by the team; for instance, the two studies by Kelly and Hellinger are shown together. To find out which authors studied a particular diagnosis or procedure (e.g., abdominal aortic aneurysm), read down the column. Also indicated are the measure of volume (HV = hospital volume or PV = physician volume) and of outcome (D = death, M = morbidity, L = long length of hospital stay, or R = readmission).

These 15 surgical procedures and medical diagnoses differ in terms of ease of analysis. Surgery is easier to study for several reasons. First, surgical procedures are generally well identified and coded both on hospital discharge abstracts and insurance claims. The occurrence of an operation is rarely in dispute, even though the choice of procedure or necessity for it may be questioned by various physicians. Only in rare cases is there a frequent miscoding of procedure, such as revision of total hip versus total hip replacement. (Random miscodings probably occur across the board. With procedures, however, one can check for the presence of a relevant diagnosis and exclude, for example, cases indicating a cholecystectomy without any gall bladder–related diagnoses.) In contrast, the determination of some medical diagnoses is often quite difficult; comparably trained clinicians may disagree on how an individual patient should be classified. For example, patients with lobar consolidation may be classified with pneumonia, pulmonary infarction, or pneumonitis associated with an underlying vasculitis. Patients with reactive airways disease may be classified with acute asthma or acute exacerbation of chronic obstructive pulmonary disease.

Second, severity of illness may vary with surgically treated patients, but it is less likely to be an important source of bias in volume-outcome studies than it is for medically treated patients. This is particularly true for procedures that are typically scheduled, such as total hip replacement. Although the degree of impairment in mobility and the presence and severity of chronic comorbidities, such as hypertension and diabetes, may vary, few surgeons would perform elective surgery for patients with acute medical illnesses. Thus the relative absence of adequate measures of severity will probably have a greater effect on analysis of medical than surgical admissions. Variability in rate of medical admissions across towns and states may be associated with differences in severity or case complexity that may, in turn, influence outcomes (Wennberg and Gittelsohn 1973; Wennberg and Gittelsohn 1975; Roos 1984; Paul-Shaheen, Clark, and Williams 1987). In particular, if some hospitals tend to admit less sick patients, volume might increase and outcomes improve simultaneously.

Third, to some extent, the reasons for medical and surgical admissions differ in ways that influence the interpretation of a volume-outcome relationship. Surgery is often used to increase longevity or to correct a problem that interferes with the quality of life but may not be immediately life-threatening. Because the patient often is in reasonably good health on admission, short-term mortality is

Table 2.1: Studies on the Relationship between Volume and Outcome for Specific Diagnoses and Procedures

Study[a]	Abdominal Aortic Aneurysm	Acute Myocardial Infarction	Appendectomy	Biliary Tract Surgery	Cardiac Catheterization	Coronary Artery Bypass Graft Surgery	Femur Fracture	Hernia	Hysterectomy	Intestinal Operation	Newborn Diseases	Prostatectomy	Stomach Operation	Total Hip Replacement	Vascular Surgery
1. Adams et al. (1973)					HV/D										
2. Williams (1979)											HV/D				
3. Luft et al. (1979)[b]	HV/D			HV/D		HV/D						HV/D	HV/D	HV/D	HV/D
4. Luft (1980)[c]	HV/D			HV/D		HV/D				HV/D		HV/D	HV/D	HV/D	HV/D
5. Maerki et al. (1986)[d]	HV/D	HV/D	HV/D	HV/D		HV/D	HV/D	HV/D	HV/D	HV/D	HV/D	HV/D	HV/D	HV/D	
6. Luft and Hunt (1986)					HV/D										
7. Luft et al. (1987)[e]	HV/D	HV/D					HV/D				HV/D				
8. Hughes et al. (1987)			HV,PV/D,L	HV/D, HV,PV/D,L	HV/D, HV,PV/D,L	HV/D, HV,PV/D,L		HV/D, HV,PV/D,L	HV/D, HV,PV/D,L	HV/D, HV,PV/D,L	HV/D	HV/D, HV,PV/D,L	HV/D, HV,PV/D,L	HV/D, HV,PV/D,L	
9. Hughes et al. (1988)							HV/D,L								
10. Pilcher et al. (1980)	HV,PV/D														
11. Farber et al. (1981)[f]			HV/M					HV/M	HV/M	HV/M					
12. Shortell and LoGerfo (1981)		PV/D	PV/M												
13. Hertzer et al. (1984)															PV/D,M
14. Flood et al. (1984a)[g]	HV/D			HV/D			HV/D			HV/D			HV/D		

Study[a]									
15. Rosenblatt et al. (1985)									
16. Riley and Lubitz (1985)		HV/D			HV/D		HV/D		HV/D
17. Kempczinski et al. (1986)			HV/D						
18. Sloan et al. (1986)[h]		HV/D	HV/D	HV/D	HV/D		HV/D		HV/D
19. Kelly and Hellinger (1986)	HV,PV/D			HV,PV/D	HV,PV/D		HV,PV/D		PV/D,M
20. Kelly and Hellinger (1987)		HV,PV/D	HV,PV/D HV,PV/D			HV,PV/D			
21. Fowles et al. (1987)	HV,PV/D						HV,PV/R		HV,PV/D,M
22. Roos et al. (1986)	HV,PV/R		HV,PV/R	HV,PV/R		HV,PV/R			
23. Roos et al. (1987)	HV/R		HV/R	HV/R					
24. Wennberg et al. (1987)					HV/D		HV/D		
25. Showstack et al. (1987)			HV/D,L						

Abbreviations: HV = hospital volume; PV = physician volume; D = death; L = long length of hospital stay. M = morbidity; R = readmission.

[a]Studies are ordered by research team and date of first publication by the team.
[b]Luft et al. (1979) also studied open-heart surgery.
[c]Luft et al. (1980) also studied open-heart surgery.
[d]Maerki et al. (1986) also studied cirrhosis, peptic ulcer, subarachnoid hemorrhage, and tonsillectomy.
[e]Luft et al. (1987) also studied cirrhosis, subarachnoid hemorrhage, and peptic ulcer.
[f]Farber et al. (1981) also studied laminectomy and cesarean section.
[g]Flood et al. (1984) also studied amputation of lower limb, nonsurgical gallbladder diagnosis, and nonsurgical ulcer diagnosis.
[h]Sloan et al. (1986) also studied morbid obesity surgery, mastectomy, nephrectomy, and spinal fusion.
Adapted from: Office of Technology Assessment, 1988.

more likely to reflect treatment effects than the patient's underlying health. In contrast, medical admissions are more apt to be in response to immediate life-threatening problems or for palliation of terminal illnesses. In such cases, the patient's health status on admission may be a more important determinant of short-term outcomes than the quality of care rendered. Thus, for example, there are no studies of the volume-outcome relationship for medical oncology patients, although we have included in our review some studies of surgical interventions for cancer.

Chapter 3

Description of Research Studies

This chapter summarizes each of the 25 studies examined in this book. The source of the data, time period under study, and outcome measures are described, and the overall results are reviewed briefly. A discussion of the statistical methodology follows, which describes the measure of volume, the specific outcome measure, the unit of analysis, and the type of analysis performed. Studies are listed here by research group and date of publication.

1. Adams, Douglass F.; Fraser, David B.; and Abrams, Herbert L. (1973). "The Complications of Coronary Arteriography." *Circulation* 48 (3): 609–18.

Summary

The authors undertook a nationwide survey to determine the rate of complications from coronary arteriography during the period 1970–71. Analysis of responses from 173 hospitals, reviewing a total of 46,904 coronary arteriograms, considered both the angiographic technique used and the number of examinations performed at each hospital. The mortality rate in institutions performing fewer than 200 arteriograms every two years was eight times higher than that in institutions performing more than 800 arteriograms every two years. This pattern was also present for the incidence of such complications as myocardial infarction and cerebral embolism.

Method

The authors grouped institutions into four volume categories: fewer than 200, 200–499, 500–799, and more than 800 angiograms per two years. They displayed the relationship between hospital volume category and the different outcomes graphically and used chi-square tests to compare the outcomes of the lowest-volume category and the highest-volume category. A separate analysis compared two subgroups of angiograms, those performed by the brachial approach and those performed by the femoral approach. There was no adjustment for patient risk factors.

2. Williams, Ronald L. (1979). "Measuring the Effectiveness of Perinatal Medical Care." *Medical Care* 17 (2): 95–109. [Reprinted in Chapter 18]

Summary

The author examined the effectiveness of perinatal care for 3,370,338 births in 504 California hospitals in 1960 and 1965–73. The outcome measure in this study was the indirectly standardized observed-to-expected mortality ratio. This ratio was correlated significantly with many of the explanatory factors examined. Mortality ratios were significantly lower in hospitals with larger delivery services, in urban hospitals, in hospitals performing a higher percentage of cesarean sections, in those routinely recording Apgar scores, and in those having higher specialist-to-generalist ratios. Conversely, the mortality ratios were significantly higher in hospitals with large percentages of Hispanic mothers and in private, proprietary hospitals.

Method

Williams first calculated an expected infant mortality rate for each hospital, based on the distribution of that hospital's births by 19 birthweight categories, gender, race (white, Hispanic, black), and plurality (single, multiple). He then divided the actual death rate for each hospital by the expected death rate to generate the outcome variable, an indirectly standardized mortality ratio. Finally, he regressed the outcome variable against hospital volume, specified as number of annual births. Certain regressions included the squared volume term to measure a curvilinear effect. The regression analysis included numerous other hospital characteristics, such as ownership status, urban location, and cesarean section rate, as additional independent variables. The regression was weighted to account for binomial variation within hospitals with small numbers of annual births.

Note that this approach controls, in a linear fashion, for the statistical effect of urban location, cesarean section rate, and so forth, on the outcome measure. These adjustments will shift the volume-outcome curve up or down, but they will not affect its shape. For example, suppose that higher C-section rates led to better outcomes in low-volume hospitals but had no effect on outcomes in high-volume hospitals. One would have to include interaction terms in the regression to test for this effect.

3. Luft, Harold S.; Bunker, John P.; and Enthoven, Alain C. (1979). "Should Operations Be Regionalized? The Empirical Relation between Surgical Volume and Mortality." *New England Journal of Medicine* 301 (25): 1364–69. [Reprinted in Chapter 12]

Summary

This study examined mortality rates for 12 surgical procedures of varying complexity in 1,498 hospitals to determine whether there was a relationship between a hospital's surgical volume and its surgical mortality. The authors obtained data from the Commission on Professional and Hospital Activities from the years 1974 and 1975. The mortality of open-heart surgery, vascular surgery, transurethral resection of the prostate, and coronary artery bypass grafting decreased with increasing number of operations throughout the range of hospital volumes examined. For other procedures, mortality also decreased with increasing hospital volume, but the relation flattened at relatively low volume. Other procedures, such as cholecystectomy, showed no relation between volume and mortality.

Method

The authors classified hospitals into volume groups based on the average number of the specific procedures performed annually: 1, 2–4, 5–10, 11–20, 21–50, 51–100, 101–200, and more than 201 surgical procedures. Then they calculated expected death rates for each hospital, based on its mix of patients categorized by five age groups, gender, and whether single diagnoses or multiple diagnoses were coded. This subdivision yielded 20 cells ($5 \times 2 \times 2$). The authors calculated each hospital's expected death rate using cell-specific death rates for the whole sample, weighted by the proportion of each hospital's patients falling in each of the 20 cells. After plotting actual and expected death rates for patients in hospitals within each volume category, the authors interpreted the effect of volumes on outcome as the difference between the expected and actual values. Although this method offered a clear graphic representation of the relationship between volumes and outcomes, statistical testing was not performed.

4. Luft, Harold S. (1980). "The Relation between Surgical Volume and Mortality: An Exploration of Causal Factors and Alternative Models." *Medical Care*, 18 (9): 940–59. [Reprinted in Chapter 16]

Summary

This study explored the relationship between volume and postoperative mortality in relation to several other potentially important variables such as hospital size, teaching status, charges, and geographic area. The author examined 12 procedures of varying complexity in 1,498 hospitals from 1974 and 1975, using the same data as did Luft, Bunker, and Enthoven (1979). In general, the importance of volume was not decreased by inclusion of the other variables. Luft discussed alternative hypotheses concerning the causality of the relationship and proposed a preliminary simultaneous-equation approach.

Method

This study used regression techniques to explore the relationship between volume and mortality. The dependent variable was the actual-minus-expected mortality rate for each hospital. Luft calculated the expected mortality rate as in Luft, Bunker, and Enthoven (1979), using the same matrix to account for case-mix differences between hospitals. The regression was weighted to give more emphasis to hospitals with higher volumes and to patient mixes with lower expected death rates. The author specified volume as the logarithm of the current year volume, although he performed some regressions using combinations of current and previous year volume, and others using the logarithm of total volume of related procedures (such as total open-heart procedures in the equation for coronary artery bypass surgery). He included several hospital variables as additional independent variables: bed size, number of admissions, house staff size, metropolitan location, region, and hospital charges.

5. Maerki, Susan C.; Luft, Harold S.; and Hunt, Sandra S. (1986). "Selecting Categories of Patients for Regionalization: Implications of the Relationship between Volume and Outcome." *Medical Care* 24 (2): 148–58.

Summary

This article examined data for 15 diagnoses to explore the implications of regionalization policies for various categories of patients. The authors used data from the CPHA for 1972 to model actual and expected hospital death rates as a function of hospital volume. Using these estimated curves, the authors explored the implications of transferring patients from low-volume to high-volume hospitals. For all but two diagnoses, either the volume or the volume-squared coefficient (or both) was significant, an indication of improved outcomes at higher-volume hospitals. Further analysis showed large potential differences in lives saved for varying degrees of regionalization.

Method

The regression used the hospital mortality rate as the outcome variable and the expected hospital death rate, volume, and volume-squared as the independent variables. The authors determined the expected death rate by indirect standardization, using age, gender, single or multiple diagnoses, and admission blood pressure. The actual number of cells varied for each diagnoses or procedure. Each observation was weighted to account for hospitals with higher volumes and with patient mixes with lower expected death rates.

6. Luft, Harold S., and Hunt, Sandra S. (1986). "Evaluating Individual Hospital Quality through Outcome Statistics." *Journal of the American Medical Association* 255 (20): 2780–84. [Reprinted in Chapter 19]

Summary

Using 1982 CPHA data, the authors found an inverse relationship between hospital volume and patient mortality for cardiac catheterization. Small numbers of patients and relatively low rates of poor outcomes made it difficult to evaluate the performance of many hospitals. Nevertheless, examination of patterns of outcomes indicated that low-volume hospitals were more likely to have results that were worse than expected, and high-volume hospitals were more likely to have results that were better than expected. The paper discusses the limitation of using statistical methods to identify outliers.

Method

The regression analysis performed was almost identical to Luft (1980). The dependent variable was the actual-minus-expected mortality rate, where the expected mortality rate for each hospital was calculated based on its mix of patients, categorized by three age groups and presence of cardiac dysrhythmia, heart failure, single and multiple diagnoses (12 cells). The authors regressed the actual-minus-expected death rate against the log of volume, but did not include other hospital variables in the regression. They also presented probability distributions of hospitals' actual mortality rates within five volume categories.

7. Luft, Harold S., Hunt, Sandra S., and Maerki, Susan C. (1987). "The Volume-Outcome Relationship: Practice Makes Perfect or Selective Referral Patterns?" *Health Services Research* 22 (2): 157–82.

Summary

In order to explore the causal relationship between volumes and outcomes, this article examined 1972 CPHA data for 17 categories of patients from a sample of over 900 hospitals. The authors found a clear-cut relationship between volumes and outcomes for several categories of patients and developed a simultaneous-equation model to explore the relative importance of the practice-makes-perfect and selective-referral hypotheses. The results suggested that (1) both explanations are valid, and (2) the relative importance of the practice or referral explanation varies by diagnosis or procedure.

Method

This paper took two approaches to studying the relationship between volumes and outcomes. First, hospitals were divided into several volume categories. Then an actual-to-expected mortality ratio was calculated for each volume category. The expected mortality rate took into account each hospital's mix of patients categorized by age, gender, presence of multiple diagnoses, and admission blood pressure (see discussion of the study by Maerki, Luft, and Hunt [1986]). The shape of the histogram indicated the relationship. The curves were described as decreasing, L-shaped, or indeterminate. The same approach was used to examine the proportion of patients transferring into or out of hospitals in each volume category. Statistical testing of the curves was not performed.

The second approach used a simultaneous-equation model to test the causality of the relationship. To test the relationship from volumes to outcomes, the authors performed regressions with the actual-minus-expected death rate as the *dependent* variable and log volume as the *independent* variable. They derived each hospital's expected death rate as described above. They included as additional independent variables other variables such as medical school affiliation, patient transfer rate, and geographic location, which might affect patient outcomes but not volumes. The second regression in the model had log volume as the dependent variable and actual-minus-expected death rate as an independent variable, along with factors likely to influence volume but not outcomes, such as hospital size and medical staff members per bed. The regressions were weighted to account for different numbers of patients in each hospital.

8. Hughes, Robert G.; Hunt, Sandra S.; and Luft, Harold S. (1987). "Effects of Surgeon Volume and Hospital Volume on Quality of Care in Hospitals." *Medical Care* 25 (6): 489– 503. [Reprinted in Chapter 17]

Summary

This paper analyzed the influence of hospital volume and surgery by low-volume surgeons on hospital death rates and long stays. Ten surgical procedures were examined for 503,662 patients in 757 hospitals. Hospitals included in the study were subscribers to the 1982 CPHA study and respondents to the 1983 Survey of

Specialized Clinical Services. Higher hospital volume and lower proportion of patients operated on by low-volume surgeons were positively related to better patient outcomes for most procedures.

Method

In order to determine the number of poor outcomes, the authors added the number of in-hospital deaths and the number of admissions resulting in hospital stays greater than the 90th percentile length of stay for each procedure. The authors calculated the expected poor outcome rate for each hospital, using each hospital's case-mix matrix for each procedure, generally using age categories, gender, and single versus multiple diagnoses. The number of cells varied for different procedures. They expressed the results as the probability that the actual outcome would differ from the expected outcome rate, based on the Poisson distribution, the number of patients in each hospital, the actual outcome rate, and the expected outcome rate. Then they converted this figure to a Z-score, which served as the dependent variable in the regression. The effects of hospital volume and physician volume were tested simultaneously. The authors specified hospital volume as the logarithm of current volume, and surgeon volume as the proportion of patients in each hospital operated on by surgeons doing less than the median volume of the procedure. The regression equation included several other hospital and demographic variables.

9. Hughes, Robert G.; Garnick, Deborah W.; Luft, Harold S.; McPhee, Stephen J; and Hunt, Sandra S. (1988). "Hospital Volume and Patient Outcomes: The Case of Hip Fracture Patients." *Medical Care* 26 (11) 1057–67.

Summary

The authors used two sets of simultaneous equations to analyze the causal direction of the observed volume-outcome relationship for 44,905 patients with hip fractures from 704 short-term general hospitals in 1982. Hughes, Hunt, and Luft (1987) also examined this procedure using the same data. The outcome measures were mortality (expressed as in-hospital deaths) and morbidity (expressed as long hospital stays as a proxy for complications). Results showed that higher volumes of patients led to better outcomes, indicating a practice-makes-perfect effect, and hospitals with better performance attracted higher volumes, confirming a selective-referral effect. Patient and hospital factors associated with poorer outcomes were secondary diagnoses of diabetes and heart disease, public hospital ownership, medical school affiliation, location in the eastern United States, and a higher percentage of blacks in the county population.

Method

The in-hospital mortality served as the outcome measure in one set of simultaneous equations, and morbidity, defined as hospital stays longer than the 90th-percentile length of stay, served as the outcome measure in the other set. The authors used the actual mortality, expected mortality, and number of patients to generate a mortality Z-score, similar to the study by Hughes, Hunt, and Luft (1987). Similarly, the actual morbidity (measured in terms of long stays), expected morbidity, and number of patients generated a morbidity Z-score. In the equation predicting outcome, the Z-score was the dependent variable in a weighted regression with the logarithm of hospital volume and the other variables expected to account for differences in outcomes, such as proportion of patients with certain secondary diagnoses, proportion of transferred patients, and several hospital variables. In the equation predicting volume, the Z-score was an independent variable along with variables expected to account for differences in volume, such as hospital size, proportion of local population over age 64, and presence of an orthopedic department.

10. Pilcher, David B.; Davis, John H.; Ashikaga, Takamuru; Bookwalter, John; Butsch, David W.; Chase, Christopher R.; Ellman, Barry R.; Vacek, Pamela M.; and Lord, Frederick C. (1980). "Treatment of Abdominal Aortic Aneurysm in an Entire State over 7½ Years." *American Journal of Surgery* 139 (4): 487–94.

Summary

In a survey of results of abdominal aortic aneurysm resection in eight general hospitals in Vermont between 1970 and 1977 the authors examined mortality after elective and emergency surgery by hospital volume and surgeon volume. They found that mortality rates for ruptured aneurysm were significantly inversely related to hospital volume, and for elective aneurysm resection, to surgeon volume. Hospital volume group and patient characteristics such as age, presence of diabetes, coronary artery disease, and history of back pain were important factors associated with postoperative mortality.

Method

The authors divided hospitals performing aneurysm surgery into three volume categories: the university medical center (high), greater than one patient per year (middle), and less than one patient per year (low). They also divided surgeons into three groups with cutoff values of fewer than two, two to four, and more than four aneurysm patients per surgeon per year. The authors compared the mortality rate in each volume group using a chi-square test. The paper also describes a discriminant analysis of uncertain type with hospital volume group included as a variable. The data analysis examined elective and ruptured aneurysm patients separately. The hospital volume analyses did not consider any other patient case-mix variables beyond the type of aneurysm surgery (elective versus emergency).

11. Farber, Bruce F.; Kaiser, Donald L.; and Wenzel, Richard P. (1981). "Relation between Surgical Volume and Incidence of Postoperative Wound Infection." *New England Journal of Medicine* 305 (4): 200–204. [Reprinted in Chapter 9]

Summary

The authors examined the relationship between the volume of seven surgical procedures and the incidence of postoperative wound infection for 25,941 surgical procedures at 22 Virginia area hospitals between 1977 and 1979. Each hospital collected information on infections prospectively as part of a statewide infection-control program. The authors found a significant inverse relationship between the frequency of operations and the infection rate for appendectomy, herniorrhaphy, cholecystectomy, colon resection, and abdominal hysterectomy. The relationship was borderline for laminectomy and not significant for cesarean section.

Method

The authors performed a logistic regression using the binary outcome of the presence or the absence of postoperative infection. Hospital volume was expressed as the base-ten logarithm of the number of operations performed during the study period. No other patient or hospital variables were included in the analysis. The authors performed separate analyses to test hypotheses of hospital infection reporting rates and overall infection rates as a function of the number of hospital beds, to account for the potential confounding effect of hospital size. The authors displayed infection rates graphically over several volume categories for each procedure.

12. Shortell, Stephen M., and LoGerfo, James P. (1981). "Hospital Medical Staff Organization and Quality of Care: Results for Myocardial Infarction and Appendectomy." *Medical Care* 19 (10): 1041–53.

Summary

The authors examined the relationship of hospital structural characteristics, physician characteristics, and medical staff organization to outcomes for acute myocardial infarction (AMI) and appendectomy in 96 hospitals in the east-north-central United States. The authors obtained data from a 35-percent stratified sample of the hospitals in this region that subscribed to the CPHA. They found an association between lower mortality rates from AMI and a higher volume of patients treated per family practitioner or internist. The presence of a coronary care unit also lowered mortality rates. They did not observe a volume-outcome relationship for appendectomy.

Method

For AMI the outcome measured was the in-hospital mortality rate. For appendectomy, the outcome measured was the proportion of cases with normal tissue pathology. The paper expressed both outcome measures as indirectly standardized mortality (normal tissue) ratios. Standardization of AMI mortality rates was based on age category and admission blood pressure (six cells); standardization of appendectomy normal tissue rates was based on age and gender (four cells). The paper expressed physician volume as the number of patients in each diagnosis divided by the number of appropriate physicians on staff (for AMI patients—internists and family practitioners; for appendectomy patients—surgeons, and family practitioners). The authors regressed the outcome ratios for the two diagnoses against this measure of physician volume and several hospital organizational and structural characteristics.

13. Hertzer, Norman R.; Avellone, Joseph C.; Farrell, Charles J.; Plecha, Fred R.; Rhodes, Robert S.; Sharp, William V.; and Wright, George F. (1984). "The Risk of Vascular Surgery in a Metropolitan Community." *Journal of Vascular Surgery* 1 (1): 13–21.

Summary

This paper analyzed morbidity and mortality rates for 5,686 vascular surgical procedures of four types performed by 29 vascular surgeons in 27 northeastern Ohio hospitals from 1978 through 1981. Procedures examined were carotid endarterectomy, femoral-popliteal or distal bypass, abdominal aortic aneurysm repair, and aorto-femoral reconstruction. Operative mortality rates were not related to the size of the 27 hospitals studied. Annual surgeon volume significantly influenced only the mortality rate for elective abdominal aortic aneurysm resection and the amputation rate after femoropopliteal or distal revascularization.

Method

The authors divided annual surgeon experience for each procedure into three categories: fewer than 10, 10 to 25, and more than 25. The authors then compared mortality and morbidity rates in each surgeon volume group, using the chi-square test. They measured postoperative mortality as the outcome for all procedures and selected morbid outcomes for certain procedures. In addition, they performed some analyses on subgroups with procedures, such as elective and ruptured abdominal aneurysm resection, and carotid endarterectomy with and without preoperative neurologic symptoms. There were no additional factors included in the analyses to account for differences in patient risk.

14. Flood, A. B.; Scott, W. R.; and Ewy, W. (1984). "Does Practice Make Perfect? Part I: The Relation between Volume and Outcomes for Selected Diagnostic Categories. Part II: The Relation between Volume and Outcomes and Other Hospital Characteristics." *Medical Care* 22 (2): 98–114, 115–25. [Part I reprinted in Chapter 14]

Summary

The authors studied the effect of patient volume on mortality for 550,000 patients treated in more than 1,200 U.S. acute-care hospitals belonging to CPHA in 1972 for 15 surgical procedures and two medical diagnoses. For several categories of patients, high patient volume was associated with lower mortality. Additional analyses incorporated the risk level of patients. The evidence suggested a particular association between low hospital volume and poor outcomes for low-risk surgical patients.

Method

The authors calculated an expected probability of in-hospital death for each patient, using logistic equations based on each patient's outcome, demographic, and clinical information drawn from the discharge abstract. The authors compared patients in hospitals with less than the mean hospital volume for each diagnosis to those in hospitals with greater than the mean hospital volume. They used chi-square tests to determine the difference between the actual number of deaths and the expected number of deaths in the two volume categories. Further analyses sought to identify volume effects for varying levels of patient risk. Using the logistic equations, the authors grouped the patients into three risk levels chosen so that approximately one-third of the deaths fell into each category. Within each risk category, the expected mortality rate and the actual mortality rate were calculated for hospitals with greater than the mean volume and less than the mean volume.

15. Rosenblatt, Roger A.; Reinken, Judith; and Shoemack, Phil (1985). "Is Obstetrics Safe in Small Hospitals? Evidence from New Zealand's Regionalised Perinatal System." *Lancet* 2 (8452): 429–32.

Summary

The authors calculated crude and birthweight-adjusted perinatal mortality rates for all public maternity hospitals in New Zealand for the years 1978–81, according to designated hospital levels (primary, secondary, or tertiary care units) and hospital volume of deliveries. Level 1 (primary maternity care) units had lower crude and birthweight-specific perinatal mortality rates in all but the lowest birthweight categories. There was no volume threshold detectable below which obstetrical care became unsafe. The authors cited effective regionalization of perinatal services as an explanation for their findings.

Method

This article used chi-square tests to examine the relationship between hospital volumes and perinatal mortality. One analysis plotted each hospital's unadjusted perinatal mortality rate as a function of its average annual births. Another analysis calculated mortality rates across three birthweight categories (less than 1,501 grams, 1,501 to 2,499 grams, and greater than 2,499 grams) for three hospital volume categories.

16. Riley, Gerald, and Lubitz, James (1985). "Outcomes of Surgery among the Medicare Aged: Surgical Volume and Mortality." *Health Care Financing Review* 7 (1): 37–47. [Reprinted in Chapter 15]

Summary

Using 1979 and 1980 data on a 20-percent sample of Medicare beneficiaries, the authors examined the relationship between hospital surgical volume and mortality within 60 days of surgery for eight procedures. High surgical volume was associated with lower mortality for CABG surgery, transurethral resection of the prostate, hip arthroplasty (excluding total hip replacement), and resection of the intestine. No relationship was seen for cholecystectomy, total hip replacement, inguinal hernia repair, and femur fracture reduction.

Method

This study used logistic regression with mortality as the binary outcome variable for each patient observation. The specification of hospital volume was the logarithm of hospital volume. (This method differs from the one used by Kelly and Hellinger in that the transformation of the volume variable causes the value of the dependent variable, mortality, to approach 1 as volume approaches 0. Otherwise, the slope gradually decreases as volume increases.) Since the study was based on a 20-percent sample of Medicare patients, hospital volumes were estimated by multiplying by 5 the number of patients undergoing each procedure at each hospital. The regression included patient risk factors as additional independent variables: age, gender, age multiplied by gender, emergency operation (defined as operation on the same day as admission), and presence of certain procedure-specific diagnoses. Hospital and demographic variables in the regression included geographic region, Standard Metropolitan Statistical Area (SMSA) location, proprietary hospital, and bed size.

17. Kempczinski, Richard F.; Brott, Thomas G.; and Labutta, Robert J. (1986). "The Influence of Surgical Specialty and Caseload on the Results of Carotid Endarterectomy." *Journal of Vascular Surgery* 3 (6): 911–16.

Summary

This paper examined the impact of surgical specialty and operative caseload on the results of all carotid endarterectomies in the greater Cincinnati area during 1983 and 1984. In all, 61 surgeons working in 16 hospitals performed 750 operations on 656 patients. The authors observed a trend of decreasing stroke rate with increasing physician volume, although this result was not statistically significant. They found no such trend for hospital volume.

Method

The authors divided yearly surgical caseloads of surgeons into three categories (fewer than 12, 12 to 50, and more than 50 procedures). They compared mortality rates and stroke rates of the three different volume categories, using the chi-square test. There was no adjustment for differences in patient risk factors.

18. Sloan, Frank A.; Perrin, J. M.; and Valvona, F. (1986). "In-Hospital Mortality of Surgical Patients: Is There an Empiric Basis for Standard Setting?" *Surgery* 99 (4): 446–53. [Reprinted in Chapter 13]

Summary

The authors analyzed mortality data from patients undergoing one of seven surgical procedures between 1972 and 1981 from a national cohort of 521 hospitals subscribing to the CPHA. On the average, lower mortality rates were associated with higher annual hospital volumes. This decline was significant for three of the seven procedures examined when regression techniques were used. Regressions explained less than 10 percent of the variation in hospital death rates, however. Using an alternative analysis, the authors demonstrated that low mortality rates (zero deaths) were found in low-volume hospitals. For these reasons, the authors suggested that a statistical basis for minimum volume standards did not exist.

Method

Regressions were estimated with the in-hospital mortality rate as the dependent variable. The unit of observation was the hospital, and patient risk factors, expressed as the proportion of patients in each hospital with the risk factor, included patient age, gender, surgery within six hours of admission, multiple diagnoses, consultations, insurance status, and several procedure-specific diagnoses. To account for the curvilinear effect of volume on mortality, the authors included both volume and volume-squared as independent variables. Hospital characteristics included as independent variables were bed size, teaching status, and presence of particular services and residency programs. Regressions were run on the full sample of hospitals studied and on the subset of hospitals that experienced at least one death for the particular procedure. Other regressions included a variable to account for differences in state rate-setting regulations.

19. Kelly, Joyce V., and Hellinger, Fred J. (1986). "Physician and Hospital Factors Associated with Mortality of Surgical Patients." *Medical Care* 24 (9): 785–800.

Summary

This study examined the effects of both physician volume and hospital volume on hospital mortality for four categories of surgical patients: stomach cancer, peptic ulcer, colon cancer, and abdominal aortic aneurysm. Data were obtained for 1977 from the Hospital Cost and Utilization Project (HCUP), a sample of 373 short-term general, nonfederal hospitals. The results were generally consistent with an inverse relationship between hospital volume and mortality. However, there was no consistent relationship between physician volume and mortality, which suggested that the relationship reflected hospital rather than physician characteristics. Other variables, such as physician board certification and hospital medical school affiliation, were associated with lower patient mortality rates.

Method

This study used logistic regression analysis with each patient record as the unit of observation. Physician and hospital volume were both included as independent variables and expressed as simple continuous variables. The binary outcome variable that was assessed was in-hospital mortality. The authors controlled for several patient risk factors as additional independent variables: age, insurance status, number of diagnoses, and stage of disease. They also included several hospital variables as independent variables: teaching status, geographic location, charges, and total number of admissions. The analysis excluded patients with lengths of stay of one day, patients over the age of 99 or under the age of 18, and patients in proprietary hospitals.

20. Kelly, Joyce V., and Hellinger, Fred J. (1987). "Heart Disease and Hospital Deaths: An Empirical Study." *Health Services Research* 22 (3): 369–95. [Reprinted in Chapter 10]

Summary

This study examined the mortality of patients with coronary artery bypass graft surgery, cardiac catheterization, and acute myocardial infarction in short-term general hospitals included in the 1977 Hospital Cost and Utilization Project. For CABG, there were data on 26 hospitals, for cardiac catheterization, data on 39 hospitals, and for AMI, data on 146 hospitals. This study showed that patients undergoing cardiac catheterization or CABG were more likely to survive when their procedures were performed in hospitals with higher procedural volumes, but that higher physician volumes had no significant effect. For AMI patients, higher physician volume, but not hospital volume, correlated with increased survival.

Method

Study methods were identical to those used by Kelly and Hellinger (1986).

21. Fowles, Jinnet; Bunker, John P.; and Schurman, David J. (1987). "Hip Surgery Data Yield Quality Indicators." *Business and Health* 4 (8): 44–46.

Summary

The authors examined the relationship between hospital and surgeon volumes and death or major complications following total hip replacement. They studied 1,324 procedures performed on Medicare patients in northern California during 1982. These cases were followed through their claims histories for 22 to 32 months. Mortality within 90 days and readmissions requiring major or minor revision surgery were recorded. The results indicated that patients who died or had major complications were more likely to have been operated on by low-volume surgeons. This trend was also apparent for patients operated on at low-volume hospitals, although it was not statistically significant.

Method

The authors did not describe the statistical method used in the article. A pilot study by the authors used two sample *t*-tests to compare the mean surgeon (or hospital) volume for patients who died or had complications with those who did not. The analysis did not take into account patient case mix or hospital characteristics.

22. Roos, Leslie L.; Cageorge, Sandra M.; Roos, Noralou P.; and Danzinger, Rudy (1986). "Centralization, Certification, and Monitoring: Readmissions and Complications after Surgery." *Medical Care* 24 (11): 1044–66. [Reprinted in Chapter 8]

Summary

This paper analyzed patient, surgeon, and hospital characteristics associated with serious postdischarge complications following hysterectomy, cholecystectomy, and prostatectomy. The authors studied patients age 25 and older in Manitoba, Canada, between 1974 and 1976. They found a significant inverse association between physician surgical volume and risk of complications after cholecystectomy. When the authors controlled for age, gender, type of surgery, and duration of anesthetic, they found that patients of surgeons performing fewer than 20 cholecystectomies per year had increased odds of readmission for complications. For prostatectomy and hysterectomy, the study found no significant associations for either physician or hospital volumes.

Method

This study used multivariate logistic regression. The outcome variable was readmission in the two-year postoperative period for surgical complications as identified by physician panels for each procedure. Both hospital and physician volume were expressed as categorical variables. Low-volume hospitals performed fewer than 100 of each operation. Low-volume surgeons for each procedure performed fewer than 20 hysterectomies, fewer than 20 cholecystectomies, and fewer than 50 prostatectomies. The analysis included several patient characteristics as independent variables: age category, residence, type of surgery, duration of anesthetic, prior admissions to the hospital, chronic diagnoses, and presence of heart disease. Other physician and hospital characteristics included in the model were teaching status and physician specialty. The individual patient was the unit of analysis. The study used stepwise regression techniques, which first included statistically significant patient covariates before hospital and physician characteristics were allowed to enter the model. The results of such a regression showed only the variables that were statistically significant; variables not entering the model were not significant.

23. Roos, Leslie L.; Roos, Noralou P.; and Sharp, Sandra M. (1987). "Monitoring Adverse Outcomes of Surgery Using Administrative Data." *Health Care Financing Review* (Annual Supplement): 5–16.

Summary

Using administrative data from Manitoba, Canada for 1972–73, 1978–79, and 1982–83, the authors traced changes in mortality, readmissions for complications, case mix, and volume of surgery in hospitals and by individual surgeons for cholecystectomy, hysterectomy, and prostatectomy. Lower hospital volume, defined as fewer than 200 procedures over two years, was associated with higher readmissions for complications for cholecystectomy and hysterectomy.

Method

Study methods were identical to those used by Roos and colleagues (1986).

24. Wennberg, John E.; Roos, Noralou P.; Sola, Loredo; Schori, Alice; and Jaffe, Ross (1987). "Use of Claims Data Systems to Evaluate Health Care Outcomes: Mortality and Reoperation Following Prostatectomy." *Journal of the American Medical Association* 257 (7): 933–36.

Summary

Claims data for 1974 to 1977 from the Maine Medicare and Manitoba (Canada) Health Services Commission files were examined for deaths within 91 days following prostatectomy in hospitals doing fewer than 40, 40 to 90, or more than 90 procedures annually. After controlling for several patient and hospital characteristics, the authors found no significant relationship between mortality and the volume of prostatectomies performed.

Method

Except for the differences noted above, study methods were the same as those used by Roos and colleagues (1986). This study did not test physician volume.

25. Showstack, Jonathan A.; Rosenfeld, Kenneth E.; Garnick, Deborah W.; Luft, Harold S.; Schaffarzick, Ralph E.; and Fowles, Jinnet (1987). "Association of Volume with Outcome of Coronary Artery Bypass Graft Sur-

gery." *Journal of the American Medical Association* 257 (6): 785–89.
[Reprinted in Chapter 11]

Summary

The authors analyzed discharge abstracts for 18,986 coronary artery bypass graft surgeries in 77 California hospitals in 1983 using multiple regression techniques. After the authors adjusted for case mix, high-volume hospitals had lower in-hospital mortality, shorter average postoperative lengths of stay, and fewer patients with extremely long stays. These effects were greatest for patients who had "nonscheduled" bypass graft surgery.

Method

This study used ordinary least squares (OLS) multivariate regression techniques. The authors performed separate regressions for two different binary outcomes: in-hospital mortality and "poor outcome," defined as patients discharged alive beyond the 90th-percentile length of stay. The authors defined four volume categories: 20–100, 101– 200, 201–350, and more than 350 cases per year. Although hospital volume category was based on the total volume of bypass surgery performed at the hospital, the regression analysis excluded patients who underwent concurrent valve surgery. Additional independent variables in the regressions included the following patient risk factors: age, gender, white race, presence of acute myocardial infarction, congestive heart failure, or angina, and other procedures such as cardiac catheterization or angioplasty. The analysis also included the date of surgery relative to hospital admission as an independent variable: scheduled patients underwent surgery on the first or second day after admission, and nonscheduled patients underwent surgery on the day of admission or three or more days after admission.

Chapter 4

Does Method Matter? The Effect of Method on Findings

To what extent can the differences in findings among studies be attributed to the analytical approach rather than to true differences in hospital settings or the underlying data? The previous chapter illustrates the wide range of methods that were used to explore the volume-outcome issue. Some authors used simple approaches; others used complex multivariate techniques. Some authors computed tests of statistical significance, and others did not. One way to find out whether analytic methods account for differences in findings would be to acquire the original data from each of the authors and examine each data set with a preferred method. However, this would be a difficult, if not impossible, task. An alternative is to apply a broad range of methods to a fixed set of data, setting aside the role of differences in time periods, geographic settings, data, and other factors. We used two 1983 data sets from California: one for patients undergoing coronary artery bypass graft surgery and one for patients undergoing cholecystectomy. The goal was to determine whether methods designed to mimic those in each of the studies would produce evidence of a volume-outcome relationship.

The two procedures were chosen to determine whether the findings are sensitive to different clinical and practice situations. The CABG surgery is a procedure of moderately high risk, with a mortality rate of 3.6 percent in California in 1983. It was performed in relatively few hospitals (76), and volumes were generally fairly high, at 243 per hospital. Cholecystectomy, a lower-risk procedure (1.2 percent mortality), was performed in a much wider spectrum of hospitals (443), and average volumes were much lower, at 69 per hospital.

The first section of this chapter provides a brief overview of the methods used in the 25 studies reviewed in this book. These studies are grouped into six major methodological approaches, although some studies used several approaches. The following sections focus on the data used to explore the effects of methods on findings, and the application of the methods to the data. The primary focus is on the identification of a volume-outcome relationship. Since there are many more combinations of plausible approaches than were used in the 25 studies, the discussion goes beyond a simple attempt at replication and is focused, instead, on the lessons to be learned from differences in findings when different approaches are used. The final section summarizes these lessons.

METHODOLOGICAL APPROACHES

Table 4.1 summarizes the methods used by the authors of the 25 articles reviewed in this book. The methods can be roughly categorized into six groups:

Group by Volume without Risk Factors, or with Minimal Splitting by Risk

The authors in the first group classified hospitals by their patient volume, with little or no explicit adjustment for risk factors across hospitals. In some cases, results were presented separately for high- and low-risk patients. The number of volume categories varied from 3 to 15. In some studies, the mortality rates for the high- and low-volume categories were compared, and, in one study, a chi-square test for linear trend was performed.

Group by Volume with Risk Adjustments

The authors of the second set of studies also compared outcomes for hospitals grouped by volume, but they took into account case-mix differences across volume categories through some type of risk adjustment. These adjustments range from simple comparison of plots of actual and expected death rates to examination of the distribution of hospitals by the likelihood that their outcomes were worse than expected given their case mix.

Group by Outcomes, then Compare Volumes

The authors of the third group of studies categorized hospitals by their outcomes and then compared average volumes of hospitals with different outcomes. This is analogous to the case-control study in epidemiology, in which characteristics of people with a certain disease were compared with the characteristics of people without the disease.

Regressions with the Hospital as the Unit of Observation

The authors in the fourth group of studies used the hospital as the unit of observation in a simple linear regression. Within this group, however, there is substantial variation in the formulation of the dependent variable and in the explanatory variables. The dependent variable was sometimes the observed death rate, while the expected death rate was included as an independent variable. In one instance, the proportions of patients with various risk factors were included as explanatory variables. In other studies, the expected death rate was taken over to the left-hand side, either by subtracting it from the actual death rate, by using the ratio of actual to expected rates, or by computing a Z-score based on observed and expected rates. Explanatory variables may be limited to various formulations of volume, such as volume alone, volume and volume-squared, or the log of volume. Other hospital characteristics, such as bed size and ownership, may also be included in the equation.

Regressions with the Patient as the Unit of Observation

The fifth set of methods involves the use of the patient as the unit of observation. Although most authors using this approach employed logistic models, one study used ordinary least squares. Again, the measure of volume varies substantially across studies; specifications included volume, log of volume, and volume categories. Furthermore, some authors used selected data sets; in two instances patients with one-day hospital stays were dropped, and in another instance the analysis was limited to a 20-percent random sample of Medicare patients.

Multiple Causal Pathways

The methods in the sixth group all tested multiple causal pathways. In some instances, this involved the simultaneous estimation of the effects of physician volume and hospital volume. Unfortunately, the California data used in this chapter do not allow us to measure physician volume, but the senior author of one of the physician-hospital volume studies reestimated his equations to allow us to compare the hospital volume effects in equations with and without physician volume. A second set of multiple causal pathways involves the simultaneous estimation of the effects of volume on outcome and the effects of outcome on volume. Again, we are fortunate to be able to present results, both published and unpublished, on those data with both simple and simultaneous models. The results of these comparisons are presented in Chapter 5, since they do not rely on the same data used in this chapter.

Table 4.1:   Methods Used in the Volume-Outcome Studies

Study	Group by Volume w/o Risk Factors or Minimal Split by Risk	Group by Volume with Risk Adjustments	Group by Outcomes then Compare Volumes
Adams, et al. (1973)	4 categ. *t*–hi vs. low		
Hertzer et al. (1984)	3-4 categ. *t*–hi vs. low		
Kempczinski et al. (1986)	3 categ. *t*–hi vs. low		
Farber et al. (1981)	~15 categ. *t*–low vs. others		
Pilcher et al. (1980)	3 categ. χ^2 for *t*–hi/low risk		
Rosenblatt et al. (1985)	3 categ. *t*–low vs. others hi/low risk		
Luft et al. (1979)		ADR, EDR plots	
Luft et al. (1987)		ADR/EDR, trans in, out, EDR	
Luft and Hunt (1986)		Distrib. of P(ADR | EDR) by vol.	
Flood et al. (1984a)		Logistic reg→EDR; cut at average volume	
Fowles et al. (1987)			Poor vs. good outcomes → volume
Sloan et al. (1986)			Low, med, hi rates → volume
Luft (1980)			
Maerki et al. (1986)			
Shortell and LoGerfo (1981)			
Williams (1979)			
Hughes et al. (1987)			
Roos et al. (1986)			
Roos et al. (1987)			
Wennberg et al. (1987)			
Showstack et al. (1987)			
Riley and Lubitz (1985)			
Kelly and Hellinger (1986)			
Kelly and Hellinger (1987)			
Hughes et al. (1988)			

Table 4.1: Continued

Regressions, Hospital as Unit of Observation	Regressions, Patient as Unit of Observation	Multiple Causal Pathways
	$log \frac{p}{1-p} = f(v)$	
		ADR EDR $= f(log\ v, \ldots)$ $log\ v = f(ADR\text{-}EDR, \ldots)$
ADR $= f(v, v^2, \%Risk, \ldots)$		
ADR-EDR $= f(log\ v, adm, \ldots)^{wtd}$		ADR-EDR $= (log\ v, \ldots)$ $log\ v = f(ADR\text{-}EDR, ops, \ldots)$
ADR $= f(EDR, v, v^2, \ldots)^{wtd}$ ADR/EDR $= f(vol, \ldots)$		
ADR/EDR $= f(v, v^2, \ldots)^{wtd}$ ADR/EDR $= f(v, v^2, \ldots)^{wtd}$ $Z(bad) = f(log\ vol, \ldots)$		$Z(bad) = f(log\ Hv, \%\ low\ MD, \ldots)$
	$log \frac{p}{1-p} = f(vlo, [vhi], risk)$ $log \frac{p}{1-p} = f(vlo, vmed, [vhi], risk)$ $log \frac{p}{1-p} = f(vlo, vmed, [vhi], risk)$ Dead $= f(v1, v2, v3, [v4], risk)$ $log \frac{p}{1-p} = f(log\ v, risk)$ 20% sample, pts>65 $log \frac{p}{1-p} = f(v, risk, hosp)$	$log \frac{p}{1-p} = f(Hv, MDv, \ldots)$
	$log \frac{p}{1-p} = f(v, risk, hosp)$ drop 1 day stays	$log \frac{p}{1-p} = f(Hv, MDv, \ldots)$
		$Z (death, LLOS) = f(log\ v, \ldots)$

DATA FOR THE COMPARATIVE ANALYSES

Patient data were selected from 1983 hospital discharge abstracts routinely collected by the California Health Facilities Commission. (The data responsibilities of the commission were subsequently taken over by the Office of Statewide Health Planning and Development.) All nonfederal, non-HMO, short-term general hospitals in the state were included in our data, which were already selected for other studies. The data were trimmed further by excluding patients thought to have been admitted for reasons other than the procedure in question. For example, a cholecystectomy patient would have to have a primary procedure of cholecystectomy or common bile duct exploration (with cholecystectomy as a secondary procedure).[1] Hospitals were also excluded if they had only one cholecystectomy patient or fewer than six CABG patients, since it was possible that such patients were miscoded.

Given these exclusions, there were 18,462 patients undergoing CABG surgery in 76 hospitals, and 30,322 patients undergoing cholecystectomies in 443 hospitals, in 1983. Since the data are based on discharges, the same person could appear more than once, although this is relatively unlikely for CABG within a given year and is implausible for cholecystectomy.

Risk factors were considered at two levels. First, each patient was placed in a high- or low-risk category, depending on the type of admission and date of surgery. All patients admitted from the emergency room or transferred from another acute hospital were considered nonscheduled and therefore, at high risk. In addition, patients who underwent surgery more than two days after admission (three if admitted on a Friday) were considered to be at high risk. Using these criteria, there were 4,733 high-risk CABG patients with an average mortality rate of 6.03 percent, in contrast to 12,689 low-risk patients with an average mortality rate of 2.50 percent. There were 10,002 high-risk cholecystectomy patients with a death rate of 2.77 percent, and 20,320 low-risk patients with a death rate of 0.48 percent.

Specific patient risk factors may also lead to differential mortality rates among hospitals. To account for them, we estimated multiple logistic regressions on all patients with a given procedure. The risk factors include gender, transfer from an acute-care hospital, age, chronic diagnoses in various organ systems, related and unrelated procedures, and for CABG patients, the presence of a catheterization on the day of surgery or a previous day during the same hospitalization. Each of these variables was also allowed to interact with the high-risk dummy. For example, having a catheterization during the admission prior to the day of the CABG has no effect on risk for patients in general, but it indicates a lower probability of death for high-risk patients. Table 4.2 presents the results of these logistic regressions for the two procedures.

Given the estimated coefficients from these regressions and the characteristics of each patient, it is possible to compute the probability of death for the patient based on the experience of all California patients in 1983. By adding together those probabilities for all patients in a given hospital, one then has an estimate of the expected number of deaths in that hospital given its case mix. If one divides the actual or observed number of deaths by the expected number, the result is analogous to the indirectly standardized mortality rate commonly used in the public health literature. That approach usually uses a matrix of risk factors, such as gender by age, to compute the probability of death for patients in each cell, and these rates are then applied to the case mix at each hospital. The matrix method allows for interaction effects, but one is limited in the number of variables that can be considered, because cell sizes get too small to be statistically reliable predictors. The logistic regression can allow for interactions, such as high risk multiplied by the other variables, but it is more difficult to explain. As long as the principal variables are included, it probably does not make much difference which approach is used.[2]

HOSPITALS GROUPED BY VOLUME WITHOUT RISK FACTORS OR MINIMAL SPLIT ON RISK

The authors of six studies compared average death rates for patients in various volume categories without adjusting for differences in risk factors.[3] It is important to note that, although the volume of patients in the hospital was used to assign patients to volume categories, attention was focused on the experience of all patients in the category, not on the death rates in hospitals within the group. Thus the mortality rate is the observed number of deaths in all hospitals in the volume group divided by the number of patients in all hospitals in the volume group.

One crucial decision in this type of approach is the number of volume categories and the selection of cutoff points. The six studies reviewed included from 3 to 15 volume categories. The articles do not indicate whether the authors examined alternative volume categories, but in each of these six, the underlying data for each hospital were available, so alternative categorizations were possible. In some other instances, hospital-specific data were not available and volume categories for a wide range of procedures had to be specified prior to examination of the data; this was the case for the study by Luft, Bunker, and Enthoven (1979) discussed in the next section. It may be useful to explore the implications of choosing different levels of detail for analysis. To illustrate, we have chosen six sets of volume groupings (see Table 4.3). Volume Grouping A has nine categories with fine detail at the low-volume end and a rather high cutoff (501+) for the top volume category. Volume Grouping B collapses the top three volume categories but is otherwise the same as Volume Grouping A. Volume Grouping C collapses the bottom six categories into three but provides a little more detail at the high end. Volume Grouping D further collapses the lower categories, so all hospitals with up to 100 patients are lumped together. In Volume Grouping E

Table 4.2:   Logistic Regressions for Risk Factor Adjustment

	CABG	
Variable	*Coefficient*	*Std. Error*
Intercept	−4.375	0.179‡
Male	−0.593	0.128‡
Transfer in	0.471	0.163†
Age 60–69	0.550	0.150‡
Age 70–79	1.062	0.161‡
Age 80 +	1.379	0.373‡
Endocrine/nutritional diagnoses	−0.528	0.237*
Blood and blood organs diagnoses	−0.354	0.497
Circulatory system diagnoses	0.009	0.122
Respiratory system diagnoses	0.255	0.233
Related cardiac procedure	2.480	0.156‡
Nonrelated procedure	0.738	0.140‡
Nonrelated procedure postop	1.924	0.174‡
Cath earlier in admission	0.086	0.153
Cath same day	0.523	0.174†
Nonelective admission	0.662	0.272*
Nonelective male	0.360	0.179*
Nonelective transfer in	−0.143	0.217
Nonelective age 60–69	0.087	0.222
Nonelective age 70–79	0.101	0.232
Nonelective age 80 +	0.505	0.464
Nonelective endocrine/nutritional	0.294	0.306
Nonelective blood and blood organs	0.421	0.615
Nonelective circulatory system	0.334	0.171
Nonelective respiratory system	−0.416	0.334
Nonelective related cardiac proc.	−0.428	0.214*
Nonelective nonrelated procedure	−0.209	0.197
Nonelective nonrelated procedure postop	−0.383	0.258
Nonelective cath earlier	−0.487	0.199*
Nonelective cath same day	−0.645	0.274*

$R = .395$; $\chi^2 = 951.33$, $29df$; $R = .483$; $\chi^2 = 1000.17$, $29df$
$* = p < .05$
$† = p < .01$
$‡ = p < .001$

there is simply a tripartite split. There are two F Groupings, representing a split at the mean volume for the procedure, 242 for CABG and 68 for cholecystectomy.

Figures 4.1 and 4.2 present graphs of the relation between actual death rate and volume category for CABG and cholecystectomy. The scales have been adjusted to be the same for all graphs within a set, to allow comparisons. In the usual situation of a given study, however, volume and outcome scales would more closely match the range of the observed points. At first glance, the sequence of

Table 4.2: Continued

	Cholecystectomy	
Variable	*Coefficient*	*Std. Error*
Intercept	−8.457	0.584‡
Male	0.419	0.214
Age 50–59	2.020	0.654†
Age 60–69	2.667	0.617‡
Age 70–79	3.195	0.615‡
Age 80+	4.337	0.623‡
Endocrine/nutritional diagnoses	0.077	0.388
Blood and blood organs diagnoses	0.582	0.555
Circulatory system diagnoses	0.315	0.239
Respiratory system diagnoses	0.565	0.390
Genitourinary system diagnoses	1.742	0.319‡
Operations on bile duct	0.442	0.251
Operations on pancreas and other biliary tract	1.166	0.391†
Nonrelated procedure	0.747	0.279†
Nonrelated procedure postop	2.334	0.308‡
Nonelective admission	2.063	0.676†
Nonelective male	0.048	0.250
Nonelective age 50–59	−0.679	0.774
Nonelective age 60–69	−0.709	0.719
Nonelective age 70–79	−0.543	0.711
Nonelective age 80+	−1.129	0.719
Nonelective endocrine/nutritional	−0.397	0.457
Nonelective blood and blood organs	−0.498	0.662
Nonelective circulatory system	0.003	0.275
Nonelective respiratory system	−0.254	0.448
Nonelective genitourinary system	−0.137	0.387
Nonelective operations on bile duct	−0.343	0.288
Nonelective operations on pancreas and other biliary tract	−0.662	0.455
Nonelective nonrelated procedure	0.238	0.314
Nonelective nonrelated procedure postop	−0.449	0.372

graphs for CABG appears to represent a vanishing relationship. Volume Groupings A, B, and C exhibit nonmonotonic relationships, but this is due to one hospital with 20 patients and no deaths, a likely occurrence for a procedure with a 3.6 percent mortality rate. If one ignores this single case, the outcomes for patients operated on in low-volume hospitals, particularly those with volumes below 100, appear to be substantially worse than for those operated on in higher-volume settings. With Volume Groupings E and F, it becomes difficult to observe

Table 4.3:   Alternative Volume Groupings

| | Volume Cutoffs | | | | | | | | |
Grouping	*1*	*2*	*3*	*4*	*5*	*6*	*7*	*8*	*9*
A	2–4	5–10	11–20	21–50	51–100	101–200	201–300	301–500	501+
B	2–4	5–10	11–20	21–50	51–100	101–200	201+		
C	2–20	21–100	101–200	201–350	351+				
D	2–100	101–200	201–350	351+					
E	2–150	151–250	251+						
F1	2–242	243+							
F2	2–68	69+							

much of a relationship because the results for these low-volume hospitals are combined with higher-volume hospitals.

The results for cholecystectomy in Figure 4.2 are quite different. Volume Grouping A, B, and C exhibit an inverted U shape with a "blip" (indicating high mortality rate) at the very low volume end. (The data underlying these graphs are presented in Appendixes 4.1 and 4.2.) Closer examination of the underlying data indicates that, even though 14 hospitals are represented in the lowest-volume group, those hospitals account for only 45 patients. The 2.2-percent mortality rate is due to one death. Precisely this type of aberration occurred for cholecystectomy in the study by Luft, Bunker, and Enthoven (1979). Therefore, if one prefers the volume categories in Volume Grouping C, there are 75 hospitals with between 2 and 20 patients and eight deaths among 820 patients. This curve suggests an inverted U, but again, one must examine the underlying data, since the very low mortality rate for the highest volume is due to one hospital with 445 patients and two deaths. Collapsing volume categories at the low end, however, can change the picture substantially. Volume Groupings D and E suggest downward-sloping curves with no hint that outcomes might be better in lower-volume hospitals. Finally, splitting the sample at the average volume of 68 produces the appearance of worsening outcomes with higher volumes.

Some studies split the patient sample into low- and high-risk groups but measured volume by the total number of patients.[4] From a policy perspective, it might be easier to redirect nonemergency admissions by adopting a policy of regionalization to refer patients to high-volume hospitals. Figures 4.3 and 4.4 present graphs of death rates for high- and low-risk patients using the same sets of volume categories shown in Figures 4.1 and 4.2. Splitting the sample for CABG patients is quite informative. Mortality rates for both low- and high-risk patients are well above average for hospitals with 21 to 50 patients per year, but there is essentially no difference in outcomes for low-risk patients in the higher-volume categories. It does appear, however, that high-risk patients are more likely to experience poor outcomes in hospitals with 51 to 100 patients.

The cholecystectomy data illustrate another problem: how to determine which differences are important. Even though high-risk patients account for only

Figure 4.1:   Average Death Rate by Volume Category, CABG

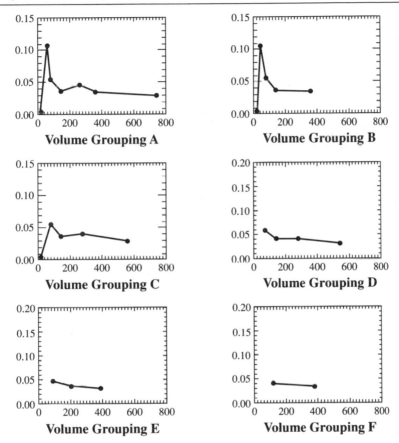

a third of the cholecystectomy patients, they account for almost three-fourths of the deaths. Therefore, the overall mortality rate for cholecystectomy is dominated by the outcomes of high-risk patients. Furthermore, even though there may be some patterns for the low-risk patients, the differences in mortality rates are unlikely to be of substantial policy importance, particularly since a regionalization policy would affect an enormous number of patients without saving a substantial number of lives.

Although these six studies simply compared observed death rates across categories, several of the authors computed tests of significance as well. Four research groups used t-tests to compare the death rates in the highest- and lowest-volume categories.[5] Pilcher and colleagues (1980) used a chi-square test for trend. If the tests are routinely applied to the volume groupings for CABG, the differences are not significant for the first three sets of volume groupings but are

Figure 4.2:   Average Death Rate by Volume Category, Cholecystectomy

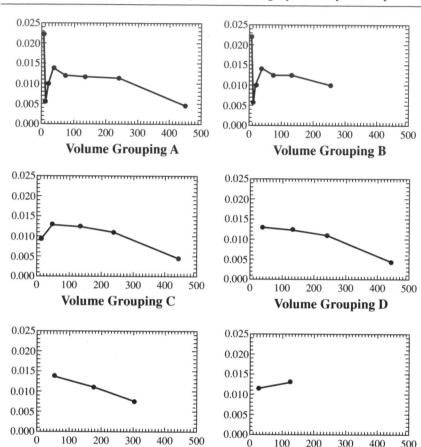

highly significant (*t*-ratios of 4.3 to 11.2) for the last three sets. Once one notices that the lowest-volume category in each of the first three sets is composed of just one hospital with 20 patients, it is obvious that this case should be either excluded or collapsed with the next lowest category. Doing either produces results indicating significant differences for all sets of volume groupings. (These tests were computed for low- and high-risk patients combined.)

The situation for cholecystectomy is quite different. None of the *t*-tests for differences between the highest- and lowest-volume categories in the six sets is significant, although Volume Grouping E is almost significant with a *t*-ratio of 1.92. However, one need not limit the testing to the high versus low categories. Rosenblatt, Reinken, and Shoemack (1985) compared middle versus low and high versus low separately. As demonstrated by the graphs, the choice of catego-

Figure 4.3:   High- and Low-Risk Death Rates by Volume Category, CABG

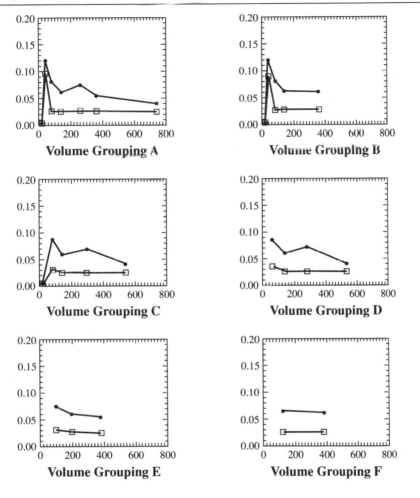

● = High-risk patients
□ = Low-risk patients

ries has a much greater impact on the shape of the curve for cholecystectomy, so simple tests of differences between pairs of categories are less meaningful.

The usefulness of the chi-square test for trend is unclear. It is essentially a measure of the extent to which the observed rates differ from what would be expected if a linear relationship were estimated with respect to volume (Fleiss 1981). For CABG these test statistics are usually significant or nearly so; for cholecystectomy they are almost always insignificant. A significant result, however, means that one can reject the null hypothesis of a linear pattern, and a large

Figure 4.4:   High- and Low-Risk Death Rates by Volume Category,
Cholecystectomy

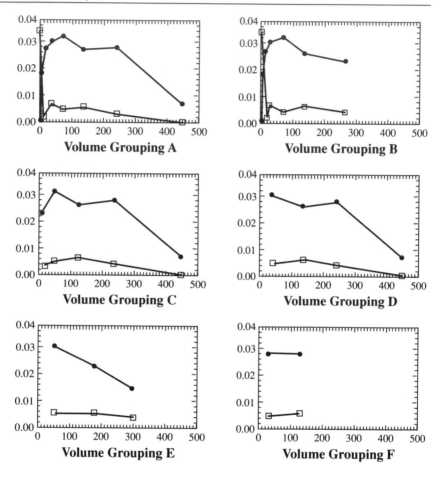

• = High-risk patients
□ = Low-risk patients

chi-square value could occur either because there is a great deal of variability or
because the curve is markedly bowed, or U-shaped. Alternatively, one may be
unable to reject the hypothesis of linearity but not know if the line is downward
sloping, flat, or upward sloping.

Group by Volume with Risk Adjustments

It is reasonable to be concerned about whether the risk of death varies among
hospitals in a nonrandom manner. In fact, many people have argued that the high-

volume referral centers will attract the highest-risk cases. Thus, even if high-volume hospitals have outcomes that are not particularly better than low-volume settings, if they have a riskier case mix, they are achieving better results than would otherwise be expected. Four studies grouped patients by the volume of their hospitals and compared actual mortality rates to what would be expected based upon the mix of patients in those hospitals. Three studies by Luft used different methods to compare actual and expected rates.[6] In each instance, however, the dependent variable was examined across a series of volume groups, as in the previous set of studies. Flood, Scott, and Ewy (1984a) split the sample of hospitals at the mean and used a chi-square test to compare the actual and expected mortality.[7]

Luft, Bunker, and Enthoven (1979) simply plotted actual and expected death rates for patients in each volume group, while Luft, Hunt, and Maerki (1987) presented tables with the ratio of actual over expected deaths for each volume category.[8] Figure 4.5 presents graphs of both measures for three of the six volume groupings. The graphs at the left repeat the plot of actual death rates but also include the rates expected for patients in each volume group based upon their case mix. It is apparent that actual and expected rates are similar, and both seem to decline somewhat for the higher-volume groupings. At the very lowest volume levels, which can be seen quite clearly in Volume Grouping A, expected mortality rates are lower than for moderate-volume hospitals. These findings suggest that although the riskier patients may be steered away from the lowest-volume hospitals, they are not all necessarily ending up at the highest-volume centers. In fact, the highest-volume centers seem to have risk levels lower than those of moderate-volume hospitals. This finding is consistent with the fact that risk of death is associated with emergency operations. That is, some hospitals may achieve very high volumes because they are referral centers. For most procedures, such referrals are scheduled, so these hospitals will tend to have a lower proportion of emergency cases. These two sets of figures are combined in the graphs on the right, where there seems to be evidence that actual rates are above what would be expected for the lowest-volume categories, but there is little pattern among higher-volume categories.

Given that there are relatively few patients in the lowest-volume categories for cholecystectomy, it was tempting to dismiss the "bouncing around" of the actual death rate as being due to random fluctuations. As seen in Figure 4.6, however, the expected rates for low-volume hospitals are below the expected rates for moderate-volume hospitals, despite the fact that cholecystectomy is a low-risk procedure. More important, the one hospital with very high volume and remarkably low mortality rates also has a low expected mortality rate. Even if one lumps relatively high volume hospitals (as in the bottom pair of graphs), however, outcomes in the higher-volume hospitals are better than expected.

Splitting the hospitals at their mean volume seems to result in an inability to detect these patterns, which are most pronounced at either the very low or very high volumes. Thus, for CABG, low-volume hospitals were expected to have

Figure 4.5:   Actual and Expected Death Rates by Volume Category, CABG

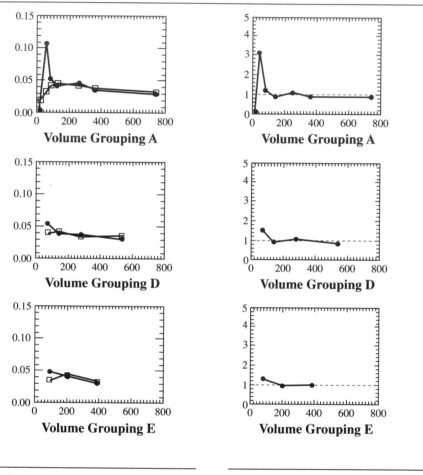

● = Actual death rate
□ = Expected death rate

● = Actual/expected deaths

212.3 deaths and 216 were actually observed, while high-volume hospitals were expected to have 451.7 deaths but only 448 were observed. Using Flood's chi-square calculations (Flood, Scott, and Ewy 1984a), this difference results in a value of .0978, which is far from significant. Similarly no significant difference was found for cholecystectomy.

Luft and Hunt (1986) examined the probability that the actual death rate for a hospital could have come from a binomial distribution with a probability equal to the expected mortality rate for that hospital.[9] Their focus was on the possibility of being able to detect hospitals with results that were significantly better or

Figure 4.6:   Actual and Expected Death Rates by Volume Category,
Cholecystectomy

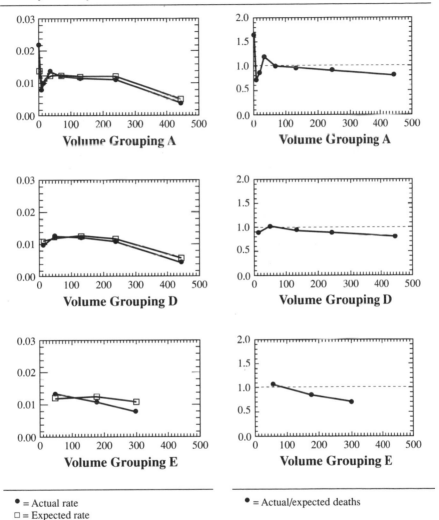

● = Actual rate
□ = Expected rate

● = Actual/expected deaths

worse than expected. They computed a Z-score based on the observed and expected number of deaths and the volume in each hospital, and examined the
number of hospitals at various volume levels falling within certain Z-score
ranges. In Figure 4.7, three sets of volume groupings are used for each of the two
procedures. Each point on a graph represents a hospital. These appear as dotted
lines because they have been grouped in volume categories. (In a later section,
the actual hospital volume will be used when the hospital is the unit of analysis,

Figure 4.7:   Distribution of Z-Scores by Volume Category

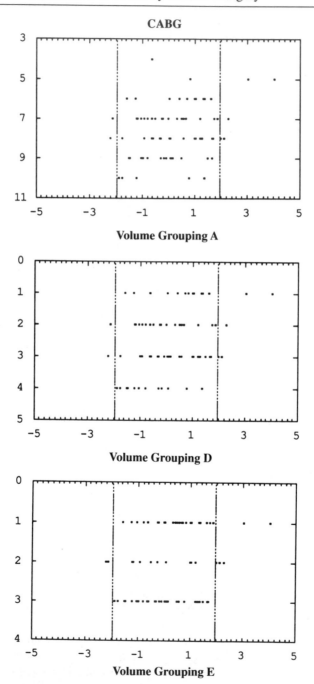

Figure 4.7: Continued

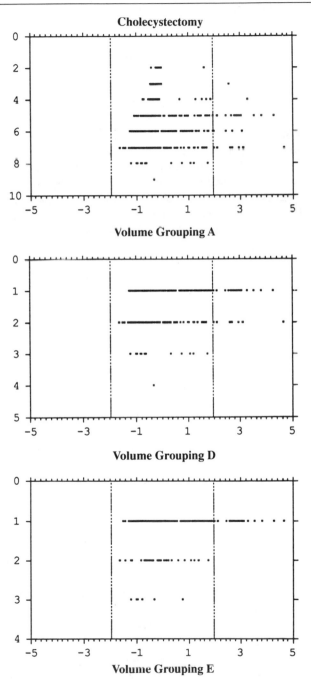

rather than the volume group.) The vertical lines are set at -1.96 and $+1.96$, representing p-values of .05. The sets of results at the left show that a vast majority of hospitals have CABG outcomes not significantly different from what would be expected from their case mix. Three hospitals have results that are significantly better than expected, and five are worse than expected. (Two hospitals with 161 and 162 patients each have almost identical Z-scores, at -2.13 and -2.12.) The very high volume groups do not have a disproportionate share of either extreme, but the "bad outliers" are concentrated in the lower-volume range. For example, of the four hospitals with volumes below 50, two have Z-scores of 3 or more.

The results for cholecystectomy are also instructive. Consistent with the earlier sets of findings, hospitals with very low volumes seem less likely to have significantly poor results, and the same is true for the highest-volume settings. What is most interesting about the cholecystectomy results, however, is that none of the 443 hospitals has a mortality rate that is significantly lower than expected. It seems that with a procedure such as cholecystectomy, which has an average death rate of about 1 percent and an average volume of 68, there just are not enough patients to demonstrate results that are significantly better than expected. This is the case even though more than half, or 234, of the hospitals had no deaths.

Group by Outcomes, then Compare Volumes

Fowles, Bunker, and Schurman (1987) and Sloan, Perrin, and Valvona (1986) first grouped by outcomes and then compared the volumes associated with those outcomes.[10] Fowles and her colleagues compared the average volumes associated with patients having either good or poor outcomes. In the context of our analysis, this is equivalent to examining the average volume of hospitals used by patients who survived versus the average volume of hospitals used by patients who died. For CABG, the 664 deceased patients were operated on in hospitals whose average volume was 333.5 with a standard deviation of 217.8; the comparable figures for the 17,798 survivors were 364.7 and 226.8. Using the t-test for the difference of two means yields a t-ratio of 3.62, which is highly significant. For cholecystectomy, there were 375 deaths in hospitals with an average volume of 108.7 and a standard deviation of 63.8. The 29,947 survivors were operated on in hospitals with slightly higher volumes (115.4 with a standard deviation of 75.1). This comparison of volumes for decedents and survivors yields a barely significant t-ratio of 2.01.

The approach used by Sloan, Perrin, and Valvona is somewhat different in that it focused on the hospital as the unit of observation. (Note, however, that the Fowles, Bunker, and Schurman approach does not require patient-level data since the numbers of dead and living patients in each hospital can be used as weights with hospital data.) They grouped hospitals into three categories: those with zero deaths, those with deaths above the 90th percentile for the death rates, and those in the middle. Average volumes were then computed for hospitals in each of the three categories. This approach is demonstrated in Table 4.4. Average volumes are markedly higher in the middle death rate category for both CABG and cholecystectomy patients. This seems to suggest an inverted U shape, but it is important to recall that we have been plotting our data with volume on the horizontal axis and outcomes on the vertical. Thus plotting average death rate against average volume gives a backward C.

The key to the difference in findings is the role of zero deaths when death rates and volumes are low. Over half the hospitals with cholecystectomy patients had no deaths, but the average volume for those hospitals was well under 100. (The figure of 115 reported for the Fowles approach is based on volumes weighted by the number of patients, so high-volume hospitals skew the mean.) Since the death rate is about 1 percent, on average less than one patient will die in each hospital, which means it is quite likely for there to be zero, one, or two deaths, even if the long-run death rate for that hospital is at the expected rate. One is faced with the problem that, with low death rates and moderate to low volumes, the absence of any deaths does not mean the hospital is performing well.

The opposite problem arises in the CABG data. The three hospitals with no deaths had 20, 87, and 161 patients. With an overall average death rate for CABG patients of 3.6 percent, it is clear that the 20-patient hospital may have "lucked out." It also becomes clear that the average patient volumes are quite high for CABG, so the expected number of deaths is about eight or nine per hospital. Even with a "true" death rate of only half the average, a hospital would report four deaths and thus be relegated to the medium death rate category.

If we use the Z-score approach discussed in the previous section, it is possible to explore whether hospitals with significantly high or low death rates have differentially high or low volumes. The Z-score takes into account both the expected rate in each hospital and the number of patients. This makes it impossible for a low-volume hospital to appear to be better than average merely because it has no deaths, although very few would have been expected anyway. Table 4.5

Table 4.4:   Comparison of Volumes by Outcome Categories

	Zero Deaths	*Medium Death Rate*	*High Death Rate*
CABG			
Death Rate Range	0	0<ADR≤.070	.070<ADR
Number of Hospitals	3	65	8
Average Volume	89.3	271.5	68.1
Average Death Rate	0	0.037	0.088
Cholecystectomy			
Death Rate Range	0	0<ADR≤.036	.036<ADR
Number of Hospitals	234	164	45
Average Volume	43.7	108.3	52.1
Average Death Rate	0	0.017	0.058

illustrates the preceding discussion. Only 8 of the 234 hospitals with no cholecystectomy deaths had *p*-values of less than .10, and these had average volumes of 147. The high volumes in these hospitals allow a zero death rate to approach significance. In contrast, the tails of the distribution for CABG are relatively "fat," because both volumes and average mortality rates are higher, so differences can be detected. Even with Z-scores, there is not a very clear pattern between outcomes and volume. In large part, this is because outcomes include a substantial random component, so categorizing hospitals by outcomes and then looking for a pattern among volumes is less likely to be fruitful than categorizing hospitals by volumes and examining outcomes.

Regressions: Hospital as the Unit of Observation

A wide range of functional forms have been used in studies focusing on the hospital as the unit of observation. The influence of case mix has been captured in several ways:

1. It has been incorporated as an independent variable with actual death rate as the dependent variable (Maerki, Luft, and Hunt 1986; and Williams 1979).

2. The actual-minus-expected death rate has been used as the dependent variable (Luft 1980; and Luft, Hunt, and Maerki 1987).

3. Actual divided by expected deaths has been used as the dependent variable (Shortell and LoGerfo 1981; and Williams 1979).

4. Patient risk factors have been measured at the hospital level (Sloan, Perrin, and Valvona 1986).

5. Z-scores based on actual and expected deaths have been used as the dependent variable (Hughes, Hunt, and Luft 1987).

Volume has been included as a simple linear variable, in quadratic form, or as a log transformation. The observations may be weighted or unweighted, and

Table 4.5: Distribution of Hospitals by Z-Scores

Z	p	CABG Hospitals	Average Patients	$\frac{ADR}{EDR}$	Cholecystectomy Hospitals	Average Patients	$\frac{ADR}{EDR}$
$Z \leq -1.96$	$p < .025$	3	186	0.381	0	—	—
$-1.96 < Z \leq 1.65$	$.025 \leq p < .050$	3	528	0.576	0	—	—
$-1.65 < Z \leq 1.28$	$.050 \leq p < .100$	3	304	0.621	8	147	0.0
$-1.28 < Z \leq 0$	$.100 \leq p < .500$	27	245	0.794	287	60	0.372
$0 < Z \leq 1.28$	$.500 \leq p < .900$	24	215	1.224	89	90	1.462
$1.28 < Z \leq 1.65$	$.900 \leq p < .950$	6	291	1.435	23	63	2.519
$1.65 < Z \leq 1.96$	$.950 \leq p < .975$	5	234	1.594	12	66	2.967
$1.96 < Z$	$.975 \leq p$	5	142	2.071	24	65	3.739

there are different formulations of the weighting variable. Finally, additional variables describing the hospital, such as its size, ownership, or medical school affiliation, may be included.

Although only eight of these many combinations are included in the literature, it may be instructive to examine a broader set of comparisons to determine not just whether each of the specific approaches used would have identified a volume-outcome relationship, but whether there are reasons to prefer one approach over another. Table 4.6 presents the results for the unweighted CABG regressions. When comparing the results of the various formulations, it is important to note that R^2 values are not comparable across different dependent variables. The first three regressions compare actual death rate as a function of expected rate and various measures of volume. The quadratic form is clearly superior to the linear form, but a log transformation is even better. The coefficient for expected death rate is highly significant, but only about .5, suggesting that, if we control for volume, hospitals with higher expected death rates tend to have somewhat better than expected outcomes, and those with easier case mixes have outcomes that are worse than expected. This finding also suggests that forcing the coefficient on the expected death rate to be 1.0 by using the difference between actual death rate (ADR) and expected death rate (EDR) as the dependent variable may be inappropriate.

Selected hospital characteristics are added in the fourth equation. These include dummy variables for public hospitals, proprietary hospitals, and medical school–affiliated hospitals, as well as three dummy variables for size: 201–300 beds, 301–350 beds, and 351 or more beds. The overall corrected R^2 increases from .147 to .301. A similar increase in corrected R^2 is observed in comparing Equations 2 and 5, but the volume-squared effect becomes insignificant. The seventh regression, which is similar to the one used by Sloan, Perrin, and Valvona (1986), drops the expected death rate variable and instead includes variables for the proportion of patients in the hospital with each of the risk factors. Thus the additional 29 variables include the items listed in Table 4.2 expressed as the percentage of patients in the hospital who, for example, are male or had a catheterization on the same day as the CABG. Surprisingly, allowing each of these factors to have an independent influence reduces the explanatory power, probably because, even though some of the variables are significant, they are unable to offset the loss in effective degrees of freedom.

The next six regressions use the ratio of actual to expected death rates as the dependent variable. The corrected R^2 values are lower than in the preceding set, but the variability of the dependent variable is also different. More important, the linear and quadratic forms of the volume variable are insignificant at conventional levels. Thus, if we were to compare Equation 4 with Equation 10, which is similar to the one estimated by Shortell and LoGerfo (1981), we might reject the notion of a volume-outcome relationship based on the latter equation but accept it based on the former.

The final set of regressions uses the difference between actual and expected

Table 4.6: Hospital Level Regressions—CABG—Unweighted

1 ADR = .0309 (.0090)‡ + .509EDR (.201)* − .0000365VOL (.0000144)* $\bar{R}^2$ = .147

2 ADR = .0413 (.0099)† + .524EDR (.196)† − .000120VOL (.000040)‡ + .106$\cdot 10^{-6}$VOL^2 (.475$\cdot 10^{-7}$)* $\bar{R}^2$ = .191

3 ADR = .0831 (.0189)‡ + .535EDR (.197)‡ − .0118LNVOL (.0032)‡ $\bar{R}^2$ = .214

4 ADR = .033 (.009)‡ + .027PUB (.011)* + .344EDR (.197) − .010PROP (.007) − .0000321VOL (.0000135)* + .012MEDS (.006) − .003BED2 (.006) + .005BED3 (.008) − .008BED4 (.007) $\bar{R}^2$ = .301

5 ADR = .0398 (.0103)‡ + .0250PUB (.0110)* + .358EDR (.196) − .0096PROP (.0074) − .0000826VOL (.0000386)* + .636$\cdot 10^{-7}$VOL^2 (.455$\cdot 10^{-7}$) + .0113MEDS (.0062) − .0034BED2 (.0058) + .0041BED3 (.0082) − .0065BED4 (.0075) $\bar{R}^2$ = .310

6 ADR = .072 (.019)‡ + .025PUB (.011)* + .393EDR (.191)* − .009PROP (.007) − .00913LNVOL (.00317)† + .010MEDS (.006) − .003BED2 (.006) + .005BED3 (.008) − .006BED4 (.007) $\bar{R}^2$ = .326

7 ADR = .0971 (.1157) + .0247PUB (.0225) − .0181PROP (.0113) − .0000715VOL (.0000635) + .408$\cdot 10^{-7}$VOL^2 (.638$\cdot 10^{-7}$) + .0083MEDS (.0088) + .0023BED2 (.0085) + .0131BED3 (.0111) + .0081BED4 (.0115) + [29vars] $\bar{R}^2$ = .238

8 ADR/EDR = 1.368 (.144)‡ − .000936VOL (.000483) $\bar{R}^2$ = .035

9 ADR/EDR = 1.699 (.219)‡ − .00347VOL (.00136)* + .0000321VOL^2 (.00000162) $\bar{R}^2$ = .072

10 ADR/EDR = 2.925 (.584)‡ − .339LNVOL (.110)† $\bar{R}^2$ = .102

Eq		Intercept	PUB	PROP	VOL / LNVOL	MEDS	VOL²	BED2	BED3	BED4	$\bar{R}^2$
11	ADR/EDR =	1.354 (.186)‡	+ .949PUB (.391)*	− .354PROP (.268)	− .000766VOL (.000484)	+ .058MEDS (.214)		− .166BED2 (.208)	+ .150BED3 (.294)	− .122BED4 (.265)	.107
12	ADR/EDR =	1.591 (.257)‡	+ .865PUB (.394)*	− .355PROP (.266)	− .00250VOL (.00139)	+ .047MEDS (.213)	+ $.210 \cdot 10^{-5}$VOL² $(.164 \cdot 10^{-5})$	− .169BED2 (.207)	+ .105BED3 (.294)	− .091BED4 (.264)	.116
13	ADR/EDR =	2.611 (.617)‡	+ .838PUB (.387)*	− .353PROP (.262)	− .274LNVOL (.114)*	+ .022MEDS (.210)		− .160BED2 (.204)	+ .160BED3 (.286)	− .067BED4 (.261)	.146
14	ADR − EDR =	.0115 (.0044)†			− .0000318VOL (.0000147)*						.047
15	ADR − EDR =	.0229 (.0066)‡			− .000118VOL (.000041)†		+ $.110 \cdot 10^{-6}$VOL² $(.490 \cdot 10^{-7})$*				.095
16	ADR − EDR =	.0633 (.0177)‡			− .0113LNVOL (.0033)‡						.123
17	ADR − EDR =	.0152 (.0076)*	+ .0302PUB (.0117)*	− .0073PROP (.0079)	− .0000817VOL (.0000413)	+ .0041MEDS (.0063)	+ $.713 \cdot 10^{-7}$VOL² $(.486 \cdot 10^{-7})$	− .0007BED2 (.0061)	+ .0061BED3 (.0087)	− .0019BED4 (.0079)	.172
18	ADR − EDR =	.0472 (.0183)*	+ .0295PUB (.0115)*	− .0072PROP (.0078)	− .0086LNVOL (.0034)*	+ .0032MEDS (.0062)		− .0005BED2 (.0060)	+ .0078BED3 (.0085)	− .0012BED4 (.0077)	.199

* = $p < .05$
† = $p < .01$
‡ = $p < .001$

rates as the dependent variable. Even though the coefficient on EDR was substantially different from 1, moving it to the left-hand side has little effect on the estimated volume-outcome relationship. Thus the coefficients on the volume variables in the last set of regressions are almost identical to those in the first set.

Many of these regression analyses incorporate a method of weighting observations based on the argument that, even if there were no true relationship between volume and outcome, the observed death rate in a given year in a hospital with many patients would be a more reliable estimate of the long-run mortality rate in that hospital than the observed rate in a hospital with few patients. Thus weights are introduced to allow the hospitals with more patients to have a greater effect on the estimated regression. None of the studies actually used the number of patients as a weight, but the two frequently used measures are roughly proportional to patients. Three of the studies used the following measure.[11]

$$\sqrt{\frac{\text{Patients}^2}{\sum\limits_{i} P_i(1 - P_i)}}$$

where Patients^2 is the square of the number of patients in the hospital and P is the probability of a "bad outcome" or death for the ith patient in the hospital.

Williams (1979) used the square root of the number of expected deaths.[12] Both measures give more weight to hospitals with more patients, and the correlation between the two measures is .762.

Table 4.7 presents the results for the same set of regressions with the weights used by Luft and colleagues. Some of the corrected R^2 values are higher and some are lower, but the interpretations of the findings are not very different. The effects of volume tend to be somewhat smaller and occasionally cross the (arbitrary) border into insignificance. Equation 2 mimics that used by Maerki, Luft, and Hunt and estimates a quadratic effect using ADR as the dependent variable. Equation 18 mimics the approach used in the other two studies (Studies 4 and 7), both of which used the difference in rates and log of volume. Again, these results suggest a volume effect. Williams used two formulation, each with a quadratic measure of volume and other hospital variables. With ADR as the dependent variable, both volume coefficients in Equation 5 are significant, but when hospital variables are included, the quadratic term loses significance. (This is also true if Williams's weights are used.) A similar pattern occurs when the ratio of actual to expected death rates (ADR/EDR) is the dependent variable. Weighting the regression does not change the inability of the Shortell and Lo-Gerfo model (Equation 10) or the Sloan, Perrin, and Valvona model (Equation 7) to detect a significant volume-outcome relationship.

The addition of the hospital-specific characteristics could confuse the analysis. The effects of hospital size per se, as measured by beds, are uniformly insignificant and would probably be dropped by an investigator carefully exploring the data. In the unweighted data, however, the coefficient for public hospitals always indicates a significantly higher mortality rate. Careful examination of the underlying data indicates, however, that one of the hospitals with very low volume and a very high mortality rate is public. This one case may account for both the significant "public" effect and the depressed volume effect. Whether it would be reasonable to exclude this one case is a judgment that must be based on more information about the hospital.

One source of controversy is whether the quadratic or log formulation is preferable. On the basis of the corrected R^2 in the unweighted regressions, the log form is preferred in each of the six sets of comparisons. In the sets of weighted regressions, the corrected R^2 values are generally within .001 of each other, and in the other two situations, they differ by .01 or less, with the log form better in one and worse in the other. To illustrate what the different functional forms imply with respect to the data, Figure 4.8 presents the data points and the estimated curves based on Equations 2 and 3 from both the unweighted and weighted regressions. The unweighted quadratic form implies a minimum at 566, and the weighted regression implies a minimum at 624. There are only three or four hospitals with volumes above those levels, and as the highest-volume hospital in 1983 had a somewhat higher than expected mortality rate, the quadratic provides a better fit at the high end. On the other hand, the log form seems to fit the data better at the low-volume end of the spectrum. It is difficult to provide a strong argument for choosing one form over the other, although the results for a single hospital at the high-volume end might deserve less weight in a policy decision than the results of the several hospitals with low volume.

Comparable regressions were estimated from the cholecystectomy data. They are not reported here because of their simple but repetitive "story." None of the 36 weighted and unweighted regressions showed a significant volume effect. In fact, there was only a handful of equations in which the t-ratios for the volume coefficients exceeded 1.0. It was not unusual for these insignificant coefficients to be the "wrong sign," indicating increasing mortality rates with volume or an inverted U shape. Clearly, if any one of these regressions was reported as part of a set of analyses on several procedures, the findings would have indicated no measurable volume-outcome relationship. This is not to say that there was a uniformly poor fit in all the regressions. When the actual death rate was the dependent variable, the expected death rate was always highly significant, which resulted in a "respectable" R^2 value in the middle of the .20 range for the unweighted regressions. With the other dependent variables, however, the corrected R^2 was often .000. The only other finding of note in these regressions is the marked improvement in the unweighted regression when the expected death rate was replaced by the proportion of patients in each risk-factor category. Examination of those results suggests that they may be attributable to the ability of a few risk-factor variables to "represent" certain hospitals with particularly high death rates.

Table 4.7: Hospital Level Regressions—CABG—Weighted

1 ADR $=$ .0224 $+$ .516EDR $-$ .134·10^4VOL $\bar{R}^2 = .139$
(.0076)† (.188)† (.718·10^5)

2 ADR $=$ .0321 $+$ .541EDR $-$ .716·10^4VOL $+$ .574·10^{-7}VOL^2 $\bar{R}^2 = .172$
(.0089)‡ (.185)† (.298·10^4)* (.287·10^{-7})*

3 ADR $=$ .057 $+$ .501EDR $-$ .0068LNVOL $\bar{R}^2 = .176$
(.017)† (.183)† (.0026)†

4 ADR $=$ .026 $+$ .412EDR $-$ .0000174VOL $\bar{R}^2 = .208$
(.008)† (.187)* (.0000075)*
$+$ .017PUB $-$ .010PROP $+$ .006MEDS $-$ .0002BED2 $+$ .005BED3 $-$ .002BED4
(.012) (.005) (.005) (.0040) (.005) (.006)

5 ADR $=$ .036 $+$ .415EDR $-$ .00007VOL $+$ .526·10^{-7}VOL^2 $\bar{R}^2 = .229$
(.010)‡ (.185)† (.00003)* (.306·10^{-7})
$+$ .0291PUB $-$ .0093PROP $+$ .0076MEDS $-$ .0008BED2 $+$ .0015BED3 $-$ .0030BED4
(.0120)* (.0054) (.0049) (.0044) (.0057) (.0059)

6 ADR $=$ .064 $+$ .404EDR $-$ .00764LNVOL $\bar{R}^2 = .239$
(.018)‡ (.183)* (.00264)†
$+$ .014PUB $-$ .010PROP $+$ .006MEDS $-$ .0003BED2 $+$ .004BED3 $-$ .002BED4
(.012) (.005) (.005) (.0040) (.005) (.006)

7 ADR $=$ .201 $-$ .0115PROP $-$ .00005VOL $+$ .418·10^{-7}VOL^2 $\bar{R}^2 = .004$
(.099)* (.0093) (.00006) (.520·10^{-7})
$+$ .0151PUB $+$ .0041MEDS $+$ .0050BED2 $+$ .0004BED3 $+$ .0028BED4 $+$ [29vars]
(.0093) (.0075) (.0069) (.0095) (.0093)

8 ADR/EDR $=$ 1.154 $-$ .00028VOL $\bar{R}^2 = .006$
(.102)‡ (.00023)

9 ADR/EDR $=$ 1.496 $-$ .000216VOL $+$ .00000186VOL^2 $\bar{R}^2 = .044$
(.200)‡ (.00098)* (.00000094)

10 ADR/EDR $=$ 1.993 $-$ .165LNVOL $\bar{R}^2 = .037$
(.480)‡ (.083)

11 ADR/EDR $=$ 1.195 (.132)‡ $+$ .529PUB (.402)* $-$ .319PROP (.184) $-$ .00038VOL (.00025) $+$ .015MEDS (.161) $-$ .028BED2 (.149) $+$ .165BED3 (.185) $+$ .005BED4 (.202) $\bar{R}^2 = .025$

12 ADR/EDR $=$ 1.476 (.230)‡ $+$ .392PUB (.409)* $-$ .00193VOL (.00107) $-$ .308PROP (.183) $+$ $.156\cdot10^{-5}\text{VOL}^2$ $(.105\cdot10^{-5})$ $+$ .069MEDS (.163) $-$ .047BED2 (.148) $+$ .073BED3 (.194) $-$ .013BED4 (.200) $\bar{R}^2 = .042$

13 ADR/EDR $=$ 2.124 (.516)‡ $+$ .428PUB (.402)* $-$ .187LNVOL (.089)* $-$ .324PROP (.182) $+$ .025MEDS (.158) $-$ .033BED2 (.147) $+$ .160BED3 (.179) $-$ .006BED4 (.199) $\bar{R}^2 = .053$

14 ADR$-$EDR $=$ .0044 (.0032) $-$ $.951\cdot10^{-5}\text{VOL}$ $(.727\cdot10^{-5})$ $\bar{R}^2 = .009$

15 ADR$-$EDR $=$ .0159 (.0063)* $-$ .0000725VOL (.0000308)* $+$ $.622\cdot10^{-7}\text{VOL}^2$ $(.296\cdot10^{-7})$* $\bar{R}^2 = .052$

16 ADR$-$EDR $=$ .0321 (.0151)* $-$ .00545LNVOL (.00262)‡ $\bar{R}^2 = .043$

17 ADR$-$EDR $=$ .0141 (.0076) $+$ .0141PUB (.0127)* $-$ .00007VOL (.00003)* $-$ .0083PROP (.0057) $+$ $.533\cdot10^{-7}\text{VOL}^2$ $(.326\cdot10^{-7})$ $+$ .0038MEDS (.0051) $-$ .0006BED2 (.00462) $+$ .0029BED3 (.0060) $-$ .0006BED4 (.0062) $\bar{R}^2 = .067$

18 ADR$-$EDR $=$ .0343 (.0161)* $+$ .0155PUB (.0126)* $-$ .00600LNVOL (.00277)* $-$ .0088PROP (.0057) $+$ .0023MEDS (.0050) $+$ .0004BED2 (.0046) $+$ .0058BED3 (.0056) $+$ .00004BED4 (.00621) $\bar{R}^2 = .073$

* $= p < .05$
† $= p < .01$
‡ $= p < .001$

Figure 4.8:   Log vs. Quadratic Formulations for CABG

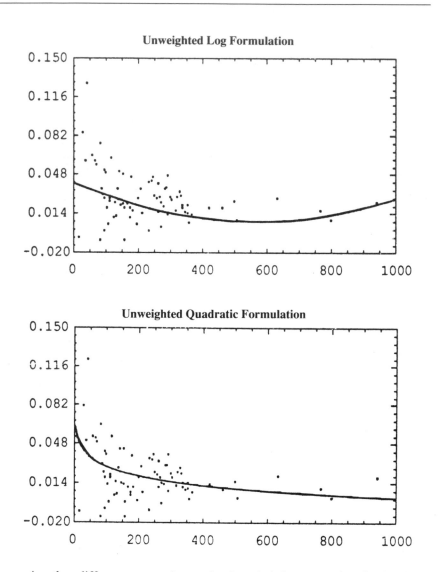

A rather different approach to using hospital data was taken by Hughes, Hunt, and Luft (1987).[13] Their study actually includes measures of both physician and hospital volume and, thus, is appropriately grouped in the last set of methods. Results based on only hospital volume are presented in Chapter 5, so the approach will be discussed here. To account for the problem of low death rates and small numbers of patients, they computed a Z-score for each hospital based on its observed and expected number of poor outcomes. Since they were con-

Figure 4.8: Continued

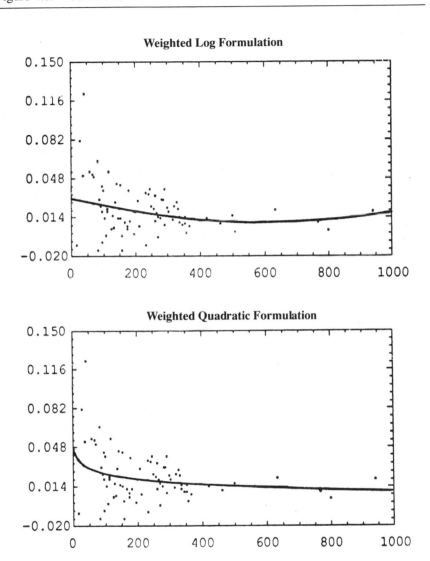

cerned that differences in mortality might be too low to be detected by referring physicians, they used a "poor outcome" measure for each patient, which is set equal to 1 if the patient dies or survives and has a hospital stay exceeding the 90th percentile for survivors. They limit their analysis to the Z-score based on the combined poor outcomes. Table 4.8, however, presents results for Z-scores based both on combined poor outcomes and on the components of poor outcomes: death and long stay. Furthermore, both unweighted and weighted results are presented. (Hughes, Hunt, and Luft weighted their regressions by a variable analogous to that used in Table 4.7. This procedure implies different weights for each dependent variable, however, so to allow a comparison of results, the weight used in this table are the square roots of the numbers of patients.)

It is quite clear that the poor-outcome measure largely reflects the effects of long-stay patients. Although there are substantially more such patients (by definition, 10 percent of the survivors, in contrast to death rates of 3.6 percent and 1.2 percent for CABG and cholecystectomy, respectively), deaths could still have dominated the combined index if the number of long stays in a hospital tended to be close to the expected number. Of course, if there is a comparable amount of variability in both groups, the long-stay component will dominate the total. A significant volume effect is found for both procedures based on the poor-outcome measure. However, there is no effect for Z (died) for cholecystectomy in the weighted regression, and the sign is in the wrong direction (positive) in the unweighted cholecystectomy regression. For CABG, there is a volume effect in all the regressions, although it is substantially larger for measures including long stays as a poor outcome. As was the case for the earlier sets of regressions, weighting has little effect on the CABG coefficients. Weighting, however, results in substantial changes for the cholecystectomy regressions.

There are several lessons to be learned from using the hospital as the unit of observation in these regressions. At least for these two procedures and this data set, the results are quite robust, regardless of the particular dependent variable, formulation of the volume variable, inclusion of hospital characteristics, or weighting. For CABG, 14 of the 19 unweighted regressions on mortality (including the Z-score formulation) have significant volume coefficients, and most of the others are nearly significant. The results are similar for the weighted regressions. For cholecystectomy, volume has a significant effect only in the unweighted Z-score regression, and then it is of the wrong sign. Thus almost any of the regression approaches would have detected a relationship for the CABG patients, although it might have been rejected in some instances if a strict .05 significance level was required. None of the regression approaches would have found the hypothesized relationship for cholecystectomy patients.

This is not to say that differences in approach had no effect. The addition of hospital characteristics sometimes weakens the estimated volume effect. This finding, however, is based on the CABG data, in which there are relatively few hospitals (76), and some with special characteristics also have extremely high mortality rates and low volumes. Thus this finding may not be generalizable, but it would be wise to be concerned about such problems when the number of hospitals is small. More important, one should ask whether the policy interest is in the effect of volume independent of other hospital characteristics. For example, certificate-of-need regulations usually specify a minimum volume for open-heart units, but these regulations do not take into account "adjustments" for ownership, hospital size, or teaching status.

Table 4.8: Hospital Level Regressions—Z-Scores

	Constant	LNVOL	PUB	PROP	MEDS	BED 2	BED 3	BED 4	
CABG—unweighted									
Z (DIED) =	2.854 (1.031)†	+ .467 (.190)*	+ .800 (.646)	− .556 (.437)	+ .114 (.350)	+ .102 (.340)	+ .282 (.478)	+ .066 (.436)	$\bar{R}^2$ = .098
Z(LLOS) =	6.205 (1.385)‡	− 1.292 (.255)‡	+ 1.266 (.867)	+ .243 (.587)	+ .209 (.471)	+ .923 (.457)*	+ 1.354 (.642)*	+ 1.898 (.586)	$\bar{R}^2$ = .587
Z (DIED or LLOS) =	6.161 (1.345)‡	− 1.268 (.248)	+ 1.350 (.842)	− .049 (.570)	+ .214 (.457)	+ .869 (.444)	+ 1.347 (.624)*	+ 1.744 (.569)†	$\bar{R}^2$ = .397
CABG—weighted									
Z (DIED) =	3.193 (1.254)*	− .550 (.217)*	+ .443 (.968)	− .663 (.450)	− .133 (.374)	+ .340 (.358)	+ .944 (.440)	+ .480 (.472)	$\bar{R}^2$ = .136
Z (LLOS) =	6.778 (1.838)‡	− 1.405 (.317)‡	+ 1.097 (1.419)	+ .172 (.660)	− .147 (.549)	+ .844 (.524)	+ 1.667 (.645)*	+ 2.709 (.692)‡	$\bar{R}^2$ = .352
Z (DIED or LLOS) =	6.677 (1.823)‡	− 1.375 (.315)‡	+ 1.148 (1.408)	− .128 (.654)	− .206 (.544)	+ .851 (.520)	+ 1.894 (.640)†	+ 2.620 (.687)‡	$\bar{R}^2$ = .345
Cholecystectomy—unweighted									
Z (DIED) =	−.131 (.198)	+ .164 (.054)‡	+ .059 (.192)	+ .060 (.100)	+ .001 (.169)	+ .087 (.104)	+ .147 (.179)		$\bar{R}^2$ = .027
Z (LLOS) =	.892 (.207)‡	− .118 (.056)*	+ .024 (.201)	+ .417 (.105)‡	+ .473 (.177)	− .101 (.109)	+ .019 (.187)		$\bar{R}^2$ = .051
Z (DIED or LLOS) =	.932 (.200)‡	− .135 (.054)*	+ .107 (.194)	+ .363 (.101)	+ .411 (.170)*	− .087 (.105)	+ .059 (.180)		$\bar{R}^2$ = .049
Cholecystectomy—weighted									
Z (DIED) =	.764 (.326)*	− .040 (.074)	+ .238 (.190)	− .100 (.119)	− .157 (.141)	+ .144 (.103)	+ .137 (.141)		$\bar{R}^2$ = .327
Z(LLOS) =	1.737 (.345)‡	− .303 (.078)‡	+ .160 (.201)	+ .297 (.126)*	+ .568 (.149)‡	− .205 (.109)	− .184 (.150)		$\bar{R}^2$ = .234
Z (DIED or LLOS) =	1.788 (.333)‡	− .318 (.076)‡	− .323 (.194)	+ .203 (.122)	+ .434† (.144)	− .180 (.105)	− .159 (.145)		$\bar{R}^2$ = .220

*=p<.05   †=p<.01   ‡=p<.001

It is difficult to state a clear preference among the various formulations of the volume measure or dependent variable. Some may prefer the log or quadratic form for volume, for theoretical or policy reasons, but there is no strong empirical basis for choosing one over the other, to judge from these CABG data. The choice of dependent variable will have a marked impact on explanatory power, but this difference is largely determined by whether the expected death rate is on the right or left side of the equation. This is not to say, however, that such decisions are irrelevant in certain situations. For example, suppose one were interested in the volume associated with the minimum mortality rate from equations ignoring hospital characteristics. From the unweighted regressions with a quadratic term for volume, the "optimal volumes" are 566, 541, and 536 if we use ADR, the ratio of actual to expected death rate (ADR/EDR), and the difference between actual and expected death rate (ADR–EDR) as the dependent variables, respectively. From the weighted regressions, the values are 624, 581, and 583. It appears that allowing the expected death rate to have an independent effect on outcomes results in a higher "optimal volume," and this effect is somewhat greater in the weighted regressions. For most purposes, these differences should be inconsequential, but they might be important in some circumstances.

Regressions: Patient as the Unit of Observation

Several studies used the patient as the unit of observation and included a measure of volume in the equation. Farber, Kaiser and Wenzel (1981), Kelly and Hellinger (1987), Roos et al. (1986), and Riley and Lubitz (1985) all estimated logistic regressions, while Showstack et al. (1987) used ordinary least squares. However, there are other differences in the specification of the models.

We reproduced the various approaches in Table 4.9 using the CABG data because no effects were apparent for cholecystectomy. Farber, Kaiser, and Wenzel (1981) used a logistic regression on volume, but mentioned no patient risk factors.[14] Although the explanatory power is quite low, there was a highly significant volume effect. This result is consistent with the other findings using different approaches, which indicated a volume relationship for CABG without such risk factors held constant, as in Equation A1. When patient risk factors are added, as in Equation A2, the volume coefficient becomes smaller and is not quite significant.

Kelly and Hellinger (1987) included both patient risk factors and hospital characteristics, as in Equation A3.[15] This modification leaves the volume coefficient insignificant. In fact, Kelly and Hellinger excluded patients with less than a two-day stay, arguing that patients with one-day stays are quite different and their outcomes may largely reflect preadmission health status. For CABG, this exclusion implies dropping 88 patients or 0.48 percent of the sample, but since all but 6 of these patients died, this number represents 12.35 percent of the deaths. In this case, the exclusion results in a small reduction in the volume coefficient and an increase in its standard error. Thus the figures in A3 might be taken to suggest a volume effect, but those in A4 would not.

Roos and colleagues (1986) sometimes used several categories of volumes and sometimes just two.[16] If four volume categories are used, representing 6–100, 101–200, 201–350, and 351 or more patients, with the last being the omitted category, then all three of the lower-volume categories have higher mortality rates than those in the highest-volume hospitals. Patients in the lowest-volume hospitals have a much higher risk of death, those in hospitals with volumes of 201–350 have significantly elevated risks, and those in hospitals with volumes of 101–200 have little difference in risk, after controlling for patient risk factors. Although this pattern may seem strange, it is quite apparent in the simple graphical presentation in the middle panels of Figure 4.5. On the other hand, if just two volume groups are used (as in Equation A6 in Table 4.9), with a split at the mean volume of 242, then no volume effect is seen.

Riley and Lubitz (1985) used the log of volume, as in Equation A7, and given the earlier sets of findings, it is not surprising that the coefficient is somewhat more significant than its analog in A2.[17] Although they used this form, they were limited by their data set to a 20-percent sample of Medicare patients. (Because of the restricted data set, some of the risk-factor variables had to be omitted.) If we limit our data to patients 65 and over, as in A8, the volume effect is still apparent. Since Riley and Lubitz used the patient as the unit of analysis, the sampling should have little impact. Had they used the hospital, the sampling would have been far more likely to drop low-volume hospitals and retain higher-volume settings, thereby resulting in some potential for bias.

Although computational costs have been falling over time, logistic regressions on large numbers of patients can still be expensive. Showstack and colleagues (1987) reported on ordinary least squares regressions with a model similar to B5 (Table 4.9).[18] The coefficients in logistic and OLS regressions are not directly comparable, but the "story" is essentially the same, with significantly higher likelihood of death for patients in low- and high-volume hospitals compared to those in settings with very high volumes. More important, the conclusions reached from the OLS and logistic regressions are substantively the same.

SUMMARY AND IMPLICATIONS

The preceding sections have examined the results obtained from applying a wide variety of techniques that are similar to, but not limited to, those used in the published studies of the volume-outcome relationship. It is apparent that, for a given set of data, the findings will depend to some degree on the approaches used. A simple counting of results is not appropriate, since minor variations were often included to allow comparisons in which one thing was changed at a time, rather than simply to mimic the set of widely varying approaches in the literature.

Table 4.9:   Volume Coefficients in Patient Level Regressions

Logistic regressions

A1		$-$ .000661VOL (.000190)‡	
A2		$-$ .000374VOL (.000205)	
A3		$-$ .000404VOL (.000211)	
A4		$-$ .000367VOL (.000226)	
A5	.629LOW (.171)‡	$+$ .077MED (.128)	$+$ .296HIGH (.100)‡
A6	.032LOWHALF (.092)		
A7	$-$ .192LNVOL (.068)*		
A8	$-$ .210LNVOL (.083)*		

Ordinary least squares

B1		$-$ .0000211VOL (.0000060)‡	
B2		$-$ .0000103VOL (.0000059)	
B3		$-$ .0000117VOL (.0000063)	
B4		$-$ .00000943VOL (.00000527)	
B5	.0224LOW (.0062)‡	$+$ .0014MED (.0039)	$+$ .0082HIGH (.0030)†
B6	.00102LOWHALF (.00295)		
B7	$-$ .00582LNVOL (.00213)†		
B8	$-$ .00989LNVOL (.00399)*		

$* = p < .05$ $† = p < .01$ $‡ = p < .001$

Table 4.10 extracts the simulated findings for each of the approaches actually used and also presents the authors' original findings for CABG or cholecystectomy. In a few instances, it is difficult to determine exactly how the findings would have been interpreted. For example, in some cases a visual inspection might indicate a downward-sloping relationship, but the tests of significance did not quite meet standard levels. In these instances, we have listed the more conservative interpretation first and discussed the problem in the notes. We

Table 4.9: Continued

	$\bar{R}^2$	χ^2	
	.0019	12.84	1DF
+ (29 patient variables)	.1568	954.74	30DF
+ (29 patient and 6 hospital variables)	.1568	969.38	36DF
+ (29 patient and 6 hospital variables— patients with stays of 2 + days)	.1608	903.64	36DF
+ (29 patient variables)	.1584	969.34	32DF
+ (29 patient variables)	.1560	951.45	30DF
+ (29 patient variables)	.1568	959.20	30DF
+ (20 patient variables—7253 patients aged 65 + only)	.1289	441.33	21DF
	.0006		
+ (29 patient variables)	.0852		
+ (29 patient and 6 hospital variables)	.0856		
+ (29 patient and 6 hospital variables— patients with stays of 2 + days)	.0812		
+ (29 patient variables)	.0858		
+ (29 patient variables)	.0850		
+ (29 patient variables)	.0854		
+ (20 patient variables—7253 patients aged 65 + only)	.0922		

should also emphasize that the simulated results are a somewhat naive approximation of what generally occurs in research studies. For example, the inclusion of hospital-specific variables often added little to the regression equation but resulted in the volume coefficient changing from significant to insignificant. It is likely that in the "real world" of empirical research, a simplified equation would be reported with the significant findings.

To illustrate the findings in Table 4.10, Figure 4.9 summarizes the interpretations for the two procedures. In each case there are 26 simulated results, and the articles actually included 10 CABG findings and 11 cholecystectomy findings. We do not really have a "gold standard" or true knowledge of the volume-outcome relationship for either procedure, nor is it reasonable to assume that findings from the 1983 California data should even approximate findings from other settings, some of which do not even focus on mortality. In spite of this caveat, there is substantial consistency for the CABG data. Twenty of the 26 simulated findings support a "classic" volume-outcome relationship in which outcomes are worse in low-volume hospitals. (The six exceptions are the most interesting cases and will be discussed below.) Furthermore, 9 of the 10 actual findings support this interpretation. Only one of these used 1983 California data, although with some minor differences in exclusions and risk factors. For cholecystectomy, the results are almost inverted; 20 of the simulations show no effect, as do 3 of the 11 actual findings.

An examination of the patterns of results leads to some insights about the influence of method on findings. The simulated findings for CABG are quite consistent in indicating a relationship, yet there are six exceptions. One is a very close call: using a tripartite categorization, there appears to be a relationship, but the pairwise t-tests used by Rosenblatt, Reinken, and Shoemack (1985) barely fail the standard significance tests. Likewise, the approaches taken by Shortell and LoGerfo (1981) and Williams (1979), which rely on the ratio of actual to expected deaths in hospital-level regressions yield volume coefficients that are not quite significant. The other two negative results, with approaches used by Flood, Scott, and Ewy (1984a) and Roos and colleagues (1986), use a high-versus low-volume categorization that seems too insensitive for the CABG relationship, in which the poorest outcomes seem concentrated at the very low volume levels. The final exception is the comparison of volumes for hospitals categorized by outcomes, as reported by Sloan, Perrin, and Valvona (1986). Both the simulated and actual findings are in the form of a "greater than" sign ($>$), lending support to the explanation given above concerning the sensitivity of the approach to the classification of outcomes. The remaining findings are also informative. All six of the approaches indicating an L-shaped relationship gave the same result with the simulated data. Of the two approaches with reported U-shaped curves, one yielded the same pattern and the other a downward slope ($\searrow$) because the coefficient for the quadratic term was not significant.

The situation for cholecystectomy is quite different. The simulated results suggest there is little evidence of a volume-outcome relationship, but there are six exceptions to this pattern. Fowles, Bunker, and Schurman (1987) compared the average volumes of hospitals for survivors and decedents, and even though the differences are relatively small, the large sample size allows this case-control approach to detect such a difference. The Sloan, Perrin, and Valvona (1986) approach to analyzing volumes according to outcome groups yields the same findings as was the case for CABG. The other four "exceptions" all indicate a downward-sloping relationship. Three rely on visual inspection of the data, and one combines inspection with *t*-tests among categories. This result suggests that the cholecystectomy data from California may not be entirely devoid of a volume-outcome relationship, but it might be a subtle one and may be detectable only by focusing on selected parts of the data. Alternatively, one might argue that no general relationship exists and that sufficiently determined mining of any set of random numbers will identify patterns in subsets of the data.

Eight of the 11 actual cholecystectomy findings indicated a relationship. Of these eight, however, two by Farber, Kaiser, and Wenzel (1987) and one by Roos and colleagues (1986) focused on complications rather than death, and the Hughes, Hunt and Luft (1987) study combined death and long stay. The others used data from hospitals across the nation in the early 1970s. One may want to be cautious in interpreting the available data as supporting the notion of a volume-outcome relationship for cholecystectomy mortality in the 1980s.

In general, this exercise suggests that the published findings are relatively insensitive to the differences in methods used, although there are some important exceptions. For example, if one believes the California CABG data support the existence of a volume-outcome relationship, the various methods could have misled the reader to believe that there was no relationship in only 6 of 26 times; and in three of those instances, it would have been a close call. The nature of the functional form is more sensitive to method because most approaches do not allow the comparison of alternative forms. The situation is somewhat more complex for cholecystectomy. Twenty of the 26 approaches indicate no relationship, and most of the others suggest a less than powerful connection between volume and outcome, but we do not know whether a relationship really exists or is artifactual.

Although there is general consistency among methods in determining whether a relationship exists, this does not mean that method does not matter. For example, if just one of the 26 CABG simulations was chosen at random to provide evidence for the existence of a volume-outcome relationship, there would be a 6 in 26 chance of giving the "wrong" conclusion. This would be the case even though the data are drawn from a reasonable number of hospitals and a large number of patients, so tests of significance could be taken to be reliable. Most people would not "bet the farm" on the results of a single study, and this discussion suggests that even multiple studies using the same methods should be treated with some caution. The lack of easy comparability across studies with varying methods is offset by increasing confidence in the general "bottom line," if it is consistent across the vast majority of the approaches.

The methods investigated range from simple categorization by volume to fairly sophisticated regression models. This set of comparisons does not indicate a clear superiority of one form over the other. Each has unique problems, advantages, and disadvantages, although some lessons can be learned from our investigation. If the necessary data are available, risk-factor adjustments should be included in the analysis. This is possible with any of the general approaches.

In the examination of outcomes across volume categories, it may be sufficient

Table 4.10: Simulated and Reported Findings for CABG and Cholecystectomy

Method	CABG			Cholecystectomy		
	Simulated	Reported	Notes	Simulated	Reported	Notes
Adams, et al. (1973) 4 categories, t-test high vs. low risk	∟	NA	1	—	NA	2
Hertzer et al. (1984) 3–4 categories, t-test high vs. low risk	∟	NA	1	—	NA	2
Kempczinski et al. (1986) 3 categories, t-tests, high vs. low risk	∟	NA	1	—	NA	2
Farber et al. (1981) up to 15 categories	⊤	NA	3	/ ⊃	∟	4
Pilcher et al. (1980) 3 categories χ^2, high vs. low risk	∟	NA	5	—	NA	6
Rosenblatt et al. (1985) 3 categories, t-tests, high vs. low risk	—	NA	7	—	NA	8
Luft et al. (1979) ADR, EDR plots	∟	∟	9	/	—	10
Luft et al. (1987) ADR/EDR by volume	∟	/	11	/	/	12
Luft & Hunt (1986) Distribution of Z-scores	∟	NA	13	—	NA	14
Flood et al. (1984a) Actual vs. Expected, χ^2	⊡	NA	15	⊡	⊡	15
Fowles et al. (1987) Compare volumes by outcomes	∧	∧	16	∧	NA	17
Sloan et al. (1986) Compare volumes by hospital outcomes	/	NA	18	—	NA	19
Sloan et al. (1986) Hospital ADR $= f(v, v^2,$ pt risk factors)	⊃	⊃	20	—	NA	21
Luft (1980) Hospital ADR-EDR $= f(log\ v, ...)$wtd	⊃	∟	22	—	NA	21
Maerki et al. (1986) Hospital: ADR $= f($EDR, v, $v^2)$wtd	⊃	⊃	23	—	NA	21
Shortell & LoGerfo (1981) Hospital: ADR/EDR $= f(v, ...)$	—	NA	24	—	NA	21
Williams (1979) Hospital: ADR/EDR $= f(v, v^2, ...)$wtd	—	NA	25	—	NA	21
Williams (1979) Hospital: ADR $= f($EDR, $v, v^2, ...)$wtd	/	NA	26	⊤	—	28
Hughes et al. (1987) Hospital: Z-score $= f(log\ v, ...)$wtd	∟	∟	27	—	∟	30
Farber et al. (1981) Patient: $log\ \frac{p}{1-p} = f(v)$	∟	NA	29	—	—	30
Kelly & Hellinger (1986) Patient: $log\ \frac{p}{1-p} = f(v,$ risk factors, hosp$)$	∟	∟	31	—	NA	33
Roos et al. (1986) Patient: $log\ \frac{p}{1-p} = f(v$low, risk factors$)$	—	NA	32	—	⊡	35
Roos et al. (1987) Patient: $log\ \frac{p}{1-p} = f(v1, v2, v3,$ risk factors$)$	∟	NA	34	—	—	30
Wennberg et al. (1987) Patient: $log\ \frac{p}{1-p} = f(v1, v2, v3,$ risk factors$)$	∟	NA	32	—	NA	30
Showstack et al. (1987) Patient: Dead $= f(v1, v2, v3,$ risk factors$)$	∟	∟	36	—	NA	30
Riley & Lubitz (1985) Patient: $log\ \frac{p}{1-p} = f(log\ v,$ risk factors$)$	∟	∟	37	—	—	30

NA indicates no results available

— indicates an insignificant relationship

⊓ indicates two groupings, with worse outcomes at lower volumes

/ indicates a downward sloping linear relation

∪ indicates a U-shaped curve with worsening outcomes above a certain volume

∟ indicates an L-shaped curve, with poor outcomes at low volumes and little change at higher volumes

⊂ indicates worse outcomes at moderate volumes

∧ indicates very good and very poor outcomes at low volumes, moderate outcomes at moderate volumes

1. Based on Figure 4.1D, with four volume categories. The *t*-test merely compares the highest and lowest categories and thus would have to be coded as downward sloping.

2. Figure 4.2D suggests a downward-sloping curve, but it would probably be noticed that the highest volume category includes only one hospital. Figures 4.2A and 4.2B, would probably be interpreted as "no clear pattern." This interpretation would be supported by *t*-tests.

3. Figure 4.1A suggests a ∟ shape.

4. Figure 4.2A suggests a ﹨ shape, on the assumption that outcomes in the very lowest volume settings were visually combined. Figure 4.2C suggests an inverted U. Note that the Farber study focuses on wound infections, not mortality.

5. Figure 4.3E suggests an ∟ curve for high-risk patients and little effect for low-risk patients. The hypothesis of linearity would not be rejected for either group of patients.

6. Figure 4.4E suggests a downward sloping pattern for high-risk patients and little effect for low-risk patients. The hypothesis of linearity would not be rejected for either group of patients.

7. Although Figure 4.3E suggests an ∟ curve, the pairwise *t*-tests are not significant at the .05 level. The comparison between the low- and high-volume groups for high-risk patients yields a *z* (or *t*) value of 1.93 which is certainly close enough to be discussed.

8. Figure 4.4E supports a downward-sloping curve. The difference between low- and high-volume groups for the high-risk patients is significant at the .05 level. The other comparisons are not statistically significant.

9. Figure 4.5A indicates substantially higher than expected mortality in the lowest-volume hospitals, with no clear pattern thereafter. The authors used fixed volume categories for all procedures.

10. Figure 4.6A suggests no clear pattern.

11. Figure 4.5B indicates higher actual/expected deaths in the lowest-volume group. The authors used different volume categories for each procedure.

12. Figure 4.6B suggests a ﹨ or ∩ curve. The very low volume group would probably have been discounted.

13. Figures 4.7A and 4.7C suggest a much greater risk of a low-volume hospital having significantly worse than expected outcomes while the highest volume settings are neither better nor worse than expected.

14. Figures 4.7B and 4.7D suggest the hospitals with significantly poor results are concentrated in the low-to-middle ranges, but there are very few high-volume hospitals.

Continued

Table 4.10: Continued

15. When the samples are split at the mean volumes, there is almost no difference between the observed and expected number of deaths for either CABG or cholecystectomy.

16. The mean volume for CABG survivors is 365 vs. a mean hospital volume of 334 for those who died. This yields a highly significant difference.

17. The mean volume for cholecystectomy survivors is 115 vs. 109 for decedants. This yields a difference significant at the .05 level.

18. The hospitals with zero deaths have an average volume of 89, those with the highest death rate (average of 6.8%) have an average of 68 and moderate death rate hospitals (3.7%) have volumes averaging 272.

19. Hospitals with no deaths have an average volume of 44, those with the highest death rates (5.0% average) have volumes averaging 52, and those with moderate death rates (1.5%) have volumes averaging 108.

20. The coefficient for v is significant but that for v^2 is not.

21. None of the cholecystectomy volume coefficients were significant.

22. See Table 4.7, Equation 18.

23. See Table 4.7, Equation 2.

24. See Table 4.6, Equation 11. The coefficient for volume is negative, but not significant.

25. See Table 4.7, Equation 12. The coefficients are consistent with a U shape but neither is significant.

26. See Table 4.7, Equation 5. The coefficient for volume is negative and significant, that for volume^2 is positive but not significant.

27. See Table 4.8, Equations 4 and 6. The former indicates a significant volume relation for mortality alone, the latter indicates significant volume relation for mortality and long stays. The Hughes paper uses an equation including surgeon volume, but the results for an equation without physician volume are presented in Chapter 5, Table 5.4.

28. See Table 4.8, Equations 10 and 12. The former indicates an insignificant volume coefficient for mortality alone and the latter a significant effect for mortality and long stays. The results for the Hughes model with physician volume indicated no hospital effect; without physician volume there is a significant hospital coefficient for poor outcomes. See Chapter 5, Table 5.4.

29. See Table 4.9, Equation A1. Note that a linear volume coefficient in a logistic repression implies a curvilinear relation.

30. None of the cholecystectomy regressions had significant volume effects.

31. See Table 4.9, Equation A4. The reported equation included a measure of physician volume.

32. The coefficient for the "low volume" dummy was quite insignificant.

33. The coefficient reported in the paper indicates significantly higher readmission rates for hospitals with volumes below 100.

34. See Table 4.9, Equation A5.

35. The paper actually uses three volume categories (one omitted) and readmissions.

36. See Table 4.9, Equation B5.

37. See Table 4.9, Equation A8.

Figure 4.9: Summary of Simulated and Reported Findings

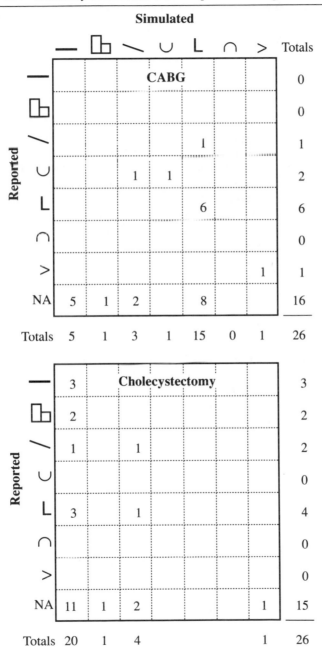

to plot actual divided by expected deaths, preferably with confidence intervals. The addition of confidence intervals to the analysis would make the interpretation of "patterns" across categories less idiosyncratic. Similar plots of the actual and expected death rates may be informative if they indicate a nonuniform pattern of risk across volume categories. Such risk differentials may suggest selective referral of patients toward or away from certain types of hospitals.

The choice of volume categories is more problematic. In a few instances, there are externally set volume levels that can be used, but in general, categories are merely devices for grouping enough hospitals so that the number of patients is sufficiently large to give a stable estimate of the mortality rate. One could devise a criterion that would rank hospitals by volume and proceed down the list, beginning with the smallest, until the requisite number of patients was included, then begin with the next category, and so forth. A simple application of this rule would result in an equal number of patients in each category, but given the skewed distribution of volumes, the lowest category would be very broad and would include a very large number of hospitals, while the highest-volume categories might include only one or two hospitals. Thus it is important to combine statistical guidelines and a sense of how the data are to be used. Regardless of how the categories are designed, however, one should examine the hospital data to determine whether one or two hospitals are outliers that dominate the estimates for their categories.

Regression approaches can also be sensitive to specific decisions concerning the interpretation of findings and the formulation of the model. Although the "eyeball analysis" of categories might appear to be relatively unscientific, a slavish devotion to the .05 level of statistical significance may be equally inappropriate. Several of the "miscalls" in the simulations arose from situations in which a coefficient was just short of statistical significance. When viewed alone, such a result may not be enough to reject the null hypothesis of no relationship, but if one has already developed a prior hypothesis of a relationship based on other studies, then a marginally insignificant coefficient (of the correct sign) is hardly cause to reject the notion. In fact, if one were to undertake a more formal meta-analysis and combine the statistical results, then the "insignificant result" would actually strengthen the overall confidence in the relationship.

Just as one should test the robustness of the choice of categories, it is important to examine alternative functional forms in regressions. Since there is no clear theoretical preference for linear, log, quadratic, or other functional forms, one should examine several forms to determine the best fit. Likewise, the choice of the dependent variable should also be explored. Weighting the observations, however, does make intuitive and statistical sense. Although there might not be a clearly preferred set of weights, the choice among reasonable weights is not likely to make much difference.

At least for the data examined in this chapter, quite similar conclusions were reached with hospital- and patient-level regressions. (The logistic and OLS coefficients cannot be compared directly. Nevertheless, if one were to compare the weighted hospital results with the OLS patient results [Equation 1 on Table 4.7 with Equation B2 on Table 4.9, and Equation 3 on Table 4.7 with Equation B7 on Table 4.9], the volume effects are very similar.) The choice of approach may be far more dependent on the larger context of the questions being asked. For example, if one is trying to understand why some hospitals have high volumes and other have low volumes, while at the same time estimating the effects of volume on outcomes, then the hospital is the natural unit of observation. If one is concerned about the influence of selected hospital variables, then it is important to keep in mind the fact that even though there may be tens of thousands of observations in a patient data set, the true number of degrees of freedom for hospital variables is much lower.

It is also important that both the analysis and its interpretation be sensitive to the requirements of different applications. For example, if one questions whether a relationship exists between volume and outcome, it is certainly reasonable to include various patient risk factors. Whether one should include other variables, such as hospital ownership or teaching status, is less clear. For example, if the data are to be used for regulatory guidelines, then unless such hospital-specific variables are also included in the guidelines, a simpler model including only volume and risk factors is appropriate. On the other hand, if one is attempting to understand what *underlies* the volume-outcome relationship, then it is reasonable to use a wide range of hospital variables, including factors such as quality review programs, organizational structure, staff skills, and the like. If this is done well, however, and the correct explanations are found, then the "volume" effect may disappear—but this is not to say it does not exist. Rather, it is a proxy for a series of factors not generally or easily measured.

Regardless of the types of models and approaches to be used, it is important to be extraordinarily careful in the analysis and interpretation of the data. Estimates may be sensitive to one or two data points that may be outliers, either because of unusual but true occurrences, or because of coding or other errors. Errors can also occur in the steps required in the analysis. Furthermore, one cannot assume that errors in large data sets are unimportant because they will be swamped by the "true data." In the analyses of the data in this chapter, two occasions of "minor" errors in the cholecystectomy data created significant volume effects. Had those analyses been done in a vacuum, without their jarring inconsistency with other analyses of the same data, the errors might not have been identified.

It would probably be best for a researcher to examine a new set of data quite carefully, to proceed with some simple breakdowns by categories, and then to use regression models to include additional variables. A step-by-step approach could first identify relationships in the data and point to the most appropriate functional form. Using a combination of approaches can also help in interpreting the results for others. Thus one could use a fairly complex model in exploring the underlying relationships but fall back on simple categorical findings in a section on implications for policymakers, focusing on the results for patients in low-, moderate-, or high-volume hospitals. The presentation of findings with alternative methods is also likely to be more convincing to a broader range of readers and will facilitate the comparison of findings with those of other studies.

NOTES

1. For a further discussion of the selection criteria, see Luft et al. (1990).
2. See, for example, DesHarnais et al. (1988).
3. See Adams, Fraser, and Abrams (1973); Hertzer et al. (1984); Pilcher et al. (1980); Kempczinski, Brott, and Labutta (1986); Rosenblatt, Reinken, and Shoemack (1985); and Farber, Kaiser, and Wenzel (1981).
4. See, for example, Pilcher et al. (1980) and Rosenblatt, Reinken, and Shoemack (1985).
5. See Adams, Fraser, and Abrams (1973); Hertzer et al. (1984); Kempczinski, Brott, and Labutta (1986); and Rosenblatt, Reinken, and Shoemack (1985).
6. See Luft, Bunker, and Enthoven (1979); Luft and Hunt (1986); and Luft, Hunt, and Maerki (1987).
7. Part I of Flood, Scott, and Ewy (1984a) is reprinted in Chapter 14 of this volume.
8. See reprint of Luft, Bunker, and Enthoven (1979) in Chapter 12 of this volume.
9. Luft and Hunt (1986) is reprinted in Chapter 19 of this volume.
10. See reprint of Sloan, Perrin, and Valvona (1986) in Chapter 13 of this volume.
11. See Luft (1980); Luft, Hunt, and Maerki (1987); and Maerki, Luft, and Hunt (1986).
12. See reprint of Williams (1979) in Chapter 18 of this volume.
13. The study by Hughes, Hunt, and Luft (1987)is reprinted in Chapter 17 of this volume.
14. The study by Farber, Kaiser, and Wenzel (1981) is reprinted in Chapter 9 of this volume.
15. See reprint of Kelly and Hellinger (1987) in Chapter 10 of this volume.
16. See reprint of Roos et al. (1986) in Chapter 8 of this volume.
17. See reprint of Riley and Lubitz (1985) in Chapter 15 of this volume.
18. The study by Showstack et al. (1987) is reprinted in Chapter 11 of this volume.

Appendix 4.1: Mortality Rates by Volume Group—CABG

Group	Volume Category	Number of Hospitals	All Patients		Nonelective		Elective	
			Patients	Death Rate	Patients	Death Rate	Patients	Death Rate
A	6–20	1	20	.000	10	.000	10	.000
	21–50	3	115	.104	51	.118	64	.094
	51–100	10	848	.051	388	.082	460	.024
	101–200	22	3,202	.038	1,244	.059	1,958	.025
	201–300	20	5,167	.040	1,541	.073	3,626	.026
	301–500	15	5,462	.033	1,606	.052	3,856	.024
	501+	5	3,648	.028	893	.041	2,755	.024
B	6–20	1	20	.000	10	.000	10	.000
	21–50	3	115	.104	51	.118	64	.094
	51–100	10	848	.051	388	.082	460	.024
	101–200	22	3,202	.038	1,244	.059	1,958	.025
	201+	40	14,277	.034	4,040	.058	10,237	.025
C	6–20	1	20	.000	10	.000	10	.000
	21–100	13	963	.057	439	.087	524	.032
	101–200	22	3,202	.038	1,244	.059	1,958	.025
	201–350	28	7,807	.038	2,223	.072	5,584	.025
	351+	12	6,470	.029	1,817	.040	4,653	.025
D	6–100	14	983	.056	449	.085	534	.032
	101–200	22	3,202	.038	1,244	.059	1,958	.025
	201–350	28	7,807	.038	2,223	.072	5,584	.025
	351+	12	6,470	.029	1,817	.040	4,653	.025
E	6–150	26	2,465	.047	1,015	.073	1,450	.029
	151–250	18	3,554	.039	1,272	.061	2,282	.026
	251+	32	12,443	.033	3,446	.056	8,997	.024
F	6–242	41	5,279	.041	2,064	.065	3,215	.025
	243+	35	13,183	.034	3,669	.058	9,514	.025

Appendix 4.2: Mortality Rates by Volume Group—Cholecystectomy

Group	Volume Category	Number of Hospitals	All Patients		Nonelective		Elective	
			Patients	Death Rate	Patients	Death Rate	Patients	Death Rate
A	2–4	14	45	.022	15	.000	30	.033
	5–10	23	172	.006	55	.018	117	.000
	11–20	38	603	.010	185	.027	418	.002
	21–50	138	4,666	.014	1,489	.030	3,177	.007
	51–100	124	9,090	.012	2,950	.031	6,140	.003
	101–200	93	12,402	.012	4,126	.026	8,276	.006
	201–300	12	2,899	.011	895	.028	2,004	.003
	301+	1	445	.004	287	.007	158	.000
B	2–4	14	45	.022	15	.000	30	.033
	5–10	23	172	.006	55	.018	117	.000
	11–20	38	603	.010	185	.027	418	.002
	21–50	138	4,666	.014	1,489	.030	3,177	.007
	51–100	124	9,090	.012	2,950	.031	6,140	.003
	101–200	93	12,402	.012	4,126	.026	8,276	.006
	201+	13	3,344	.010	1,182	.023	2,162	.003
C	2–20	75	820	.010	255	.024	565	.004
	21–100	262	13,756	.013	4,439	.031	9,317	.005
	101–200	93	12,402	.012	4,126	.026	8,276	.006
	201–300	12	2,899	.011	895	.028	2,004	.003
	301+	1	445	.004	287	.007	158	.000
D	2–100	337	14,576	.013	4,694	.030	9,882	.004
	101–200	93	12,402	.012	4,126	.026	8,276	.006
	201–300	12	2,899	.011	895	.028	2,004	.003
	351+	1	445	.004	287	.007	158	.000
E	2–150	403	22,448	.013	7,352	.030	15,096	.005
	151–250	34	6,052	.011	2,002	.022	4,050	.005
	251+	6	1,822	.008	648	.015	1,174	.003
F	2–68	273	9,134	.012	2,843	.028	6,291	.004
	69+	170	21,188	.013	7,159	.028	14,029	.005

Chapter 5

Summary of Research Findings

There are sufficient studies concerning the volume-outcome relationship that we can focus on patterns of results, rather than solely on findings for each of the 25 studies or the sets of findings for selected procedures and diagnoses. However, there is no particular reason to believe that a volume-outcome relationship is present for all procedures and diagnoses. Therefore, we should focus not just on how universal the relationship appears to be, but on whether the situations in which it is found (or not found) tend to form a pattern. Since we do not have clear hypotheses about potential patterns across procedures or methods, this analysis must be considered exploratory. In other words, the validity of any apparent patterns must be checked with new data and analyses.

It is difficult to formally combine or compare results of several studies because their methods differ. For example, it is impossible to compare directly the findings of a study contrasting mortality rates for hospitals with volumes above or below an arbitrary cutoff with another study estimating the influence of the log of volume on outcomes, while at the same time controlling for numerous hospital characteristics and referral effects. To overcome this difficulty, we chose a "minimalist" approach and, upon review of each study, categorized the findings for each diagnosis or procedure according to the implicit shape of the volume-outcome relationship curve. When possible, we used the authors' "bottom line" interpretations of their own data, even though other results reported earlier in the study, such as bivariate correlations, might have been different.

SUMMARIZING FINDINGS

Depending on the specification of the volume variable, findings fall into six categories: (1) dichotomous results showing lower rates of poor outcomes in high-volume settings; (2) a negative linear relationship also showing lower poor outcome rates in high-volume settings; (3) a U-shaped relationship; (4) an inverse logarithmic form, with large reductions in the rates of poor outcomes at low volumes and a relative flattening at high volumes; (5) a flat curve, indicating no significant relationship; and (6) an increasing rate of poor outcomes with higher volumes.[1] The methods used in the various studies influence the categories into which the findings fall. For example, a dichotomous finding could result from a study that used two volume categories or many volume categories. Table 5.1 indicates categories of findings that were possible using various measures of volume. Although having many volume categories is the most flexible approach in the sense that it can "fit" any curve, this also demands the greatest reader discretion. It is not always important how a finding is classified among the first four groups of research findings, since all imply worse outcomes among low-volume settings. For some purposes, however, readers may want to know whether poor outcomes were found in only the very lowest-volume hospitals. However, none of the studies really tested alternative formulations.[2]

Table 5.2 summarizes the results of this categorization of findings for hospital volume; Table 5.3 for physician volume. These tables should be read along with Table 2.1, which lists the 25 studies and shows the diagnoses and procedures examined in each. For example, results for abdominal aortic aneurysm are shown in the first column of Table 5.2.

When a single study includes two methods (e.g., dichotomous and continuous volume variables) or differentiates between two subcategories of a procedure (e.g., ruptured aneurysm surgery and elective aneurysm surgery), the results are counted separately (and represented by a lower-case letter). As an example, Table 5.2 shows that seven studies (with nine sets of results) compared hospital volume

Table 5.1:   Categories of Research Findings and Methods of Specifying Volume

	Discontinuous Measures		*Continuous Measures*		
Research Findings	*Two Volume Categories, High vs. Low*	*Many Volume Categories*	*Volume*	*Volume, Volume²*	*log Volume*
1. Dichotomous ⌐	✓	✓	NA	NA	NA
2. Negative linear \	NA	✓	✓	✓	NA
3. U-shaped U	NA	✓	NA	✓	NA
4. Inverse log L	NA	✓	NA	NA	✓
5. "Flat" —	✓	✓	✓	✓	✓
6. Increasing /	✓	✓	✓	✓	✓

NA = not applicable

Table 5.2:   The Hospital-Volume/Outcome Relationship: Summary of Research Findings by Specific Diagnoses or Procedures

Shape of the Curve*	Abdominal Aortic Aneurysm	Acute Myocardial Infarction	Appendectomy	Biliary Tract Surgery	Cardiac Catheterization	Coronary Artery Bypass Surgery	Femur Fracture	Hernia	Hysterectomy	Intestinal Operation	Newborn Diseases	Prostatectomy	Stomach Operation	Total Hip Replacement	Vascular Surgery
1. ⊓	14			14,23	1,5	7a,25h			23	14		7a	7a	7a	3
2. /	5,7a,10d	7a	5,7a	5,7a	7a	5,18			5,7a	5,7a	2,5	5	5	5,18	4
3. U		5													
4. L	3,4,19	7c	8,11	3e,3f, 4e,4f, 4g,7c, 11	6,8,20	3,4,8, 16,20, 25i,25j	9l,9m	7a,8,11	7c,8,11	3,4,7c, 8,11,16	7a,7c	3,4,8,16	3n	3,4,7c, 8,16r	
5. —	7c,10b	20	7c	3g,8, 16,22		7c,25k	5,7a, 7c,14, 16	5,7c,16	18,22	19		7c,22,24	3o,4n, 4o,7c, 8,14, 19p,19q	16s,21t, 21u	
6. /															

*Note: The curves in this table illustrate the following relationships between volume and outcome:
1. Volume grouped into two categories, with lower rates of poor outcomes at higher volumes;
2. Downward-sloping line (negative linear relationship), with lower rates of poor outcomes at higher volumes;
3. U-shaped curve, with higher rates of poor outcomes at lower volumes, lower rates of poor outcomes in intermediate volume ranges, and higher rates of poor outcomes at higher volumes;
4. L-shaped curve (inverse logarithmic form), with large reductions in rates of poor outcomes as volume increases from low levels and little change at higher volumes;
5. Flat, indicating no significant relationship between volume and outcome; and
6. Upward-sloping line (positive linear relationship), with higher rates of poor outcomes at higher volumes.

The numbers in the entries for this table refer to the study numbers in Table 2.1. The meanings of the letters in the entries are as follows:

a. Analysis using volume categories
b. Ruptured aneurysm surgery
c. Analysis using regressions
d. Elective aneurysm surgery
e. Cholecystectomy with common bile duct exploration
f. Other biliary tract surgery
g. Cholecystectomy alone
h. Nonscheduled CABG, death outcome
i. Scheduled CABG, poor outcome
j. Nonscheduled CABG, poor outcome
k. Scheduled CABG, death outcome

l. Femur fracture, death outcome
m. Femur fracture, poor outcome
n. Vagotomy and/or pyloroplasty for duodenal ulcer
o. Vagotomy, all
p. Stomach operations, cancer diagnosis
q. Stomach operations, ulcer diagnosis
r. Other hip arthoplasty
s. Total hip replacement
t. Total hip replacement, death outcome
u. Total hip replacement, major complications

Adapted from: Office of Technology Assessment, 1988.

Table 5.3: The Physician-Volume/Outcome Relationship: Summary of Research Findings by Specific Diagnoses or Procedures

Shape of the Curve*	Abdominal Aortic Aneurysm	Acute Myocardial Infarction	Appendectomy	Biliary Tract Surgery	Cardiac Catheterization	Coronary Artery Bypass Graft Surgery	Hernia	Hysterectomy	Intestinal Operation	Prostatectomy	Stomach Operation	Total Hip Replacement	Vascular Surgery
1. ⌐	12		8	22	8		8			8			
2. /	10a											21e	13g
3. U													
4. L		20											
5. —	10b,19			8,23	20	20		8,22,23	8,19	22	8,19c,19d	8,21f	13h,13i, 13j,17
6. /						8							

*Note: The curves in this table illustrate the following relationships between volume and outcome:
1. Volume grouped into two categories, with lower rates of poor outcomes at higher volumes;
2. Downward-sloping line (negative linear relationship), with lower rates of poor outcomes at higher volumes;
3. U-shaped curve, with higher rates of poor outcomes at lower volumes, lower rates of poor outcomes in intermediate volume ranges, and higher rates of poor outcomes at higher volumes;
4. L-shaped curve (inverse logarithmic form), with large reductions in rates of poor outcomes as volume increases from low levels and little change at higher volumes;
5. Flat, indicating no significant relationship between volume and outcome; and
6. Upward-sloping line (positive linear relationship), with higher rates of poor outcomes at higher volumes.

The numbers in the entries for this table refer to the study numbers in Table 2.1. The meanings of the letters in the entries are as follows:

a. Elective aneurysm surgery
b. Ruptured aneurysm surgery
c. Stomach operations, cancer diagnosis
d. Stomach operations, ulcer diagnosis
e. Postoperative deaths
f. Major complications
g. Femoral popliteal bypass, amputation outcome
h. Carotid endarterectomy
i. Aortofemoral bypass
j. Femoral popliteal bypass, death outcome

and abdominal aortic aneurysm. None found a U-shaped curve. Rather, all the studies showed poorer outcomes at lower volumes. Using regression analysis, Luft, Hunt, and Maerki (1987) showed an insignificant (flat) relationship (see Study 7c in Table 5.2); however, when they used categories the same authors showed a downward-sloping relationship (Study 7a).

When reviewing data such as these, which cover many procedures and diagnoses so that each cell has only a few observations, one is torn between "lumping" to provide a "gestalt" and "splitting" to explain differences. For example, it is often important to distinguish the *type* of surgery, as in the case of biliary tract surgery, in which the volume-outcome relationship may be valid only for more complex surgery that combines cholecystectomy with common bile duct exploration and other operations on the biliary tract. For coronary artery bypass graft surgery, the hospital volume–mortality relationship may be driven primarily by emergency rather than scheduled patients (see Studies 25h and 25k in Table 5.2). Similarly, Pilcher and his colleagues (1980) showed a volume-outcome relationship for elective but not emergency aneurysm surgery (see Studies 10b and 10d in Table 5.2). Although it is relatively easy to make this observation for the procedures in which several types of surgery are distinguished in the data, one can only speculate on what would be found if other patient groupings were split into subcategories.

Upon examining Tables 5.2 and 5.3, we see that far more studies relate to hospital volume than to physician volume, and that many more studies of physician volume than of hospital volume showed no effect. There are three possible reasons for these differences. First, the early studies in the literature focused on hospital volume, since physician volume data are more difficult to obtain. Thus there have been more opportunities to undertake hospital studies. Second, even when physician data are available, it is difficult to identify which physician is truly responsible for a patient when several specialists and consultants are involved in a case. This difficulty tends to exclude studies of physician volume in medical diagnoses. Third, the small number of studies increases the importance of methodological differences. For example, Kelly and Hellinger (1987) found no surgeon volume-outcome relationship for cardiac catheterization when low-volume providers were omitted from their study.[3] But Hughes, Hunt, and Luft (1987), who focused on low-volume providers, found worse outcomes associated with low-volume angiographers.[4]

None of the regression studies explicitly tested a log volume (L-shaped curve) against a volume-squared (U-shaped curve), and with the exception of research by Williams (1979) and Rosenblatt, Reinken, and Shoemack (1985) on perinatal outcomes, we found no studies that explicitly discussed the *observation* of increased mortality in very high volume settings.[5] (Some studies did discuss the possibility of worsening outcomes implicit in the *estimated* relationship.) Therefore, it is possible to lump the first four types of results together, since they all support the notion of worse outcomes in low-volume settings. (This is not necessarily the same as saying that more is better). The pattern of results shown on Figure 5.1 shows (1) worse results at low volumes, or (2) no effect. For abdominal aortic aneurysm, the seven sets of results indicating worse outcomes at lower volumes (*y*-axis) outweigh the two sets of results showing no relationship (*x*-axis). For the 12 diagnoses and procedures in the upper left part of the graph, more studies show a volume-outcome relationship than no relationship. Only 2 of the 15 patient groupings, femur fracture and stomach operation, have more findings of no effect than of worse outcomes at lower volumes. Worse outcomes are demonstrated at lower volumes in 11 of 13 studies for CABG, 10 of 11 for intestinal operations, 8 of 11 for total hip replacement, and all 6 for cardiac catheterization.

EXPLANATIONS FOR NO ESTIMATED EFFECT

It is interesting that the nature of the dependent variable has very little influence on the interpretation of whether a volume-outcome relationship exists. Of the 121 findings for hospital volume, 96 use death alone as the dependent variable, and 70 percent of these show an effect. The remaining 25 studies use either morbidity or poor outcomes including death. Of these, 72 percent demonstrate an effect. We do not mean to suggest that the outcome measure is irrelevant, but it does not account for the variability in finding a volume-outcome relationship.

Although detailed analyses of the methods used by each study are necessary to understand why results differ for a single diagnosis or procedure (see Chapter 6), several important factors help explain inconsistencies among studies: (1) physician versus hospital volume, (2) causal linkages from volume to outcome or outcome to volume, and (3) the problem of detecting an effect if the rate of poor outcomes is low and the sample size is small.

Physician versus Hospital Volume

Relatively little work has been done to distinguish various causal linkages in the volume-outcome relationship. High-volume hospitals are often institutions in which physicians also have high volumes, and it may be the physician volume that truly matters. Therefore, it is critical to distinguish hospital and physician effects. Of the 121 findings concerning the effect of hospital volume on outcomes, 99 tested hospital volume without including physician volume, and 22 tested hospital volume and physician volume concurrently. Almost three-fourths of the 99 studies of hospital volume alone indicated a hospital effect, but only about half of the studies testing hospital and physician effects concurrently indicated a hospital effect.

Of the 22 findings examining both physician and hospital effects, 13 found a hospital effect and two of the nine with no hospital effect found a physician

Figure 5.1: Number of Findings Showing Either Worse Outcomes at Low Hospital Volume or No Effect, by Diagnosis or Procedure (from Table 5.2)

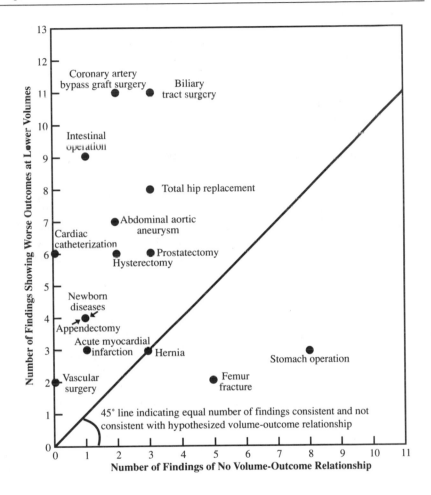

effect. Thus, of the 22 studies testing both variables, 15 showed one or both volume effects, a proportion more consistent with the hospital-only studies. To find out whether testing two volume effects simultaneously would explain some of the negative results, we asked Robert Hughes to reanalyze the Hughes, Hunt, and Luft (1987) data. When estimated together in the original study, hospital volume was not related to outcomes for cholecystectomy and stomach operations. When Hughes tested hospital volume only, cholecystectomy outcomes became significantly related to volume. When he tested physician volume only, many more of the procedures showed a significant relation between volume and outcome.

It appears that, in some instances, a measured hospital effect may be substituting for an untested physician effect. Alternatively, the high collinearity between physician and hospital volume may make it impossible to detect true effects if both exist. One should note that the proportion of patients operated on by the low-volume surgeons reported in the Hughes paper is probably less correlated with hospital volume than are simple counts of physician and hospital volume. Given the paucity of physician studies, one should reserve final judgment on this issue.

Volume Effects versus Selective Referrals

As was previously discussed, although volume may not determine outcome, it may serve as a marker for hospitals or physicians with special skills whose performance attracts a disproportionate share of referrals. When one attempts to test, in a simultaneous-equation model, both the effect of volume on outcomes and the effect of outcomes on volume, one may observe statistically significant effects for only one causal path. Even if the results indicate only an effect of outcome on volume in such a model, a simple test of volume as a function of outcome alone would probably show a relationship. As indicated in Chapter 6, Luft, Hunt, and Maerki (1987) sometimes failed to find an effect of volume on outcome even though, using the same data, Maerki, Luft, and Hunt (1986) found a highly significant effect in a single-equation model, albeit with many fewer independent variables.

To test whether the simultaneous-equation estimates are obscuring what would be perceived as volume-outcome effects in simpler models, Table 5.4 presents results from three studies, each of which analyzed several diagnoses or procedures. Luft (1980) presented both single-equation and simultaneous-equation estimates.[6] Luft, Hunt, and Maerki (1987) estimated only a simultaneous equation, but also presented categorical results. Hughes and his colleagues (1988) presented only simultaneous-equation results, but subsequently provided us with single-equation results based on the same data. The first approach to these results is to examine the pattern of effects *within* the simultaneous equations. In 10 of the 18 instances in which there is no significant negative effect of volume on outcome, there is a significant negative effect of outcome on volume. Thus, if one requires either a volume or a referral effect, it is present in 23 of the 31 instances. If we look more carefully at the remaining eight studies, we see that half of these exhibit the expected volume-outcome effect in the single-equation situation. The four that never show an effect are two stomach procedures (vagotomy, vagotomy and/or pyloroplasty), other biliary tract surgery, and subarachnoid hemorrhage. The last exhibits positive coefficients in all three situations.

Power to Detect an Effect

In designing any research study, one should undertake a power test (ideally in advance) to determine the likelihood of detecting an effect if one truly exists. This test depends on the sample size and the overall likelihood of the outcome being measured. None of the studies reviewed indicated that a power test was done beforehand, and there are often insufficient data in the published studies to do the formal computations after the fact.

Indeed, there are substantial differences among studies in the number of patients involved and the average poor-outcome (or mortality) rate. To provide a sense of the importance of the power issue, Figure 5.2 plots each of the findings for total hip replacement according to its volume-outcome effect for hospital volume. Of the ten findings, seven (shown as solid dots) show an effect and three (which are open dots) do not. In what we might call the "low-power corner of the plot," the three results that showed no effect were based on analyses of small numbers of patients (fewer than 1,000 patients in two studies and 10,000 in the third) and showed low rates of poor outcomes (under 5 percent death rates). (In practice, one should also consider the number of hospitals in each study, but that would be too complicated for a simple presentation.) These studies probably had insufficient power to detect an effect unless it was very large. In short, because of the design of the studies, the "mixed" results for total hip replacement (Table 5.2) are not surprising. Nor does the absence of a significant finding for these

Table 5.4: Results from Studies Using Simultaneous Equations

Pattern of Effects within Simultaneous Equations

Effect of Outcome on Volume	Effect of Volume on Outcome		Total
	Significant Negative	*Not Negative*	*Total*
Significant negative	5	10	15
Not negative	8	8	16
	13	18	31

Single Equation vs. Simultaneous Equation Results Using the Same Data

Single Equation	Simultaneous Equation Results	
	Significant Effect of Volume or Outcome	*No Effects in Expected Direction*
Significant volume	20	4
No negative effect	3	4
	23	8

Figure 5.2:   Findings of Worse Outcomes for Patients Undergoing
Total Hip Replacement in Low Volume Hospitals by Number of
Patients in the Study and Overall Poor Outcome Rate

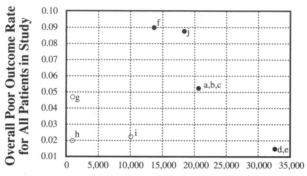

● = Worse outcome in low volume hospitals

○ = No effect

The studies corresponding with the plotted points are as follows:

   a. Luft, Hunt, and Maerki (1987), analysis using regression
   b. Luft, Hunt, and Maerki (1987), analysis using volume categories
   c. Maerki, Luft, and Hunt (1986)
   d. Luft, Bunker, and Enthoven (1979)
   e. Luft (1980)
   f. Hughes, Hunt, and Luft (1987)
   g. Fowles, Bunker, and Schurman (1987), major complication
   h. Fowles, Bunker, and Schurman (1987), death outcome
   i. Riley and Lubitz (1985), total hip replacement
   j. Riley and Lubitz (1985), other hip arthroplasty

three studies add much doubt to the notion that a volume-outcome relationship
exists.

SUMMARY

Table 5.5 presents a summary of the findings of similar graphs and analyses for
each of the diagnoses and procedures. For example, for abdominal aortic
aneurysm, seven studies reported a volume-outcome effect; two did not, and of
these two, one was in the low-power corner. Since we did not attempt to do power
calculations, the determination that a study is in the low-power corner (that is,
that it found low volumes and low poor-outcome rates) is somewhat subjective. A
few studies were dropped because the number of patients or the average outcome
rates could not be determined from the published report. Despite these caveats,
the results are quite striking.

   In addition to noting whether a study falls in the low-power corner, we note

Table 5.5:   Hospital Volume Effects and Explanations for the Lack of an Effect

	Effect of Hospital Volume		If No Effect, the Reason Is:			
	Yes	*No*	*In Low-Power Corner*	*Significant in Single Equation*	*Significant w/o MD Volume*	*Other*
Abdominal aortic aneurysm	7	2	1	1	—	—
Vascular surgery	2	0	—	—	—	—
Biliary tract surgery	11	4	3	1	1	—
Appendectomy	4	1	—	1	—	—
Cardiac catheterization	6	0	—	—	—	—
CABG	11	2	1	1	—	1
Total hip replacement	8	3	2	—	—	—
Prostate surgery	6	3	2	1	—	5
Stomach operations	3	8	2	1	—	—
Intestinal operations	9	1	1	—	—	1
Hysterectomy	6	2	1	—	—	—
Acute myocardial infarction	3	1	1	—	—	—
Newborns	4	1	—	—	—	1
Femur fracture	2	5	—	—	—	5
Hernia	3	3	2	—	—	1

whether a "no effect" finding arises either from a simultaneous-equation model in which a simple volume-outcome test indicated a significant effect or from the reanalysis by Hughes, in which a hospital effect was found when physician volume was dropped.

With two noteworthy exceptions, the findings indicating no effect are associated either with low power or with one of the two studies with other methodological explanations. The two important exceptions are stomach operations and fracture of the femur, both of which also stand out because of a very low proportion of total findings indicating a volume-outcome relationship.

Taken together, the available studies provide rather substantial evidence of a relationship between hospital volume and patient outcomes for most of the procedures and diagnoses that have been studied. But the volume-outcome relationship is not universal. For stomach operations and fracture of the femur, the evidence of a relationship is mixed, with the majority of studies indicating no effect. With the exception of these two patient groups, nearly all the other findings that suggest the lack of a relationship either (1) have low statistical power, (2) demonstrate a volume-outcome effect if one omits the linkage from outcome to volume, or (3) are part of larger analyses in which a physician-volume effect is found or a hospital effect is found if the physician variable is dropped.

It is far more difficult to summarize answers to the other main questions. The published findings on physician volume are far more equivocal than those on hospital volume. This may reflect the absence of a true effect or the difficulties in measuring physician volume, both of which result in bias in estimates (toward zero) and reduce the number of significant findings. The data in Table 5.5, however, suggest that collinearity between physician and hospital volume may be an important problem. The issue of causal linkages is even more problematic because, with the exception of Dranove's (1984) letter on the issue, all the work supporting the notion of selective referral has been done by Luft and his colleagues. Although some of their work (e.g., Luft, Hunt, and Maerki 1987) attempts to use evidence to supplement simultaneous-equation models, some readers remain skeptical. At this point, we encourage readers to be open-minded about the possibility of selective referrals in addition to experience effects.

NOTES

1. One set of findings by Sloan, Perrin, and Valvona (1986) approximates a "greater than" sign (>) and thus is impossible to classify in this schema. Their other findings fit a U-shaped pattern and are included in the table.
2. This issue is discussed more fully in Chapter 4.
3. See reprint of Kelly and Hellinger (1987) in Chapter 10 of this volume.
4. Hughes, Hunt, and Luft (1987) is reprinted in Chapter 17 of this volume.
5. See reprint of Williams (1979) in Chapter 18 of this volume.
6. See reprint of Luft (1980) in Chapter 16 of this volume.

Chapter 6

Diagnosis- and Procedure-Specific Research Results

Regardless of the methodological differences among studies, one might reach the same qualitative conclusion with respect to a volume-outcome relationship. However, one should not assume that the cause of the observed relationship is present for all hospitalized patients. The observed effect may arise from surgical or anesthetic techniques, and hence be absent in medical cases. It may appear only in diagnoses or procedures handled by sub-specialists, rather than by primary care or generalist physicians (perhaps because of a referral effect). It may only appear in high-risk cases, perhaps because only for such cases does the system collect enough experience to detect differences in outcomes, or because only in such cases does a lack of experience matter. For these and other reasons, one must examine the findings for specific diagnoses or procedures.

In this chapter, results are summarized across studies for each diagnosis and procedure. In an attempt to reconcile differences in results across studies, the results of each study are discussed, and differences in methods, case selection, and case definition are explored. We selected diagnoses and procedures that are reported on in the literature. However, we excluded findings for diagnoses or procedures reported on by just a single study.

DIAGNOSIS- AND PROCEDURE-SPECIFIC FINDINGS

Abdominal Aortic Aneurysm

The circumscribed dilation of the abdominal aorta is called abdominal aortic aneurysm (AAA). Surgery for this condition involves resection and replacement of the aneurysm with an artificial graft. An important clinical issue in understanding outcomes of aneurysm surgery is the difference between emergency and elective surgery. Elective aneurysm repair is performed to prevent acute rupture of the aneurysm, and is considered when the aneurysm is six centimeters or greater in diameter. Emergency repair is undertaken under varying conditions, from a rapidly expanding aneurysm to frank rupture. Without surgery, a ruptured aneurysm results in virtually 100 percent mortality; emergency surgery generally saves about 50 percent of patients depending on their condition on admission. Even though elective operation is associated with much lower mortality, it is considered a high-risk operation because of the potential for catastrophic complications and the fact that virtually all patients have underlying heart disease.

Seven of the 25 studies examined the relationship between hospital volume and surgical mortality following abdominal aortic aneurysm repair; two examined the relationship between surgeon volume and surgical mortality after AAA repair.

Flood, Scott, and Ewy (1984a) examined 1972 data for 9,532 patients undergoing intra-abdominal artery surgery in 645 hospitals divided into two groups based upon the average hospital volume of 14.78.[1] Low-volume hospitals were those with 14 or fewer patients, and high-volume hospitals had 15 or more patients per year. The overall average patient mortality was 15.5 percent. A series of patient variables in a logistic regression was used to derive an expected mortality rate for each hospital. The observed/expected mortality ratios were 1.201 in low-volume hospitals and 0.913 in high-volume hospitals. This implies a 32 percent higher risk-adjusted mortality rate for patients undergoing aneurysm repair in lower-volume hospitals.

Kelly and Hellinger (1986) examined data from 999 patients undergoing abdominal aneurysm surgery in 77 hospitals. They excluded all patients with one-day hospital stays, among whom there was a 97 percent mortality rate. The overall mortality rate for patients in the study was 10.2 percent. Using logistic regression techniques to control for risk factors, they found a significant negative relationship between hospital volume and mortality. These patients were operated on by 232 surgeons. When examined in the same equation with hospital volume, surgeon volume had no effect on outcome.

Luft (1980) and Luft, Bunker, and Enthoven (1979) examined data for 4,624 patients undergoing abdominal aneurysm resection and graft in 692 hospitals and compared actual and expected death rates by volume category (controlling for patient case-mix on the basis of age, gender and the presence of multiple diagnoses).[2] They found a substantial negative relationship between hospital volume and mortality, although the death rate flattened out at relatively low volume (more than 20 patient procedures per year).

Maerki, Luft, and Hunt (1986) studied data from 6,065 patients with abdominal aortic aneurysm in 736 hospitals using 1972 data. Patients may or may not have had surgery, and the crude mortality rate was 25.2 percent. In contrast, a 15.5 percent rate was reported by Flood, Scott, and Ewy (1984a), who also analyzed data from the Commission on Professional and Hospital Activities for the same year. The difference is probably due to the fact that Maerki, Luft, and Hunt used diagnosis as the screen, which includes patients who die without surgery. The larger number of patients reported by Flood, Scott, and Ewy suggests that not all their patients with intraabdominal artery operations had aortic aneurysms. There was a significant negative relationship between volume and mortality, but not between volume-squared and mortality. In a second study, Luft, Hunt, and Maerki (1987) examined the data using a simultaneous-equation regression model, examining the effect of log volume upon the actual-minus-expected in-hospital mortality. They found that volume had an insignificant effect upon death rate but that outcome had a significant effect on volume. Using simple volume groups, they found actual divided by expected ratios of 1.15 and 1.26 for hospitals with very low and low volumes, versus 0.97 and 0.73 for hospitals with high and very high volumes.

Pilcher and colleagues (1980) examined mortality rates following abdominal aortic aneurysm repair for 294 patients in eight Vermont general hospitals over 7½ years. They found that mortality rates were significantly inversely related to hospital volume for ruptured aneurysm but not for elective aneurysm procedures. For elective procedures, there was an apparent trend, but it was not statistically significant. However, there is only one high-volume hospital in this study (the university teaching hospital). Since it had an average of 22.4 patients per year, the results do not truly reflect the effect of volume apart from other characteristics of the high-volume hospital. The other hospitals had volumes ranging from 0.5 to 4.1 patients per year.

In contrast to their findings for hospital volume, Pilcher and his associates found that, for ruptured aneurysms where emergency surgery was required, mortality was *not* significantly related to surgeon volume. For elective aneurysm repair, however, mortality was significantly inversely related to surgeon volume. Surgeons were characterized as having high volume (4 or more cases per year; 3 surgeons averaged 6.8 cases per year), medium volume (2 to 4 cases per year; 4 surgeons averaged 2.7 cases per year), or low volume (fewer than 2 cases per year; 10 surgeons averaged 0.6 cases per year). For elective aneurysm repair, mortality rates were 7 percent for high, 15 percent for medium, and 17 percent for low-volume surgeons; for ruptured aneurysm, the figures were 50 percent, 47 percent and 62 percent, respectively.

In sum, all of the studies showed a significant relationship between hospital volume and patient outcome following abdominal aortic aneurysm. (This includes Luft, Hunt, and Maerki, although they attribute the relationship to the effect of outcome on volume.) In contrast, only one of three findings in two studies showed a relationship between surgeon volume and patient outcome (for elective surgeries). These studies may actually differ more than they seem to at first glance, despite the similarity in findings. Mortality rates in studies with large samples vary from 10.2 percent to 25.2 percent, probably reflecting differences in selection criteria for inclusion in the analysis. Careful case-mix adjustment may be very important to control for the operability of the aneurysm, especially to account for the great differences in outcome between elective and emergency surgery.

The inconsistent results on the effects of surgeon volume are difficult to interpret because there are only two studies with three outcomes. It may be useful to note that Kelly and Hellinger (1986) simultaneously tested the effects of physician and hospital volume, while Pilcher and associates tested separately for physician and hospital effects. Since physician and hospital volume are correlated, Kelly and Hellinger's approach is a more conservative test. Pilcher's results may also provide some support for the selective-referral hypothesis, since high-volume surgeons have a 7 percent mortality rate for their elective patients in contrast to 15 percent to 17 percent for other surgeons. However, there is no pattern for emergency patients who, by definition, have no opportunity for selective referral.

Vascular Surgery

Vascular surgery is surgery performed on blood vessels. The authors in this section reviewed (1) several procedures for increasing blood supply to the legs by replacing vessels with prosthetic grafts, and (2) carotid endarterectomy, which is performed to reduce the risk of stroke. (Aortic aneurysm surgery, outlined above, is also a vascular procedure.) Patients are generally elderly and have preexisting heart disease, which is a major cause of mortality. For the leg revascularization procedures, there are several types of morbid outcomes, including amputation (which is rare and may be due to case selection as well as surgical quality), wound infection, or failure to palliate symptoms. For carotid endarterectomy, the major morbid risk of the procedure is stroke. Because surgery is generally not indicated during the period after a stroke, a diagnosis of stroke occurring during a hospitalization in which endarterectomy is performed may be presumed to be caused by the surgery.

Four studies focused on vascular surgery procedures. Luft (1980 and Luft, Bunker, and Enthoven (1979) studied all vascular procedures together and examined the relationship of hospital surgical volume and mortality rate. They found steadily decreasing mortality throughout the range of hospital volumes.

The remaining papers come from the surgical literature and examine the effect of surgeon volume on the outcomes of specific vascular procedures. Hertzer and colleagues (1984) studied both mortality and specific morbidity outcomes of three different vascular procedures. There was no adjustment for case-mix differences. For one procedure, femoral-popliteal bypass, the rate of amputation was negatively correlated with surgeon volume. No relationship was found for carotid endarterectomy or aortofemoral reconstruction. Kempczinski, Brott, and Labutta (1986) examined the effect of surgeon volume on mortality and stroke after carotid endarterectomy and found no significant relationship.

Both of the preceding studies collected data from areas with few physicians and relatively few patients compared to the other studies. Since they concentrated on vascular surgeons only, these studies did not assess outcomes for general surgeons with truly low volumes, who were performing vascular surgery but did not belong to vascular registries. Kempczinski, Brott, and Labutta examined 750 carotid endarterectomies performed in the Cincinnati area over a two-year period. Hertzer and his associates reviewed 650 to 2,646 operations for several vascular procedures, but the study is limited to members of the Cleveland Vascular Registry and may not be generalizable to the practice of vascular surgery in the rest of the United States. As a consequence of the low number of observations, statistical power is low and the ability to detect true differences is quite limited.

On the other hand, the spectrum of vascular procedures is broad, and to combine them into one analysis without more specific adjustment for type of procedure, as did Luft (1980) and Luft, Bunker, and Enthoven (1979) may be an oversimplification. If there are differences between high-volume hospitals and low-volume hospitals in the type and risk of vascular procedures performed, then the authors' method of case-mix adjustment will not adequately account for this. For example, certain referral hospitals may perform a high volume of technically complex but low-risk (of death) procedures, such as vascular access operations on renal failure patients. These patients will be considered average risk in any case-mix adjustment that fails to take into account the surgical procedure. In sum, this category of procedures has received little attention, and it is difficult to evaluate the current evidence.

Biliary Tract Surgery

Surgery on the bile ducts or gallbladder is biliary tract surgery. Cholecystectomy is removal of a gallbladder (the sac that stores bile, a salt that assists in digestion of fatty foods), which is diseased through the formation of gallstones (which may block the flow of bile) and/or infection or inflammation of the gallbladder itself. A more complex procedure, common duct exploration, is sometimes required to remove stones that have passed from the gallbladder. Elective cholecystectomy is performed for relief of symptoms, prevention of potentially dangerous infectious complications of gallstones, and obstruction of the bile system. Performing a cholecystectomy in an emergency situation involves a difficult clinical decision;

the increased risk of the operation during infection is weighed against the possibility of further deterioration of the patient.

We reviewed 10 studies that examined the effect of patient volumes on results of biliary tract surgery, including cholecystectomy, cholecystectomy with common bile duct exploration, and other operations on the biliary tract. All of the studies examined the effect of hospital volume; three studies also examined the effect of surgeon volume.

Findings were mixed both across and within the studies. Flood, Scott, and Ewy (1984a) used two categories of hospital volume (with a cutoff at the average hospital volume of 109 per year) and found lower mortality rates for the high-volume category. Luft, Bunker, and Enthoven (1979) graphically demonstrated similar findings for cholecystectomy with common bile duct exploration and other biliary tract surgery, but not for cholecystectomy alone. Luft (1980) examined the same three types of surgery and found a significant relationship between volumes and outcomes for all three surgeries. Maerki, Luft, and Hunt (1986) also demonstrated decreasing mortality with increasing hospital volumes for cholecystectomy. Farber, Kaiser, and Wenzel (1981) measured wound infection rates as an outcome variable and also demonstrated improved outcomes at higher operative rates.[3]

Several studies failed to find a significant relationship between volumes and outcomes. Hughes, Hunt, and Luft's analysis (1987) differed from the other studies in its use of the proportion of patients with hospital stays greater than the 90th percentile as a proxy for poor outcome.[4] Riley and Lubitz (1985) based their study on a 20-percent probability sample of Medicare patients.[5] Since the ratio of Medicare patients to all patients varies among hospitals, Medicare volume is not a good indicator of overall volume. When a 20-percent random sample of patients is used, hospitals with low volumes of patients are less likely to be represented than hospitals with high volumes. This is because a 20-percent sample has a .33 chance of eliminating all patients in a hospital with 5 patients $(.8)^5$, while the chance of all patients being eliminated from a hospital with 20 patients is only $.01(.8)^{20}$. Roos and his associates (1986) studied a much smaller database and measured readmissions for complications as an outcome variable.[6] Hospitals with greater volumes readmitted a smaller proportion of patients for complications after surgery, but the difference was not significant.

Differences in methods and case selection help to explain some of the mixed results among studies. Flood, Scott, and Ewy, (1984a) did not distinguish between different types of gallbladder operations. If, as Luft, Bunker, and Enthoven (1979) suggested, a volume-outcome relationship existed for more technically complex procedures, then most of the studies would be consistent, showing no relationship with volume for cholecystectomy alone and a significant relationship for cholecystectomy combined with other surgical procedures. The study by Maerki, Luft, and Hunt (1986) was the only one that showed a relationship for cholecystectomy alone.

Only a few of the studies allowed estimation of a volume where mortality or poor outcomes leveled off. Luft, Bunker, and Enthoven suggested that it occurred at low volumes (in the range of five to ten cases per hospital). However, at these very low volumes, and with very low expected death rates (in the order of 1 percent, a single, perhaps randomly occurring, death can produce a very high mortality rate. In fact, these authors showed a 14 percent death rate among patients in hospitals with only one patient per year, but this is due to just one death. Farber and his colleagues presented data suggesting that leveling of the infection rate occurred at 100 to 150 cases over the 29-month study period (which translates to 40–60 cases per hospital per year).

The three studies that examined physician volume had inconclusive results. Roos and his colleagues (1986) presented findings that support a volume-outcome relationship for physicians although their later findings (Roos, Roos, and Sharp 1987) and the study by Hughes, Hunt, and Luft (1987) do not. All three studies measured concurrently the effects of physician and hospital volume. However, their methods of case selection, outcome measure, and statistical methods were all different, so it is impossible to make direct comparisons.

Overall, for the category of biliary tract operations, there was mixed evidence for volume-outcome relationship. Some evidence suggested that hospitals managing more of the technically complex cases may have better patient outcomes. There have not been definitive results with respect to physician volumes.

Appendectomy

Surgical removal of the appendix is performed in response to indications of inflammation or infection of the appendix, but it is occasionally performed prophylactically during abdominal surgery for some other reason. Except for the study by Farber, Kaiser, and Wenzel (1981) all of the studies focus on appendectomy as the primary procedure. (Farber, Kaiser, and Wenzel do not specify whether or not they exclude incidental appendectomies.) Outcomes of appendectomy are dependent on the general health of the patient and the condition of the appendix at operation, which may be normal, inflamed, or ruptured. A ruptured appendix is generally associated with poorer outcomes.

Four studies examined the relationship between hospital patient volume and surgical mortality or morbidity for appendectomy. Three of the four found a significant relationship. Two studies examined the relationship between surgeon volume and postoperative mortality or morbidity; one of the two suggested a relationship.

Hughes, Hunt, and Luft (1987) studied the influence of hospital volume on mortality and long hospital stay following appendectomy for 646 hospitals and 39,545 patients. They found an overall 8.5 percent occurrence of poor outcomes (including 38 deaths) and a significant negative curvilinear relationship between volume and poor outcomes.

Maerki, Luft, and Hunt (1986) examined 80,211 patients undergoing appendectomies in 916 hospitals; they found a 0.34 percent death rate. There was a significant negative relationship between hospital volume and mortality. In a second study (Luft, Hunt, and Maerki 1987), using a simultaneous-equation regression model (which also allowed for an evaluation of the effect of outcome upon volume), these authors found the effect of log volume upon actual-minus-expected in-hospital mortality to be insignificant. However, the other equation in the model showed a significant effect of outcomes on volume. The authors found their evidence for a significant referral effect (the influence of outcome on volume) coupled with an insignificant practice-makes-perfect effect (the influence of volume on outcome) to be implausible in the case of appendectomy. They attributed this finding to the very low mortality rate, which might have led a few hospitals to dominate the regression or to the use of the number of cholecystectomy patients as a "control" variable for emergency access. (Appendectomy was used as a control variable in all the other regressions.)

Farber, Kaiser, and Wenzel (1981) studied the relationship between hospital volume and the wound infection rate following 3,671 appendectomies in 22 Virginia hospitals between 1977 and 1979. The overall mean wound infection rate was 5 percent. The authors found a significant inverse relationship between the log of the frequency of the operation and the postoperative wound infection rate.

Hughes, Hunt, and Luft (1987) also examined the relationship between surgeon volume and poor outcomes (mortality and/or long stay) following appendectomy. They found a median annual surgeon volume of six patients. In a regression holding hospital volume constant, there was a significant positive relationship between the proportion of patients operated on by surgeons with fewer than six cases and poor outcomes. Shortell and LoGerfo (1981) found no relationship when they studied the rate of normal appendix removal as a function of average number of appendectomies per family practitioner or surgeon.

These two studies, which offer the only test of the possible effect of surgeon volume on appendectomy outcomes, also provide a clear example of the potential problems in comparing studies. Hughes, Hunt, and Luft used patient outcomes as the dependent variable, albeit with a combination of deaths and long stays as a proxy for complications. They also focus on the impact of low-volume surgeons (those performing fewer than six appendectomies a year). In contrast, Shortell and LoGerfo examined the rate of normal appendix removal, not patient outcomes. The proportion of normal appendices should not be too low, since that would suggest an overly conservative approach (which involves placing the patient at risk of a ruptured appendix), nor too high, since that might mean that the healthy patient is at risk for poor surgical outcomes (Neutra 1977). Thus it is not clear whether a linear model is appropriate. Furthermore, the proportion of normal appendices is really a measure of the surgeon's diagnostic skill and risk tolerance, not technical skill. In terms of volume, the average rate of appendectomies per family practitioner and general surgeon fails to distinguish hospitals in which (1) all the practitioners have average volumes from (2) those in which a high average is due to a single high-volume surgeon and where many patients are operated on by a large number of low-volume practitioners. Given these differences, it is impossible to determine whether the two sets of findings are really contradictory.

Only Shortell and LoGerfo's study takes into account whether the appendix was normal, inflamed, or ruptured. Because the condition of the appendix is related to the risk of poor outcomes, and because the clinical criteria used to decide whether to operate affects both the volume of surgery and the findings, this potentially important case-mix variable often goes unmeasured. In other words, a low threshold for operation will increase volume and decrease the poor-outcome rate (because the additional patients did not need the operation), regardless of the quality of care rendered.

Cardiac Catheterization and Angiography

This procedure involves the insertion of a probe into the heart via a large vein or artery in order to measure heart function and coronary vessel anatomy. It is generally performed for diagnostic purposes, although it is being used more often in conjunction with other procedures, such as angioplasty, for therapeutic purposes. Death, heart attack, injury to the blood vessels of the heart, and stroke are the major complications. A large majority of patients undergo the procedure in elective evaluation of chest pain due to coronary artery disease. However, increasing numbers of patients are undergoing the procedure during an acute heart attack or in the convalescent period after heart attack. These patients are generally at increased risk of poor outcomes compared to elective patients.

For cardiac catheterization and angiography, six studies examined the relationship between hospital volume and patient outcome, and two studies examined the relationship between physician volume and mortality. Five studies concluded that there is a significant negative relationship between hospital volume and mortality or other complications following cardiac catheterization.

Hughes, Hunt, and Luft (1987) examined the relationship between hospital volume and in-hospital mortality or long (more than 12 day) hospital stay for 76,584 patients undergoing cardiac catheterization in 150 hospitals during 1982. Of the 8,364 patients with poor outcomes, 896 died. They found a significant negative relationship between higher patient volumes (measured as log volume) and poor outcomes.

Kelly and Hellinger (1986) who studied 4,835 patients undergoing cardiac catheterization in 39 hospitals in 1977, found a 0.8 percent death rate. Mean hospital volume was 399 procedures per year. Hospital volume was significantly negatively related to mortality.

Luft and Hunt (1986) studied 149 hospitals in 1982 using regression analysis.[7] They found a significant negative relationship between volume and in-hospital mortality. A similar pattern was evident both for mortality rate by volume category and the likelihood that outcomes were equal to the case-mix—adjusted expected rate. That is, for low-volume hospitals, none were significantly better than expected, although many were significantly worse than expected.

Maerki, Luft, and Hunt (1986), who studied 26,678 patients undergoing cardiac catheterization in 360 hospitals in 1972, found a 1.8-percent death rate and a highly significant negative relationship between volume and in-hospital mortality. They estimated that 339 deaths, or 14 deaths per 1,000 patients, could have been averted by redirecting patients from low-volume to high-volume hospitals.

Adams, Fraser, and Abrams (1973) reported on the complications of coronary arteriography among 46,904 patients at 173 different institutions. They found a 0.45-percent death rate, a 0.61-percent rate of myocardial infarction, a 1.28-percent rate of ventricular fibrillation or serious arrythmia, and a 1.44-percent rate of arterial thrombosis. When they stratified institutions into four different volume categories, their results were generally consistent, with decreasing numbers of complications in higher-volume institutions. The mortality rate in institutions performing fewer than 200 examinations per two years was eight times higher than that in institutions performing more than 800 procedures per two years.

There has been only one inconclusive study. Luft, Hunt, and Maerki (1987) examined the relationship between log hospital volume and actual-minus-expected death rate. Using a simultaneous-equation regression model for 360 hospitals with 26,678 patients undergoing cardiac catheterization in 1972, they found no significant relationship between volume and outcome. However, these are the same authors who, using the same data, demonstrated a highly significant negative effect of volume on outcome (Maerki, Luft, and Hunt, 1986). The major difference between the two studies is that Luft, Hunt and Maerki used a simultaneous-equation model that attributed almost all of the correlation between volume and outcome to the influence of outcome on volume.

Only two studies examined the effect of angiographer volume upon mortality after cardiac catheterization. Hughes, Hunt, and Luft (1987) showed a significant effect of being treated by a physician with less than the median number of patients upon two outcomes: death and long hospital stay. However, Kelly and Hellinger (1986) focused on physician volume and patient deaths after excluding patients with one-day hospital stays, and they showed no significant effect.

It is difficult to determine the effects of these methodological differences, but they may account for the inconsistent findings. For example, the mortality rate in Kelly and Hellinger's study is 0.8 percent, in contrast to a poor-outcome rate of 10.9 percent in the Hughes, Hunt, and Luft's study. (Note, however, that the Hughes, Hunt and Luft's mortality rate of 1.20 percent was comparable to that of Kelly and Hellinger.) Kelly and Hellinger studied 39 hospitals with 145 physicians and 4,835 patients; this implies an average physician volume 33.3, quite close to Hughes, Hunt, and Luft's average of 28.6. The volume distribution in Hughes, Hunt, and Luft's data is skewed. The median number of procedures per physician was only 11 and the standard deviation was 46.9. Furthermore, only 12.2 percent of all the patients were treated by physicians with below-median patient loads. Since Kelly and Hellinger's analysis focused on the patient as the unit of observation, this means that very little weight is given to low-volume physicians in the regression, reducing their ability to detect an effect by low-volume physicians. In contrast, Hughes, Hunt, and Luft focused on the importance of low- versus high-volume physicians.

Coronary Artery Bypass Graft

Coronary artery bypass graft (CABG) surgery is a procedure in which coronary arteries blocked by atherosclerotic fatty deposits or clots are bypassed using blood vessels taken from other parts of the body. Because of the special facilities and staff required to take care of CABG patients (cardiac surgeons, bypass pump technicians, intensive care units), the operation tends to be performed only in larger hospitals. For many reasons, a team approach has developed in most hospitals for both the intraoperative and postoperative management of the patient. Although one surgeon is nominally the attending surgeon, the operation and subsequent management are carried out by several attending surgeons and/or fellows. Since some hospitals have only one surgical team performing CABG surgery, there may be no distinguishable effect of physician volume separable from hospital volume.

There are ten sets of findings concerning the relationship between hospital volume and patient outcome following CABG surgery. Two studies simultaneously tested for physician volume effects. Two studies each have two sets of findings: Showstack and his colleagues (1987) presented findings for both scheduled and nonscheduled procedures; Sloan, Perrin, and Valvona (1986) presented findings based on both regressions and categories.[8] Eight of the studies exhibit either an L- or a U-shaped curve, two show a downward-sloping relationship, one shows essentially no relationship, and one a backward C.

Showstack and his colleagues (1987) found a relatively flat mortality rate for scheduled CABG procedures, with substantially lower mortality rates for hospitals with more than 350 procedures per year. If the dependent variable was total poor outcomes, including mortality and very long hospital stays, then outcomes were significantly better in hospitals with 201 patients or more. Kelly and Hellinger (1987) excluded patients with one-day stays and found a negative effect of volume on mortality.[9] One-day stay patients were among those counted as nonscheduled operations in Showstack's study. Luft, Hunt, and Maerki (1987), using data from 1972, found an L-shaped curve using volume categories, but essentially no significant effect of volume on death rate in a simultaneous-equation model. Instead, they found a significant effect of low death rates leading to higher volumes, or a referral effect.

Overall, there seems to be substantial evidence that outcomes are significantly worse in hospitals with low volumes of patients undergoing CABG. Some studies indicated poorer outcomes in hospitals with volumes of under 100 procedures per year; others found that outcomes are markedly better in institutions with over 200 patients per year. Two studies suggested an upturn in mortality at very high volumes, in the range of 215 procedures (using 1972 data) to 479–510 procedures (using 1981 data).[10] However, neither study explored whether the mortality curve actually rises. That is, quadratic equations were used in the regressions and, even if some hospitals had volumes above the volume associated with the estimated minimum mortality rate, it was not shown whether the mortality rate was actually higher in those hospitals or whether the upturn was based on a handful of observations.

Two studies tested the effects of surgeon volume on the outcomes of patients undergoing CABG. Kelly and Hellinger (1986) found that physician volume was positively but not significantly related to mortality, after controlling for hospital volume (which had a significant negative effect). Hughes, Hunt, and Luft (1987) used a composite poor-outcome measure (a Z-score reflecting the difference between observed and expected outcomes, controlling for hospital volume), which summed the in-hospital deaths and the percentage of live discharges staying in the hospital longer than the 90th-percentile length of stay for CABG surgery. This composite poor-outcome measure was negatively associated with the proportion of patients operated on by *low*-volume surgeons, implying better results. Although this implication is the opposite of what one would expect, it is consistent with Kelly and Hellinger's results.

Both studies were problematic. Kelly and Hellinger included only 26 hospitals, and there was a fairly even spread of surgeon volumes among the 99 physicians performing CABG surgery throughout the range of 1 to 248 operations. Hughes, Hunt, and Luft reported on 120 hospitals with 800 surgeons; the median number of procedures per surgeon per year was 12. Even with this low median number, they found a very high correlation between the proportion of patients operated on by surgeons with 12 or fewer procedures and hospital volume. Thus the authors discounted their findings both on the grounds of multicollinearity and because possible measurement errors resulting from the frequent use of surgical teams in CABG surgery make the identification of surgeon-specific volume more difficult.

Total Hip Replacement

The replacement of a diseased ball-and-socket joint, where the femur (the long bone of the upper leg) inserts into the pelvis (hip), is performed primarily to improve dysfunction caused by arthritis. However, it is sometimes performed to correct specific types of hip fracture. Hip arthroplasty is another type of operation in which less than a total hip replacement is performed to restore the integrity and function of the joint; it is generally performed to repair femur fractures.

Six of the eight studies reporting results on total hip replacement and hospital volume were done by researchers at the Institute for Health Policy Studies at the University of California, San Francisco, using data from 1972, 1974, 1975, or 1982 from the discharge abstract service of the Commission on Professional and Hospital Activities. The six studies all showed higher in-hospital mortality in hospitals with lower annual volumes. For "other hip arthroplasty" (as opposed to total hip arthroplasty, which is the same as replacement), Riley and Lubitz (1985) also reported higher in-hospital death rates in low-volume hospitals, using the Medicare patient as the unit of analysis. For total hip replacement, the effect of volume on 60-day postoperative mortality was insignificant.

Fowles, Bunker, and Schurman (1987) studied 1,324 total hip replacement procedures performed on Medicare patients by 399 surgeons in northern California in 1980. The authors used two sample *t*-tests to compare physician volumes for patients who died with those for patients who survived; results showed that mean surgeon volumes were lower for the patients who died. However, regression analysis showed nether physician nor hospital volume having a significant effect on mortality or complications when both were included in the regression. (One problem with this analysis was that billing data were used to identify individual physicians, yet groups of physicians sometimes billed under a single number. This would cause some low-volume surgeons to appear to have high volumes.) Hughes, Hunt, and Luft (1987) also failed to show a significant effect of surgeon volume on outcomes, despite a significant effect of hospital volume on outcomes.

While the bulk of the evidence on total hip replacement has been reported by one research group, their findings are strengthened by the fact that their analytic techniques have varied from descriptive graphs, to single-equation regressions, to simultaneous-equation regression models. Moreover, the results have been corroborated by another study that used the entire universe of U.S. hospitals (Riley and Lubitz 1985).

Prostatectomy

Surgical removal of the male prostate gland is necessary when the gland is enlarged and blocking the free flow of urine. Transurethral prostatectomy (TURP) is performed through an instrument inserted through the penis. It should not be confused with open prostatectomy, which is accomplished by open incision through the abdomen or perineum. The TURP procedure is generally performed for benign growth of the prostate, but it is also used for palliation of symptoms caused by cancer. In addition, some patients who undergo TURP for benign disease may be found to have cancer; they may have a subsequent reoperation of the open type. Several of the studies that examined prostatectomy excluded cancer patients because their patterns of treatment and outcomes are likely to be quite different than patterns for other patients.

Eight studies with nine findings examined the volume-outcome relationship for prostatectomy; six studies examined transurethral prostatectomy (TURP) alone, while Roos and his associates (1986) and Wennberg and his associates (1987) studied prostatectomy of all types. Six of nine findings suggested a significant volume-outcome relationship for hospitals. One of the studies found that the relationship was also significant for physician volumes.

In the studies by Wennberg and by Roos, three findings did not show a significant relationship. Wennberg and his colleagues reviewed data on 4,576 patients for death within 90 days and showed an increased risk of mortality in lower-volume hospitals, although the odds ratios did not reach statistical significance. Roos and his colleagues, who studied 2,943 patients for complications during two years after surgery leading to readmission, did not show an increased risk or poor outcomes in low-volume hospitals. However, these two studies had relatively small sample sizes, making their results more subject to a Type II error (or acceptance of a null hypothesis when, in fact, an alternate hypothesis is true.) The other study that did not show a relationship was actually a test of the causal relationship between volumes and outcomes (Luft, Hunt, and Maerki 1987). It showed a selective-referral effect that was significant although the practice-makes-perfect effect was not.

If a volume-outcome relationship exists, we must also determine whether there is a volume where minimum mortality is achieved. Visual inspection of Luft, Bunker, and Enthoven's (1979) data suggests that mortality continues to decline throughout the whole range of hospital volumes. The methodology of the other studies does not allow us to calculate the flat of the curve.

Hughes, Hunt, and Luft (1987) showed a relationship for physician volumes using the proportion of patients in the hospital treated by physicians who saw fewer than seven patients, the median number. (The mean number of TURPs per surgeon was 12.8.) The outcome variable was the proportion of patients with long hospital stays, since the number of deaths was quite low. When Roos and his colleagues used stepwise logistic regression, they found that a variable measuring whether the physician volume was over 50 per year had no effect. As noted above, this study had a much smaller sample size than did Hughes's study.

For prostatectomy, then, the six studies that used large data bases showed a relationship between higher volumes and lower death and complications. There was no strong evidence that mortality drops at a specific volume of procedures. Studies of physician volume were not conclusive.

Stomach Operations

Stomach operations are performed for a variety of conditions, including cancer and peptic ulcer. These operations are performed by general surgeons, who perform several types of operations on the stomach and other abdominal organs. In recent years, due to the changing epidemiology of stomach disorders and improved medical treatment, there has been a great overall decrease in the number of stomach operations performed. Compared to other diagnoses in this review, there are many fewer patients in this category.

Seven studies examined the relationship of volume to various operations on the stomach, and two studies examined physician and hospital volume concurrently. There were several different categories of stomach operations and diagnoses in the different studies, ranging from all stomach operations, to stomach cancer operations, to stomach ulcer operations, to specific procedures such as vagotomy or pyloroplasty.

Maerki, Luft, and Hunt (1986) examined all stomach operations and found lower in-hospital mortality associated with higher hospital volumes. The study controlled for several patient covariates. However, it did not account for type of surgery, despite the broad risk range of various types of stomach procedures. If high-volume and low volume hospitals differ with respect to the type and risk of operations performed, then this could potentially confound their findings.

The other six studies showed no statistically significant correlation between volumes and outcomes. These studies all examined more specific diagnoses and procedures. Luft, Bunker, and Enthoven (1979) showed that mortality for patients undergoing vagotomy and/or pyloroplasty declined from about 2 percent in hospitals with two to four cases per year to under 1 percent for hospitals with higher volumes. Luft's analysis of the same data conducted with regression techniques, however, showed no statistically significant volume effect (Luft 1980). In general, these studies have suffered from a relative lack of statistical power compared to studies of other diagnoses, perhaps because stomach procedures are much less commonly performed than the other procedures.

In sum, a procedure-specific approach to studying volumes and outcomes for stomach operations failed to show a relationship. The single study that showed a volume-outcome relationship grouped all stomach procedures together, perhaps explaining the result.

Intestinal Operations

Operations on the large and small intestines are performed for conditions such as cancer, inflammatory bowel disease, infarction, and bleeding. The majority of the studies examined different types of colon resection, mostly for the diagnosis of cancer. These operations are common and routine in most hospitals. They are performed by general surgeons and, more recently, by an emerging subspecialty of colon and rectal surgeons. In addition to mortality, the major type of morbid outcome of intestinal surgery is postoperative infection in either the abdominal cavity or the incision.

Nine studies examined intestinal operations. Several groupings of procedures were used in the various papers, ranging from colon resection to all intestinal operations. All studies examined the relationship of hospital volume to patient outcomes, and two studies examined physician and hospital volume concurrently.

Eight of the nine studies showed a statistically significant decrease in poor outcomes with an increase in hospital volume. With the exception of Farber, Kaiser, and Wenzel (1981), all the studies included some measure to account for case mix, and several of the studies also accounted for hospital variables. The two studies that examined physician volume did not find a significant relationship.

Kelly and Hellinger (1986) did not find a significant relationship for hospital volume. However, the sample size for this study was only 2,612, with a mean outcome (death) rate of 0.065. (The smallest sample size among the other eight studies was 17,872.) The direction of the relationship between volume and outcome was consistent with the other studies, but it was not statistically significant. Its results might be explicable by a Type II error, a failure to detect an actual difference due to the small sample size.

Two studies looked for the volume at which mortality or complications reached a minimum value, but the cutoff could be observed only by visual examination of the data and not by statistical tests. Luft, Bunker, and Enthoven (1979) suggested that this minimum volume was about 50 to 100 cases per hospital per year. The study by Farber, Kaiser, and Wenzel (1981) suggested that the infection rate declined from 100 to 200 cases per hospital measured over a 2½ year period (or an annual volume of about 80 cases per hospital).

In sum, the research strongly supports a volume-outcome relationship for intestinal surgery and hospitals, but the evidence is inconclusive for physician volume. The question of minimum volumes is uncertain, but the two studies that addressed the question yielded similar results.

Hysterectomy

Surgical removal of the uterus is performed for many different clinical conditions, including cancer, benign tumors such as fibroid tumors, excessive bleeding, and infection. It is also commonly performed in conjunction with operations for cancer of the colon and rectum, where its removal aids in more complete cancer eradication. Other procedures, such as removal of ovaries and bladder-support procedures, are commonly performed concurrently. These procedures do not add much additional risk of poor outcomes, but they may increase the length of stay. A vaginal hysterectomy, as opposed to an abdominal hysterectomy, is sometimes carried out in low-risk patients without cancer who wish to avoid an abdominal incision.

In general, the seven groups of authors who studied hysterectomy reported a significant relationship between low hospital volume and poor outcomes, but insignificant results for physician volume and poor outcomes. These studies varied substantially in their design and implementation, including differences in time period, patient selection, unit of analysis, and statistical methods.

Luft, Hunt, and Maerki (1987) and Maerki, Luft, and Hunt (1986) selected the 180,464 patients who underwent vaginal or abdominal hysterectomies in hospitals subscribing to the discharge abstract service of the Commission on Professional and Hospital Activities in 1972, while Hughes, Hunt, and Luft (1987) studied the 105,550 patients undergoing vaginal or abdominal hysterec tomy in a subsample of CPHA hospitals in 1982. Sloan, Perrin, and Valvona (1986) also studied women in a subsample of CPHA hospitals between 1972 and 1981. Farber, Kaiser, and Wenzel studied 517 women in 22 hospitals in Virginia between 1977 and 1979 and limited their analysis to women who underwent abdominal hysterectomy. Finally, Roos and his colleagues (1986, 1987) studied women hospitalized for vaginal or abdominal hysterectomy in Winnepeg, Can ada, between 1974 and 1976 in their first study, and between 1982 and 1983 in the second study. Patients with cancer diagnoses were excluded. The study by Hughes, Hunt, and Luft and both studies by Roos included physician volume; the others were limited to hospital volume.

In addition to the differences in patient selection, a variety of analytic methods were used. Luft, Hunt, and Maerki used a simultaneous-equation model to examine the effect of volume on outcomes (i.e., practice makes perfect) and the effect of outcomes on volumes (i.e., selective referral). This study estimated the effect of the log of volume on the difference between actual death rate and case-mix–adjusted death rates. Hughes, Hunt, and Luft examined the effect of the log of hospital volume on a Z-score derived from the probability of observed bad outcomes being different from expected outcomes. Sloan, Perrin, and Val vona studied the average volume in three categories defined as having low (zero), medium (greater than zero and less than 0.3 percent), or high (over 0.3 percent) death rates. They showed a lower mean volume for both the low- and high-mortality groups. They also estimated regressions with in-hospital mortality as the dependent variable and a series of hospital and patient-specific independent variables. Hospital volume was not significant. However, their regression in cluded hospital bed size as an independent variable. Since hospital size and volume are often related, including both can lead to insignificant coefficients. None of the other studies that examined hysterectomy included bed size as a control variable.

Other outcomes besides mortality have also been studied. Farber, Kaiser, and Wenzel used a logistic regression in which postoperative wound infection was found to be significantly related to hospital volume. However, they did not adjust for any patient factors. The analyses by Roos and colleagues used logistic regression to study readmission for complications as a function of physician hospital volume. In their 1986 study hospital volume was not found to be a significant predictor of outcome. However, the stepwise regression technique used in their study allowed variables that might be collinear with hospital volume to enter first into the regression. In their final model, a variable signifying rural location, which is highly correlated with hospital volume, was a significant predictor of outcome. In their 1987 study, without hospital location in the model, hospital volume was a significant predictor of outcomes.

Finally, in the two studies of the effect of physician volumes on outcomes, both Hughes, Hunt, and Luft and Roos and his team (1986) reported insignificant effects.

In sum, the studies that failed to show a significant relationship for hysterectomy may have included variables correlated with hospital volume. Because hysterectomy has such a low mortality rate, the inclusion of such variables further reduced the power of these studies to detect an effect solely due to hospital volume.

Acute Myocardial Infarction

Commonly referred to as heart attack, acute myocardial infarction (AMI) is damage to the heart muscle due to lack of blood supply, usually as a result of occlusion (blockage) of a coronary artery. Most heart attacks are emergencies; the patient is rushed to the nearest hospital or to the hospital designated by emergency transport protocols. However, sometimes patients who are hospitalized for other conditions, such as pneumonia or cancer, suffer heart attacks while in the hospital. These two groups, emergency heart attacks and patients hospitalized for other reasons, represent two very different types of patients and probable outcomes. Therefore, proper identification of AMI patients is critical to the accurate assessment of outcomes of these patients. Approximately 60 percent of the mortality from AMI occurs before patients reach the hospital. Thus, differences in emergency transport and resuscitation capabilities would affect hospital mortality rates if sicker patients survived and were admitted to the hospital. It is also important to keep in mind that treatment for AMI is evolving rapidly; more aggressive treatment in the early convalescent stage of AMI, including procedures such as angioplasty and bypass, may increase the short-term mortality of patients but lead to better long-term outcomes.

Acute myocardial infarction was studied by three groups of authors using data from 1972, 1973, and 1977. Kelly and Hellinger (1987) tested both physician and hospital effects, they found only physician effects. Studies by Maerki, Luft, and Hunt (1986) and Luft, Hunt, and Maerki (1987) reported hospital effects only. Shortell and LoGerfo (1981) tested physician effects.

All four studies used in-hospital mortality as the indicator of outcome and measured hospital volume or physician volume or both. Kelly and Hellinger's study found a significant association between lower physician volume and higher in-hospital mortality, using 1977 data from 146 short-term general hospitals. In their study, however, hospital volume was not significantly associated with outcomes. Shortell and LoGerfo also reported that hospitals treating fewer than 60 AMI patients per family practitioner or internist had higher adjusted mortality rates than hospitals treating more than 60 patients per family practitioner or internist. Actual physician volumes were not ascertained, and this result may have reflected either a hospital volume effect or an effect of staffing patterns. For example, if physicians were affiliated with several hospitals, this would markedly reduce the ratio, even if physician volumes were unchanged. Luft, Hunt, and Maerki showed a significant association between higher hospital volume and lower death rates. Maerki, Luft, and Hunt confirmed this result using the same data and a slightly different model.

In general, a study of patients with medical diagnoses leaves more to the discretion of the researcher than does a study of patients with surgical procedures, in which selection is based on whether the patient underwent the relevant procedure. Luft, Hunt, and Maerki and Maerki, Luft, and Hunt selected all patients with acute myocardial infarction; Kelly and Hellinger included only patients who did not undergo surgery and who were diagnosed with cardiac arrest or post-myocardial infarction syndrome. Shortell and LoGerfo included patients with several coronary conditions involving acute myocardial infarction, ischemic heart disease, and disorders of the heart rhythm. In addition, they excluded the 3 percent of patients who were discharged alive within five days as having been erroneously miscoded as AMI patients. Very few patients would have been discharged this quickly after such a short stay in 1973, and these patients may have had one of the other conditions included in the study selection criteria. Because they included patients who may not have had heart attacks, clinical discretion in admission of patients could have affected the outcomes. Kelly and Hellinger excluded patients with one-day hospital stays since their mortality rates were high and determinants of their mortality were likely to have been different from determinants of mortality for those who survived the first day of hospitalization.

These selection and exclusion rules can affect both the outcome and volume variables in each analysis. Studies that exclude more seriously ill or emergency cases will have lower overall death rates. While Kelly and Hellinger may not have decreased the total volume very much by excluding patients with one-day hospital stays, they probably disproportionately excluded patients who might have benefited from effective emergency cardiac care. This may explain, in part, why they failed to show a relationship between hospital volume and in-hospital mortality.

It is important to bear in mind that emergency heart attack victims and patients who have heart attacks while hospitalized for other reasons represent two very different types of patients and probable outcomes. The adjustments for age, gender, and stage of illness used in these studies probably did not adequately differentiate between these two groups of patients.

All of the authors reported some association between physician or hospital volume and in-hospital mortality rates. However, the differences in patient selection, the emergency nature of this condition, and the fact that all the data are more than ten years old, make it difficult to compare findings, particularly given the rapid changes in treatment for AMI.

Perinatal Illness

Perinatal illness refers to specific conditions of newborns and includes respiratory distress syndrome, a condition associated with prematurity and resulting in inadequate development and function of a newborn's lungs. Some of the research reviewed here only examined the mortality rate of newborns. Examination of volume-outcome relationships for newborns is difficult for two reasons. First, very sick infants are often transferred to special neonatal intensive-care units. Unless the data can track the infants through the system, it is difficult to attribute the poor outcome to a particular provider. Second, there are at least two physicians, the delivering obstetrician and the neonatologist, who may influence the outcome of neonates. Without more precise data as to causes of illness and mortality in infants, it may be difficult to attribute outcomes to any physician.

Four studies examined the relationship between hospital volume and perinatal mortality, but none to date have examined the relationship between physician volume and perinatal mortality.

Maerki, Luft, and Hunt (1986) used 1972 data from CPHA to study the relationship between hospital volume in 770 hospitals and mortality from respiratory distress syndrome among 16,373 newborns. After controlling for case severity (using birthweight), the hospital's actual perinatal death rate was modeled as a function of the hospital's expected death rate and its volume, expressed both as volume and volume-squared. Both volume and volume-squared were highly significant.

In a second study (Luft, Hunt, and Maerki 1987), these authors used a simultaneous-equation regression model to examine the effect of log volume upon the actual-minus-expected in-hospital death rate for newborns with respiratory distress syndrome. They found a significant negative effect of volume upon mortality.

Williams (1979) studied the effectiveness of perinatal care for 3,370,338 births in 504 California hospitals in 1960 and between 1965 and 1973.[11] He found a U-shaped curve relating hospital volume (number of births) to perinatal mortality (defined as fetal deaths of 20 or more weeks gestation plus neonatal deaths of less than 28 days age). Both the number of births and the square of the number of births were significantly correlated with the standardized perinatal mortality rate. It is important to note that Williams identified all deaths irrespective of where they occurred but that he measured volume at the hospital of birth. The U-shaped curve reached a minimum at 2,850 annual births; adjusted perinatal mortality rates ranged from 0.46 to 3.74 per 1,000 births.

Finally, Rosenblatt, Reinken, and Shoemack (1985) examined the relationship between perinatal mortality rates and hospital volume in the highly regionalized maternity care system in New Zealand between 1978 and 1981. The authors examined 206,054 births, stratified by birthweight, in 111 hospitals, stratified into those providing primary, secondary, or tertiary levels of care. Crude perinatal mortality rates (defined as fetal deaths after 28 weeks gestation and early neonatal deaths before seven days age) increased with hospital volume; birthweight-adjusted perinatal mortality rates show the smaller hospitals having the lowest rates, with a significant linear trend for infants over 2,500 grams. There was no detectable volume threshold below which obstetrical care was judged to be unsafe. The authors offered two explanations for the finding of increasing perinatal mortality with higher hospital volumes, which were opposite most of the other volume-outcome studies. First, there was already regionalization of high-risk births, in which mothers of high-risk infants were referred to larger centers. Second, stratifying by birthweight might not have completely accounted for this risk, and thus higher mortality rates persisted even after adjustment. These data point to the clear influence of regionalization and why one must be alert to its potential effects in other diagnoses and procedures.

Fracture of the Femur

The femur is the long bone of the upper leg, which extends from the pelvis to the knee. Fracture of the femur is a major cause of morbidity and mortality in the elderly. Besides being a marker for other chronic diseases, such as osteoporosis, the fracture results in prolonged bed rest and immobility, which sometimes lead to medical complications. Surgery to repair the fracture is chosen based on the type of fracture and the extent of recovery expected.

The relationship between volume and outcome was insignificant in three out of four studies of fracture of the femur. The three groups of investigators studying this problem used different analytic techniques, time periods, and populations. In several instances, the results were suggestive but insignificant. Flood, Scott, and Ewy (1984a) found a lower, but insignificantly so, mortality rate in high-volume hospitals for patients with surgery for hip fractures without other trauma. Maerki, Luft, and Hunt (1986) found coefficients consistent with a U-shaped relationship, but neither are significant. Luft, Hunt, and Maerki (1987) found an insignificant effect of volume on outcome but a significant effect of outcome on volume for femur fracture patients.

The differences in results between the study by Hughes and his colleagues (1988), which reported an effect, and the study by Riley and Lubitz (1985), which did not, illustrate the potential problems in decisions with respect to patient selection. Riley and Lubitz selected Medicare patients who had *procedures* of closed or open reduction of fracture of the femur. Hughes and his colleagues used data from 1982 on selected patients with *diagnosis* of fracture of the upper end of femur. They included 12.6 percent of patients who had a primary diagnosis of fracture of femur but had no surgery. These patients might have been high-risk cases with poor prognoses, so surgery was avoided. Moreover, Riley and Lubitz might have underrepresented low-volume hospitals in their analyses because they estimated hospital volumes based on a 20-percent sample of Medicare records. Although the sampling was random, it implies that low-volume hospitals are far more likely to have been dropped than high-volume hospitals.

In these studies, average hospital volume ranges from 34 to 45 patients per year. The mortality rates reported in these studies were high (ranging from 5.0 percent to 9.1 percent), perhaps because fracture of the femur generally occurs in elderly patients. Therefore, their poor outcomes might be related more to general frailty than to the quality of treatment for their fractured hip.

Hernia

Surgery to repair hernia, a defect in the abdominal wall in the groin area, is a common operation with very low risk of mortality. Many hernia operations are now performed on an outpatient basis. Because the mortality rate is so low, one does not expect to see a volume-outcome relationship if one measures only mortality as an outcome.

Five studies with six findings examined a volume-outcome relationship for hernia surgery. One of the studies looked at both hospital volumes and physician volumes, whereas the other studies looked only at hospital volumes.

Three studies showed an association between patient volumes and outcomes; two of them measured outcomes other than mortality. Farber, Kaiser, and Wenzel (1981) measured postoperative infection rates but did not adjust for case mix. However, for an elective operation such as hernia repair, case-mix differences may not be significant. Hughes, Hunt, and Luft (1987) used the sum of deaths and long hospital stays as the outcome measure. Since deaths were so rare, the combined outcome essentially measured long hospital stays. However, the low (1 percent) wound infection rate in the Farber, Kaiser, and Wenzel study suggests that Hughes, Hunt, and Luft's combined measure of poor outcome, which identified 10 percent of patients as having poor outcomes, might not correlate well with actual complications.

In a separate analysis of the 1972 CPHA data used by Maerki, Luft, and Hunt in 1986, Luft, Hunt, and Maerki (1987) showed declining mortality with increasing hospital volume when the data were divided into volume categories. However, this part of the analysis is not tested statistically. In a simultaneous-equation model designed to test the relationship of volumes to outcomes versus outcomes to volumes, the coefficients were insignificant for both equations.

Riley and Lubitz (1985) found no relationship between hospital volumes and in-hospital deaths. However, the sampling scheme may have seriously affected their results. A sample of only 20 percent of Medicare patients receiving the procedure was included in the study. Thus hospitals with very low volumes may have been excluded entirely if they operated on one or only a few Medicare patients. In addition, hernia surgery is uncommon among Medicare patients, so the estimate of hospital volume may have been inaccurate.

Interpretation of the studies to estimate an effect size or flat of the curve is difficult. Although there was a statistically significant regression coefficient in the study by Farber, Kaiser, and Wenzel, visual representation of the data shows a wide variation in infection rates, which makes it difficult to identify a volume at which the infection rate stopped declining. However, a general lowering in the infection rate is observable in the range of 80 to 150 annual cases per hospital. In the research by Maerki, Luft, and Hunt, only the volume-squared regression coefficient was significant, making the interpretation of the flat of the curve unclear, but suggesting that it lies beyond 380 cases per hospital.

The one study that examined surgeon volume, which was conducted by Hughes, Hunt, and Luft (1987), must be viewed as a preliminary result because the method of assessing surgeon volume was indirect. Although it found significant hospital and surgeon volume effects, these results should be interpreted cautiously, given the lack of other evidence and the fact that the outcome measure largely reflects long stays.

In sum, the results of volume-outcome studies for hernia repair are mixed, with serious methodological differences between studies making it difficult to reconcile differences in results. Studies measuring mortality outcomes either showed no association or did not statistically test their result. The low death rate may preclude the detection of an effect in studies relying only on mortality. In addition, serious complications of hernia surgery that could potentially lead to death are extremely rare relative to other operations, so that mortality may be a very insensitive measure of any quality component regarding hernia surgery.

NOTES

1. Part I of Flood, Scott, and Ewy (1984a) is reprinted in Chapter 14 of this volume.
2. See Luft (1980), reprinted in Chapter 16 of this volume, and Luft, Bunker, and Enthoven (1979), reprinted in Chapter 12 of this volume.
3. See reprint of Farber, Kaiser, and Wenzel (1981) in Chapter 9 of this volume.
4. See reprint of Hughes, Hunt, and Luft (1987) in Chapter 17 of this volume.
5. See reprint of Riley and Lubitz (1985) in Chapter 15 of this volume.
6. See reprint of Roos et al. (1986) in Chapter 8 of this volume.
7. The study by Luft and Hunt (1986) is reprinted in Chapter 19 of this volume.
8. The study by Showstack et al. (1987) is reprinted in Chapter 11 of this volume.
9. See reprint of Kelly and Hellinger (1987) in Chapter 10 of this volume.
10. See Luft, Hunt, and Maerki (1986) and Sloan, Perrin, and Valvona (1987).
11. See reprint of Williams (1979) in Chapter 18 of this volume.

Chapter 7

Future Research and Policy Options

The literature reviewed in this book suggests that although there is a relationship between volume and outcome, there is no consensus about the causal pathways. In addition, the work to date has had an academic focus; investigators have explored various analytical questions and have not developed sets of estimates that are directly useful for consumers and policymakers. Furthermore, the research often reflects constraints imposed by the availability of data rather than a carefully mapped set of studies to address all the relevant questions. Thus, although we can be fairly certain about the existence of a relationship between volume and outcome for certain types of surgery, more research is necessary in several areas before one can draw implications with confidence. This chapter outlines areas that need further research and the policy options that can be drawn from existing research.

FUTURE RESEARCH

Functional Form

Although many studies indicate the presence of a volume-outcome relationship, the wide range of analytic methods and specification of variables makes it difficult to determine whether poor outcomes are concentrated at very low volumes or whether improved outcomes are seen throughout the observed range of volumes. Although the issue of which "functional form" to use to specify the volume variable may seem to be rather obscure, it lies at the heart of whether recommendations should be to "seek the highest volume center" or to "avoid places with fewer than x patients."

In theory, the research task is not very difficult (nor very exciting, which may explain why it has not been undertaken). One would *merely* define a set of relevant procedures and diagnoses, develop risk factors to adjust for case mix and severity differences among hospitals, and then determine the shape that best represents the volume-outcome curve. This simple description of the task omits several important factors. First, the purpose of this work is not to understand the factors giving rise to the volume-outcome relationship, so complex models are neither needed nor desirable. Instead, one is merely addressing the policymaker or citizen's question, that is, whether a high-volume hospital is preferable for a procedure. If so, what volume is safe? Clearly, an answer to such a question should be accompanied by multiple caveats, but it is not useful to present the results of a relationship estimated with other factors, such as teaching status, ownership, specialized equipment, and medical staff organization variables, held constant. Since the people who pose simple questions would never be able to apply the "complex" answer, one should offer the simple answer with the appropriate cautions.

Second, although determination of the functional form should be directed primarily toward results that are useful to a lay audience, the results will also help to set the stage for more sophisticated research. Once there is a comprehensive review of the volume-outcome data across a wide range of procedures and diagnoses, future research is more likely to use a single functional form, thereby making it easier to compare results. More important, if one identifies patterns across procedures and diagnoses as being either L-shaped, downward sloping, or upward sloping, this can direct future analyses toward an understanding of why those patterns occur.

Outcome Measures and Data Sets

This review did not focus on differences in findings with respect to outcome measures, partly because the vast majority of studies used in-hospital mortality as a measure. However, we know that for some conditions, such as oncology care, this is an absurd measure. Therefore, a wide range of medical diagnoses have been omitted from study. Moreover, the hospital is no longer the sole source of major medical intervention and treatment. Significant procedures such as cardiac catheterization are increasingly being performed on an outpatient basis, so hospital discharge data not only omit many patients, but the ones who are included in the data are increasingly the sickest patients, who are too risky to be treated on an outpatient basis. Even when treated in a hospital, patients are now being discharged much more rapidly to facilities that provide less-intensive care, again resulting in a bias in hospital-based data.

Substantial research is required to determine what is gained and what is lost with various outcome measures for various procedures and diagnoses. This work may best begin with questions about how the results will ultimately be used. For example, if we are interested in improving outcomes from the patient's perspective, we may want some solid information on how patients value various outcomes. For example, would it be best to be in Hospital A, in which 1 percent of patients die postoperatively, 0.5 percent end up in a constant vegetative state, and 98.5 percent recover completely, or in Hospital B; in which 1.3 percent of the patients die postoperatively but all the survivors recover completely? Is death on the operating table better, worse, or no different than death of complications ten days after the operation? Are complications themselves a major outcome to be avoided, even though there is no difference in six-month mortality?

It is important to note that even though we are arguing for a patient-oriented perspective in the *choice of outcome measures*, this is not the same as asking for patient perspectives on the *quality of care*. Although there are many definitions of quality, most of them include measures of structure, process, outcome, and increasingly, patient satisfaction (Davies and Ware 1988). They assume that medical care providers should be offering the best care possible given the available technology. Studies of the volume-outcome relationship are designed to help understand the boundaries of the available technology. For example, if outcomes in low-volume settings are worse because the staff is unable to acquire and maintain appropriate levels of expertise, it may be that limited technology makes it inadvisable to treat certain patients in low-volume settings. Given those technological constraints, one may still find some high-volume hospitals with poor outcomes because of quality problems. In that case, a different solution is necessary.

Once the important outcome measures have been identified—and there may be several, with different ones preferred for different diagnoses—then they should be compared. For example, although some hospitals have relatively high mortality rates but low complication rates, the differences in these measures may not be important if the focus of the study is on the volume-outcome relationship, rather than on the scoring of individual hospitals. On the other hand, if one observes markedly different relationships using different outcomes, then it is important to investigate further. (It is likely that the various outcome measures will give the same general results, but one can imagine situations in which there are consistent differences. For instance, suppose that high-volume teaching hospitals have a more actively intervening staff. Patients who might die quickly in low-volume hospitals are resuscitated and eventually discharged to nursing homes. In this case, the estimated volume-outcome relationship would depend on the outcome measure.)

In the future, it is unlikely that there will be one all-purpose data set for analysis. There are too many trade-offs between the cost of data collection, accuracy, and clinical detail to settle for a "one size fits all" approach. However, if someone first investigates the relationships among findings based upon different data sets and outcomes, then it will be possible to compare the results of various studies in a way that is quite difficult now.

Physician Volume

The evidence of a relationship between physician volume and patient outcomes is far less clear than for hospital volume and patient outcomes, yet it is certainly plausible that such a relationship exists. The available data are sparse, often conflicting, and difficult to compare. Prior research has been constrained in part, by the availability of data, which has often made it impossible to develop physician-specific volumes and outcomes. Some newly available data sets include an encrypted physician license number, which will allow the accumulation of volumes across hospitals and thus open up a new area of investigation (Hannan et al. 1989).

Better physician-identifier data, however, will not be enough to solve some of the methodological problems. For example, far more detailed information will be necessary to track the volume or experience of all the physicians involved in a case, including consultants, anesthesiologists, and others who may be as important as the attending physician and principal surgeon. In some instances, the involvement of a certain type of consultant is actually an indication that complications have set in, so one will have to pay particular attention to the whole process of care, and not just treat the hospital episode as a "black box," as has so often been the case (Garnick et al. 1989).

The Role of Selective Referrals

We are convinced of the plausibility of a causal pathway whereby higher volumes arise from selective referrals to hospitals and physicians with better-than-average outcomes. This is not to say that higher volumes do not also lead to better outcomes. The two effects may vary in importance across diagnoses and procedures. As the primary researchers arguing for the plausibility of the selective-referral model, we have tried to be fair in the presentation of findings. We know of no direct evidence refuting the notion, but some unconscious biases may be present. It is therefore important that others investigate this question. It is more than just an academic issue, since without a better understanding of the causal pathways, it is difficult to choose among the policy options discussed below.

Patterns over Time

Both causal pathways have an important time dimension. What is the speed with which changes in outcomes have an effect on referrals? Can a hospital that replaces a poor-quality surgeon with a good one increase its volume, or is a poor reputation difficult to erase? Likewise, for how long can a hospital (or physician) with deteriorating outcomes maintain old referral sources?

To some extent, the time dimension distinguishes the scale effect from the experience effect. If an individual or organization forgets past experience very quickly, then accumulated experience is largely irrelevant and one need only focus on current volume or scale. On the other hand, if there is no forgetting, then accumulated experience may matter in addition to current volume. One can see how these factors may vary across procedures and diagnoses. For example, high volume may hone technical skills but accumulated experience may aid in diagnostic expertise. Organizations may be able to establish work rules and procedures to institutionalize accumulated experience.

Clinical Explanations

Finally, there is a need for a series of very detailed studies to explore precisely what factors account for the differences in outcomes. Such studies would probably rely upon careful chart review from various settings to determine the relative importance of errors of commission and omission, differences in technique, monitoring, support, and the like. It would explore the ways in which physicians and hospitals are chosen. It would also explore organizational factors leading to better or worse outcomes. It is probable that the importance of various factors will depend on the procedure or diagnosis studied. Without such studies the volume-outcome relationship will remain a "black box" that is easily rejected by skeptical clinicians. Furthermore, if the factors leading to poor outcomes are identified, one may then be able to design interventions to improve the quality of care, not just methods to label institutions or groups.

POLICY OPTIONS

Even with these substantial gaps in our knowledge about the underlying relationships, there are still several policy options that are worthy of consideration. In discussing these, it is important to consider the incentive effects of policies. For example, the publication of mortality statistics is likely to have several consequences, some intended, some not. Knowing that their outcomes will be made public, many hospitals will quickly try to identify quality-of-care problems and correct them. Some hospitals, however, may attempt to avoid admitting certain patients or to encourage the transfer of other patients, especially if one less death may have important "public relations" consequences. The following list of five policy options is roughly ordered in terms of the increasing ability of hospitals (and the increasing incentives to hospitals) to manipulate the data or otherwise behave in undesirable ways.

Public Education

General public education about the existence of the volume-outcome relationship is a rather simple recommendation. Even if the causal linkages are not clear, it seems reasonable to argue that, in the absence of other evidence, hospitals with high volumes are preferable to those with very low volumes. Upon receiving a referral for a specialized procedure, the informed consumer may then ask the referring primary care physician about the volume and quality of the proposed specialist and hospital, given the relevant alternatives. There are no new data collection requirements and the potential costs are low. One could easily see it implemented through articles in the lay press.

The public education strategy would take somewhat different approaches, depending on the relative importance of the volume versus referral effects. If volume is the key factor, then referral to the high-volume center, or at least away from a very low volume center, makes sense. While one could undertake publication of hospital or physician-specific volumes (see below), it is difficult to make such information directly relevant to the patient. For example, a hospital may be a high-volume provider of open-heart surgery but a relatively low-volume source of the particular type of open-heart surgery required by a certain patient. This type of more specific information might be acquired by a primary care physician and interpreted for the patient. If high volumes already reflect selective referrals to the better sources of care, then increased patient sensitivity to quality will build on an existing pattern of behavior. In this instance, however, the message should be to encourage the primary care physician to make quality-sensitive referrals, not just to seek the higher-volume centers. Of course, the high-volume centers are likely to be good places to start looking for better quality.

Physician Education

A second level of intervention might be directed toward physicians through their specialty associations and continuing-education programs. Specialty associations might collect volume and outcome information in their areas and make it available to physicians. Primary care physician associations might take on the responsibility for assembling, interpreting, and disseminating the information to their members. In particular, they could focus on factors that would improve their ability to refer patients selectively to settings and physicians with better outcomes. It may be necessary to clarify whether such educational efforts by local specialty associations would raise antitrust problems. By keeping the data "within the profession," this strategy may reduce opposition to any discussion of relative outcomes. In fact, the first step might be the collection and feedback of information *within* the specialty groups. Some very low volume providers may not realize where they "stand on the curve" and may choose to cease performing that procedure. Wennberg and his colleagues (1977) have demonstrated the effectiveness of feedback approaches in settings controlled by the physicians themselves.

Suppose that the local specialty association was to cooperate in identifying those patient factors thought to be important in adjusting for case-mix differences among hospitals. If the volume, outcome, and case-mix data were then collected and fed back to the physicians and hospitals without identifiers, the results would probably have far more credibility than if done by outsiders. If there were important differences in outcomes among some of the providers, those with the worst outcomes would probably undertake corrective actions. Simultaneously, some primary care physicians would probably begin to ask the specialists to whom they refer patients about the outcomes of patients in their settings.

Hospital-Specific Volumes

A third level of intervention would be the compulsory routine collection and publication of hospital-specific volume information. For states with mandatory hospital abstract reporting requirements, this is a rather simple task. One could clearly not publish data for all hospitals and all procedures and diagnoses, but relevant data should be made available to interested parties. Selected hospital-specific information could be printed in local newspapers. California Blue Shield has already compiled a list of hospitals with their coronary artery bypass graft surgery volumes. Some consumer organizations and magazines have done the same (Center for the Study of Services 1987). The *Los Angeles Times* has published a series of articles on hospital volumes (Steinbrook 1988).

Hospital-specific volumes should be published in a way that does not imply the existence of a sharp threshold unless it is clear that outcomes are markedly worse below this threshold than above the threshold. For example, one might say that volumes in the 200+ level are associated with mortality rates that are average or below average, volumes below 100 are associated with death rates that are significantly higher than average, and volumes in the 100 to 200 range are in an intermediate category. Publication of volumes might give hospitals an incentive to increase admissions, but such pressures would be far greater if the addition of a few cases meant the continuance of a certificate of need (see below) or a move from "unacceptable" to "acceptable" in volume categories.

Regulations Requiring Minimum Volumes

Currently, some state certificate-of-need laws require the projection of a certain minimum need for hospital procedures such as coronary artery bypass graft surgery and imply the potential loss of the certificate if need if minimum volume levels are not maintained. Such a policy is probably unwise for at least two reasons. First, it makes the retention of something very valuable (the ability to continue in a specific line of business) contingent on a measure (volume) that is merely a proxy for something very important (quality). Second, if decisions depend on the maintenance of a specific minimum volume, then there are enormous pressures to make sure that treatment is given to at least that number of patients. One can imagine memos from hospital administrators to the medical staff pointing out that unless another 20 patients are admitted or operated on before the end of the fiscal year, the unit will be closed down. This could lead to a more relaxed set of standards for the appropriateness of admission or surgery. In contrast to the discussion above, with respect to publication of volume levels, it is difficult for regulatory procedures to allow for flexibility and "soft" incentives.

Selective Contracting

A fifth policy application of the volume-outcome relationship is in the realm of selective contracting. Insurers, HMOs, and agents such as Medicaid programs may wish to steer the patients for whom they are responsible to those providers who are likely to achieve better outcomes. If reliable outcome data were available, either through routinely collected sources or through carefully structured bids, then such information might be used by contractors. For high-volume hospitals, outcome data include only a small chance component, so it is reasonable to require evidence on their own track record. For low-volume hospitals, however, such outcome data tend to be too unreliable. A hospital with just a few patients may have had no deaths, but this is not very useful as evidence of its quality. Even with poor outcome rates at two or three times the average, a very low volume hospital will usually not be considered a statistical outlier.

On the other hand, if outcome data are unavailable or too subject to manipulation, then volume may be a proxy for quality. For example, suppose an agency announced that it was going to utilize hospital discharge abstracts to determine death rates for the purposes of contracting. A hospital with a high inpatient death rate may monitor patients for complications and transfer those at risk of death, thereby improving its own statistics. It would be far more difficult to manipulate volume figures, and it is unlikely that many hospitals could attempt such a strategy without detection. Of course, if one is to use volume as an indicator of quality, one must first take account of the influence of selective contracts on volume.

Additional policy recommendations depend on a better understanding of the observed relationships. For example, if increasing volumes does lead to improved outcomes, then the argument for explicit regionalization strategies becomes far stronger. If hospital volume is far more important then physician volume, then one would argue against the peripatetic surgeon. On the other hand, if physician volume is the crucial variable, then one may want to encourage "circuit riding" with many low-volume hospitals sharing a single high-volume physician. If hospital malpractice claims are associated with volume, then malpractice insurance premiums should be adjusted to reflect this risk factor. However, these and other options must await future research.

Part II
Lessons from Specific Studies

Chapter 8

Posthospital Outcomes

The quality of medical care provided during a hospitalization cannot necessarily be completely evaluated during that hospitalization. Surgical incisions may not heal fully (leading to readmission), or a prostatectomy may be followed by postdischarge bleeding complications that result in continued office visits and procedures such as catheterizations. The Canadian system of universal health insurance and centralized claims allows researchers to track the medical care utilization of individual patients through time. Complications that occur subsequent to the initial hospitalization for an illness may be assessed.

Roos and his colleagues followed selected groups of surgical patients using a Canadian claims data base. Patients with cancer diagnoses were excluded, because they were likely to require further treatment and hospitalization, regardless of the quality of initial treatment. The data base allowed the researchers to know whether a patient was readmitted to the hospital after treatment and for what diagnosis or procedures. Physician panels decided whether certain diagnoses or procedures represented complications, and for what period after surgery the complication was likely to occur. This is a crucial step in analysis of the data, because the longer the posthospitalization "window," the greater the chance that a readmission was for a problem unrelated to the original hospitalization. Unfortunately, these unrelated admissions may not be randomly distributed. There is a substantial amount of literature suggesting wide variations in admission rates among small geographic areas. (Paul-Shaheen, Clark, and Williams 1987).

The potential yield from such an analysis of readmissions is quite high. For example, the mortality rates within six weeks of discharge ranged from 0.02 percent to 1.2 percent, and mortality within two years was in the range of 0.45 percent to 11.5 percent. In contrast, the readmission rates due to complications were in the range of 3 percent to 9 percent, but the readmission rates for other reasons were four to eight times as high. Although Roos and his colleagues focused on overall readmission rates, it would not be especially difficult to explore the reasons for readmissions and thereby provide useful clinical feedback to the physicians and hospitals.

Another advantage of claims data is that the prehospitalization medical care, both inpatient and outpatient, may be used to adjust for severity of illness. In this study, hospitalization in the two years preceding surgery was a significant predictor of readmission complications for both hysterectomy and cholecystectomy. Claims for outpatient visits indicating presence of chronic illness may be more accurate than the coding of coexisting conditions on the hospital discharge abstract. On the abstracts, chronic diagnoses are more apt to be omitted if the patient has many acute diagnoses (Jencks, Williams, and Kay 1988).

Other data sets have been used to identify deaths occurring outside the hospital within a certain period of time after admission. For example, Williams (1979) used linked birth and death certificate data to measure infant mortality, and Riley and Lubitz (1985) used Medicare eligibility files to determine death within 30 days.[1] Newborns at risk of death are frequently transferred to more specialized facilities, so it is critical that any outcome study for neonates go beyond the initial hospitalization. Similarly, for terminally ill patients, hospitals may have differing discharge practices depending on the availability of nursing home or hospice beds. Following patients for a specific period after admission or date of surgery would eliminate biases due to these factors.

When attempting to do a study using posthospital outcomes, one must address a series of issues. For example, does one begin the window from the date of admission, the date of the operation, or the date of discharge? With a two-year window such as the one used by Roos and his colleagues, this difference does not matter much, but with a shorter window, such as that used by Riley and Lubitz, it may have a substantial effect if some hospitals have very long postoperative stays. The difference is especially important for patients who may need to be discharged to a nursing home. In some areas, nursing home beds are unavailable, so patients are kept in the hospital for weeks or even months. In extreme cases, such as in New York City, the in-hospital mortality rate for some Medicare patients is higher than their mortality rate within 30 days of admission. The Roos study used a fixed window from the date of discharge, which ignores all complications (and deaths) during the initial admission. The study also excluded deaths from the list of complications unless they were associated with an admission for a complication. This decision was probably made because it is often difficult to attribute the cause of death. Nevertheless, it raises the issue of whether one should attempt to score complications in terms of their severity in order to get a weighted measure of outcomes.

NOTE

1. See reprints of Williams (1979) and Riley and Lubitz (1985) in Chapters 18 and 15 of this volume.

Centralization, Certification, and Monitoring

Readmissions and Complications after Surgery

Leslie L. Roos, Jr.
Sandra M. Cageorge
Noralou P. Roos
Rudy Danzinger

Several investigators have stressed the need to study the predictors of adverse outcomes following common surgical procedures.[1,2] Some research has emphasized variables measured at the hospital level (e.g., volume of surgery done in the hospital). Other studies have suggested that the focus should be on the individual surgeon's qualifications and experience. Policy directions depend both on which variables are important and on what sorts of policies are feasible to implement. Focusing on *where* a given procedure is performed highlights a concern for centralization; a centralized approach suggests that only certain hospitals (often tertiary centers) should be allowed to do the given surgery. Emphasizing *who* should perform a particular operation implies certification; physicians might be designated as appropriate on the basis of educational qualifications, experience with surgery, and so forth. Finally, monitoring involves identifying particular hospitals that, regardless of their characteristics, appear to have relatively poor (or relatively good) results.

Complications leading to hospital readmissions were chosen as the outcome measure because of their frequency, their substantive importance, and their ease of identification from health insurance data bases. As Bunker and Fowles[3] have stressed, "Claims data are potentially valuable as a source of epidemiological information on the quality of hospital care provided to the population as a whole." Such data bases are most valuable in surmounting some of the logistic difficulties associated with doing research on postoperative morbidity.[4] In contrast to almost all studies cited below, the Manitoba data permit following patients beyond their initial hospital stay and identifying complications leading to readmission in a hospital other than that of their original surgery. Extensive information on these complications has been presented elsewhere.[5]

Reprinted from *Medical Care* 24, no. 11 (1986): 1044–66, with permission from The J. B. Lippincott Company.

Supported in part by National Health Research and Development Project No. 6607-1197-44 and by Career Scientist Awards Nos. 6607-1314-48 and 6607-1001-22 to Leslie L. Roos and Noralou P. Roos, respectively.

The relationship between surgical volume, on the one hand, and associated mortality and morbidity, on the other, has received considerable attention.[6-10] For a number of procedures, the more operations performed, the lower an institution's morbidity and mortality rates. These findings have suggested concentrating these surgical procedures in high-volume centers, thus supporting a policy of centralization.[11] But if high-volume hospitals do deliver higher-quality care, is it because the surgeon has more experience, because the hospital team (including surgeon, anesthetist, and nursing staff) is better trained, or because these hospitals are treating lower-risk patients?

Physician experience with a particular procedure has been emphasized by several investigators.[12,13] Some have suggested a certification strategy: surgical privileges should be more restricted, with limits on the procedures that general practitioners would be allowed to perform.[14] However, Couch et al.[15] have found costly and unnecessary surgical mishaps even among patients operated on by board-certified surgeons. Moreover, because family physicians tend to perform less complicated procedures on less ill patients,[16-19] the extent to which restriction of surgical privileges is necessary to maintain quality is not clear. Because the importance of surgical qualification and certification has not been clearly demonstrated,[20-22] Mainen[23] has emphasized the need for studies addressing surgical outcome "as a function of the training, experience, and certification status of the surgical provider."

Since hysterectomy, cholecystectomy, and prostatectomy are largely elective operations varying substantially in both per capita rates and indications for use, these procedures seem particularly appropriate to study.[24] Surgical volume has been found to be important for both cholecystectomy and prostatectomy; considering all gallbladder operations, Flood et al.[8] found low surgical volume to be associated with higher postoperative mortality. Luft et al.'s research[7] showed no relationship between surgical mortality and surgical volume for cholecystectomy without common bile duct exploration, but low surgical volume and high mortality were related for transurethral resection of the prostate and (to a lesser degree) for cholecystectomy with incision of the common bile duct. Several authors[8,10] suggest that postoperative morbidity is a more sensitive indicator of outcome than postoperative mortality. Farber et al.[10] found a higher probability of postoperative wound infections following hysterectomy and following simple cholecystectomy in low-volume hospitals; prostatectomy was not included in the study.

Patient risk factors need to be taken into account. Thus, although Flood et al.[8,9] were able to control for patient health status, Farber et al.[10] could not directly consider the possibility that physicians in different hospitals might be operating on patient populations with varying risk characteristics. The influence of such factors as duration of operation, surgical approach (abdominal versus vaginal), and age on the rate of postoperative infections following hysterectomy has been demonstrated.[25-27] Similarly, research on the risk factors affecting surgery for both gallbladder disease and prostate disease has suggested the importance of type of surgery, coexisting conditions, age, and severity of disease.[28-33]

This paper focuses on patient, surgeon, and hospital characteristics associated with serious postdischarge complications of hysterectomy, cholecystectomy, and prostatectomy in Manitoba. To assess the feasibility of monitoring, an analysis of rates of readmissions for complications for individual hospitals was also conducted. Patients aged 25 and over readmitted to hospital with a complication during the 2 years following 1974–1976 surgery are studied using data from the provincial health claims system.

METHOD

Data Base

In Manitoba, all medical and hospital care, with a few minor exceptions (such as private room and cosmetic surgery), is free to the patient. There is neither coinsurance nor usage limitation (except on chiropractic care and optometrist visits). Several separate files—the registration, hospital, and medical files—are maintained for payment and control purposes by the Manitoba Health Services Commission (MHSC). This health insurance data base is characterized by universal coverage (all individuals registered in Manitoba, no matter where care is received). Nonparticipation in the Manitoba Health Plan is minimal, as residents are not obliged to pay any premiums to register for insured benefits. Hospital and medical care are documented in considerable detail as a result of the statistical reporting requirements for hospitals and the fee-for-service payment system for medical services.

The registration file contains data on the population covered, organized by family registration numbers. With minor exceptions, individuals can be uniquely specified by using birth date, sex, and initial identifiers in addition to family registration number. The medical claims file is the vehicle for paying physicians. Claims are submitted by physicians for services rendered to patients. These claims are filed on a temporal basis and contain physician's identification number, patient's identifying information, patient's residence (checked against the population registry), tariff (determined by whether the visit is a consultation, complete physical examination, regional examination, follow-up visit, and the like), and diagnosis (ICD-8 code). As described elsewhere, the claims appear to provide valid data on total patient-physician contact.[34-35] In a fee-for-service system, claims should not underestimate the volume of physician contact, and since physician practice profiles are routinely audited with detailed analyses of outlier practice patterns, a significant amount of overbilling appears unlikely.[36]

The hospital file is built on the basis of each admission and contains patient identification, dates of admission and discharge, limited information on services rendered, and one or more diagnoses. All surgical procedures are noted, as well as identification numbers of the surgeon or attending physician, consultants, and anesthetist. Surveillance artifacts are minimal, since all hospitals are legally required to submit information on all hospital stays.[37] Unique physician and hospital codes permit determining the number of operations of a given type performed by any physician (regardless of where the surgery was done) and the number performed in each hospital. As described in Appendix 3, diagnoses reported on hospital claims have been compared with those on hospital medical records and those on physician claims with satisfactory results.[35]

Readmissions for Postoperative Complications

The analysis looks at hysterectomies, cholecystectomies, and prostatectomies occurring in 1974 through 1976 using 2-year "before-operation" and 2-year "after-operation" histories; these histories provide the necessary information for categorizing patient risk factors and assessing readmissions for postoperative complications.

Readmissions for complications were identified by separate physician panels for each procedure; the coding of these complications is described in detail in Appendix 2. Postoperative hemorrhage (30% of the complications) was by far the most common problem causing readmission following hysterectomy. Other frequent complications included postoperative wound infection (15%) and incisional hernia/disruption of operative wound (13%). Vaginal enterocele was also quite common (8%); diseases of the kidney and ureter and incontinence with repair each affected 6% of the women. The most common causes of readmissions for complications following cholecystectomy included incisional hernia/disruption of operative wound (24%) and postoperative wound infection, peritonitis, and cellulitis (14%). More than 30% of the complications were related to continued gallstone disease; half of these had diagnoses of cholelithiasis (indicating a retained stone) at readmission. The most frequent complications necessitating rehospitalization following prostatectomy were readmission for revision (34%) and postoperative hemorrhage (22%). Other frequent complications included stricture of the urethra (18%), hematuria (9%), contracture of bladder sphincter (6%), and retention of urine (3%).

Exclusions and Follow-Up

For all three procedures, surgery associated with malignancy was eliminated from the analysis. Hysterectomies performed at the time of intra-abdominal hemorrhage were excluded, as were cholecystectomies following prior gallbladder surgery and prostatectomies representing revisions of prior surgery. In a few cases (from 1.5 to 2%), various types of identifier problems appear on the registry; the most frequent of these problems necessitated an adjustment in the birth year. Overall follow-up compares favorably with participation and follow-up in other longitudinal studies.[38]

The small numbers of individuals from outside the province receiving treatment in Manitoba and of Manitobans using out-of-province hospitals were not included because of possible difficulties in tracing them through time. The native Indian population was also excluded because responsibility for their health care is shared between federal and provincial authorities; their coverage in the claims system is known to be incomplete. In this 3-year analysis, only patients of "permanent" physicians, those remaining in the province for the entire 1974–1976 period, are considered.*

Information on mortality during the 2 years following surgery is presented in Table 8.1. Mortality was insufficient to allow specific analyses, although data from Manitoba and Maine have been combined to permit a longitudinal analysis of mortality following prostatectomy.[33] Many of the surgical patients who died in the 6 weeks following hospital discharge were included among those readmitted for complications; sensitivity testing (including all such deaths in the analysis) did not change the substantive results.

Cases excluded or lost to follow-up are presented in Table 8.1. Individuals were considered fully covered if they were covered for the 4 years surrounding the date of the operation or for 2 years before surgery and after surgery until death. Twenty individuals died in the 2 years following hysterectomy, 165 after cholecystectomy, and 313 after prostatectomy. Because of problems with tracing women through the Manitoba registry when a change in marital status occurs, loss to follow-up is greatest for the hysterectomy patients. Because MHSC number is assigned to the household "head," men have few registry problems. Out-of-province migration is minimal among the men (generally elderly) having prostatectomies. Other biases associated with loss to follow-up are very small.[39,40] Various types of sensitivity testing using excluded patients produced results very similar to those reported here.

Measures Used

Which factors (individually or jointly) have important effects on the probabilities of developing complications leading to readmissions after surgery? Variables dealing with physician characteristics (e.g., physician specialty and number of hysterectomies performed), hospital characteristics (number of hysterectomies done in a hospital), and patient characteristics (age, comorbidity, prior history) can be controlled simultaneously. Physician and hospital counts for surgical volume were made using all relevant procedures, not just those performed on patients passing the screens in Table 8.1.

The different measures of patient health status (with the exception of multiple diagnoses, a frequently used measure of comorbidity at the time of hospital

---

*Putting mobile physicians into various 1-year analyses made no difference in the results. For example, using only patients of "permanent" physicians reduced the number of relevant hysterectomy cases by 583.

Table 8.1: Cases Excluded and Lost to Follow-Up

	Hysterectomy	*Cholecystectomy*	*Prostatectomy*
Total number of operations noted on file	6609	9318	4232
Cases excluded:			
Patients who had prior (related) surgery	—	47	348
Patients with malignancies	587	331	663
Out-of-province residents	121	262	69
Patients lacking unique identifiers	208	270	97
Patients of surgeons not registered for entire 1974–76 period	583	374	112
N of cases remaining after all exclusions:	5110	8034	2943
Lost to follow-up or missing values:			
Patient lacking full (4-year) coverage	615	872	133
Patients with missing values	142	240	89
N of cases remaining for analysis:	4353	6922	2721
Percentage of relevant operations analyzed:	85.2	86.2	92.5
Percentage of total number of operations analyzed:	65.9	74.3	64.3
N of readmissions due to complications:	194	205	256
N of readmissions not due to complications:	753	1673	1020
N of deaths:			
Up to 42 days	1	36	32
Up to 2 years	20	165	313

admission) have been developed from health system contacts prior to the admission for surgery. Although detailed clinical research may find a statistically significant patients risk factor or two not included here,[27] the case mix measures used capture much of the variance reported in procedure-specific studies. Those patient variables from hospital and medical claims have been shown to be satisfactory measures of patient health status.[41,42]

The population structure of Manitoba suggested comparisons between Winnipeg and rural residents and hospitals. Manitoba has a population of more than 1 million people, spread across an area approximately the size of Alaska. Winnipeg, the provincial capital, includes slightly more than half the population of the province and both teaching hospitals. The second largest population center (Brandon, with a population of about 36,000) is included in the "rural" category along with the remainder of the province. Winnipeg versus rural residence and hospital location were explicitly entered in the regression equation predicting readmissions due to complications. Given that previous research has found few

differences in health status between Winnipeg and rural residents,[43] using the
case mix covariates described above, in combination with patient residence and
hospital location, should provide adequate control for patient health status. Finally, separate analyses for Winnipeg– rural residence and hospital location were
reported.

Although predictions using case mix and type of surgery variables provide
information relevant for clinical decision-making about the risks associated with
particular types of surgery,[44] this paper focuses on the hospital and physician
variables. In Canada, only board-certified physicians can list themselves as specialists. Board-eligible physicians are listed as general practitioners. Such physician factors as place of education and number of years in practice were not
included owing to their lack of importance in previous research.[45,46] Specialty
was included because of its importance in discussions of certification; moreover,
surgical workloads of specialists have been increasing while those of Manitoba
general practitioners have been declining.[18] Other physician and hospital variables were selected or not according to this criterion of substantive significance.
The variables used are presented in Table 8.2 and treated more fully in Appendix
2. Independent variables were dichotomized to permit easy calculation of odds
ratios.

Analytic Approach

Bivariate and multivariate analyses were carried out at the patient level with a
dichotomous dependent variable (readmission for complications) that is relatively
infrequent; key characteristics of the individual's surgeon (surgical volume, specialty) and hospital are included. Flood et al.[8,9] note that this approach limits the
amount of variation than can be explained in the analyses.[*] Multiple logistic
regression was used to estimate the influences of the independent variables on the
probability of readmission controlling for the effects of several variables at once.
Variables dealing with patient characteristics and statistically significant (at the
.05 level) were first chosen from a multiple logistic regression using backwards
elimination.[†] These measures were then put into a stepwise regression to ensure
consideration of relevant covariate controls before characteristics of the procedure, hospital, and surgeon were given a chance to enter the equation.

Hospital-specific analyses (illustrating a monitoring approach) were undertaken for those institutions annually averaging at least 50 hysterectomies or
prostatectomies, or 100 or more cholecystectomies annually. Individual hospitals
were added both after the "best" model was generated and after controlling for

---

[*]Analyzing data at the hospital level loses information but characteristically greatly increases the
amount of variance explained.

[†]Estimation was done by the method of maximum likelihood using the iterative procedure LOGIST of
the Statistical Analysis System, version 82.3.[47]

Table 8.2: Independent Variables Used in Logistic Regressions (Reference Level Is in Parentheses)

	Hysterectomy	*Cholecystectomy*	*Prostatectomy*
A. Patient Co-Variables			
Age	(20–39)	(20–44)	(<65)
	40–49	45–59	65–74
	50+	60+	75+
Sex	– –	(Female)	—
		Male	
Residence	(Winnipeg) Rural	for all three operations	
B. "Event" Variables			
Type of surgery	(Abdominal	(Simple cholecystectomy)	(Transurethral)
	hysterectomy)	More complex surgery	Open prostatec-
	Vaginal hysterectomy		tomy
Duration of opera-	(<8)	(<7)	(<6)
tion— units of	8+	7+	6+
anesthetic			
Multiple diagnoses	(No)	for all three operations	
	Yes		
C. Medical History During 2 Years Prior to Surgery			
Hospital admissions	(No)	for all three operations	
	Yes		
Physician visits with			
a. Chronic diagnoses	(<10)	(<8)	(<9)
	10+	8+	9+
b. Heart disease	(No)	for all three operations	
	Yes		
D. Hospital Characteristics			
Type of hospital	(Winnipeg teaching)	for all three operations	
	Winnipeg nonteaching		
	Rural		
Number of operations	(100+)	for all three operations	
at hospital per year	<100		
E. Surgeon Characteristics			
Specialty	(Gynecologist)	("Non"-general	(Urologist)
	General surgeon	practitioner)	Other
	General practitioner	General practitioner	
Number of operations	(20+)	(20+)	(50+)
performed per year	<20	<20	<50

just patient and surgical variables. Both approaches produced similar results with these data.

RESULTS

Hysterectomy

The most important bivariate predictors of complications following hysterectomies related to type of operation (vaginal hysterectomies had a higher complication rate than abdominal) and prior history (whether or not admitted to hospital in preceding 2 years, frequency of physician visits involving chronic diagnoses, and cardiovascular problems) (Appendix 1). One other patient characteristic (the presence of multiple diagnoses during the hospital stay) produced high odds ratios but, because of relatively few individuals with no multiple diagnoses, this variable did not quite reach statistical significance at the 0.05 level.

The bivariate analysis showed rural residence, rural hospitals, and surgery by a general surgeon or general practitioner to be associated with a higher complication rate following hysterectomy. Surgical volume, both among hospitals and among physicians, was also a significant predictor of probability of complications; lower-volume hospitals and physicians had readmission rates for complications about 40% higher than their counterparts performing more operations.

Many variables drop out in the multivariate analysis. Three patient variables (admission to hospital in 2 years before surgery, frequency of physician visits involving chronic diagnoses, and presence of multiple diagnoses) and type of operation were statistically significant. Physician specialty, physician surgical volume, hospital surgical volume, and hospital location are all substantially intercorrelated. When these hospital and physician variables were allowed to enter the regression equation after the significant patient covariables had entered, the only additional significant variable was hospital location (Table 8.3). If, instead, the hospital characteristics were analyzed by entering a separate dichotomous variable for each hospital averaging more than 50 hysterectomies per

Table 8.3: Results of Logistic Regression for Readmission for Complications after Hysterectomy (1974–1976)

Variable (Reference Level)	Beta	Adjusted Odds Ratio	95% Confidence Interval
Hospitalization in 2 years prior to surgery:			
(No)			
Yes	0.35	1.42	1.05–1.92
Physician visits with chronic diagnoses:			
(<10)			
10+	0.30	1.35	1.00–1.82
Multiple diagnoses at "event":			
(No)			
Yes	0.76	2.15	1.04–4.43
Type of surgery:			
(Abdominal hysterectomy)			
Vaginal hysterectomy	0.48[a]	1.62	1.19–2.21
Location of hospital:			
(Winnipeg)			
Rural	0.41	1.50	1.07–2.10

[a]All variables included were significant at $p \leqslant 0.05$; [a] indicates significance at $p \leqslant 0.01$.
Rank correlation between predicted probability and response = 0.23.

year, the resulting model contained no significant hospital variables; physician surgical volume became a significant predictor (with an adjusted odds ratio of 1.44) with little change in the coefficients of the other independent variables. In Tables 8.3 through 8.6, a positive, statistically significant beta means that the second category of a particular variable is associated with a higher risk of readmission; a negative value indicates that the first specification is so associated.

The seven hospitals in which an average of 50 or more hysterectomies were performed annually were added to the logistic regression in Table 8.3, but none of them entered into the equation when the other factors were present.

Cholecystectomy

Strong bivariate relationships were found in the analysis of complications following cholecystectomy (Appendix 1). Type of surgery was the strongest predictor, with the probability of complications after complex procedures (those involving bile duct surgery) being almost four times that following simple cholecystectomy. Among the patient variables, age, sex, prior history (admission to hospital in preceding 2 years), multiple diagnoses during the hospital stay, and rural

Table 8.4: Results of Logistic Regression for Readmission for Complications after Cholecystectomy (1974–1976)

Variable (Reference Level)	Beta	Adjusted Odds Ratio	95% Confidence Interval
Age			
(20–44)			
45–49	0.37	1.45	0.97–2.16
60 +	0.69[a]	2.00	1.37–2.93
Sex			
(Female)			
Male	0.40[a]	1.50	1.12–2.01
Hospitalization in 2 years prior to surgery			
(No)			
Yes	0.30	1.35	1.01–1.79
Type of surgery			
(Simple cholecystectomy)			
More complex surgery	1.05[a]	2.85	2.03–4.00
Number of cholecystectomies performed by surgeon annually			
(20 +)			
<20	0.62[a]	1.85	1.38–2.49
Duration of operation —units of anesthetic			
(<7)			
7 +	0.37[a]	1.45	1.06–1.98

[a]All variables included were significant at p≤0.05; [a] indicates significance at p≤0.01.
Rank correlation between predicted probability and response = 0.41.

Table 8.5: Results of Logistic Regression for Readmission for Complications after Prostatectomy (1974–1976)

Variable (Reference Level)	Beta	Adjusted Odds Ratio	95% Confidence Interval
Type of surgery:			
(Transurethral prostatectomy)			
Open prostatectomy	−0.46[a]	0.63	0.47–0.84
Physician visits with chronic diagnoses:			
(<9)			
9+	0.28	1.32	1.02–1.71

[a]All variables included were significant at p≤0.05; [a] indicates significance at p≤0.01.
Rank correlation between predicted probability and response = 0.14.

Table 8.6: Results of Logistic Regression for Readmission Not Due to Complications after Cholecystectomy (1974–1976)

Variable (Reference Level)	Beta	Adjusted Odds Ratio	95% Confidence Interval
Age			
(20–44)			
45–49	−0.25	0.78	0.67–0.90
60+	0.10[a]	1.10	0.95–1.28
Sex			
(Female)			
Male	−0.09[a]	0.92	0.80–1.04
Hospitalization in 2 years prior to surgery			
(No)			
Yes	0.61	1.83	1.63–2.06
Physician visits with			
a. Chronic diagnoses			
(<8)			
8+	0.35	1.41	1.25–1.59
b. Heart disease:			
(No)			
Yes	0.34	1.40	1.18–1.67
Multiple diagnoses at "event"			
(No)			
Yes	0.33	1.39	1.23–1.56
Patient residence			
(Winnipeg)			
Rural	0.41	1.51	1.31–1.74
Number of cholecystectomies performed			
at hospital annually			
(<100)			
100+	0.31	1.36	1.16–1.60

[a]Indicates variables were not significant at p≤0.05; all other variables were significant at p≤0.01.
Rank correlation between predicted probability and response = 0.33.

residence were all significantly associated with the probability of complications.* In contrast with the hysterectomy findings, location of hospital did not prove statistically significant in the multivariate analyses.

Although available hospital variables (type of hospital and frequency with which cholecystectomy was performed) were not significantly associated with probability of a complication in the bivariate analysis, the frequency with which a physician performed cholecystectomy was. Patients operated on by physicians averaging 20 or fewer procedures annually over the 3-year period were almost twice (1.78 times) as likely to have postoperative complications.

Age, sex, prior history (hospitalization in preceding 2 years), duration of operation, physician surgical experience, and type of operation all entered into the multivariate logistic equation (Table 8.4). As noted earlier, controlling for all other factors in the equation, individuals with the second specification were more likely to have a complication than were those with the first specification. For example, controlling for type of surgery, experience of the surgeon, and so forth, individuals aged 60 and older were twice as likely to be readmitted to hospital with a complication following cholecystectomy as were younger patients.†

When data from individual hospitals averaging 100 or more such operations yearly were entered, the logistic regression was quite robust. One of these hospitals had a significantly higher complication rate and was added into the equation. Coefficients and odds ratios for the variables in Table 8.4 were changed only very slightly by the inclusion of this hospital.

Additional analyses found generally similar predictors of readmissions for complications after simple cholecystectomies and after more complex procedures (generally involving exploration of the common bile duct). Physician surgical experience was a statistically significant predictor in both cases. Finally, the predictions of readmission for complications after cholecystectomy were developed on one subsample and applied to a second. The rank order correlation coefficient decreased very little between the first and second subsamples;[50] physician experience continued to be important in this cross-validation.

Prostatectomy

Few of the available measures helped in predicting the probability of a complication following prostatectomy. Type of procedure was the most important predic-

---

*Although not presented in these tables, a variable constructed to separate acute from elective cholecystectomies also was a good predictor of probability of readmission. A combination of diagnoses, length of stay before surgery, and day of admission distinguished cases classified as acute versus those classified as elective when checks were made using detailed admission and discharge data.[48]

†Finally, Cox regression analyses[49] produced results very similar to those presented for logistic regression. Cox regression permits including available data on individuals lost to follow-up but assumes readmissions occurring later are "better" than those occurring earlier (since more time has passed since the surgery).

tor; men who underwent an open procedure had about half (0.60 times) the likelihood of a readmission due to complication as did those who had a transurethral resection. One prior history variable (frequency of physician visits involving chronic diagnoses) was also a statistically significant predictor in the bivariate analysis. These same two variables were the only ones significant in the various multiple logistic regressions (Table 8.5).

Physician Surgical Experience

Because overall hospital admission rates are higher in rural Manitoba, rural hospitals and physicians might be more likely to generate readmissions classified as complications; because rural location is correlated with surgical volume, perhaps the relationships are confounded. Several types of analysis addressed this problem. The zero-order analysis in Appendix 1a showed physician surgical experience to be a much stronger predictor of readmission for complications after cholecystectomy than was hospital location.

Using physical rather than statistical controls presents a more stringent test because of the smaller N available for analysis of specific subsamples. Multiple regressions were run separately both for Winnipeg and rural patients and for Winnipeg and rural hospitals. The major finding—the importance of physician surgical experience in predicting readmission for complications after cholecystectomy—held in all four analyses. These results also substantially control for hospital bed utilization as a possible factor confounding the analysis. Winnipeg patients have their surgery in, and are readmitted to, Winnipeg hospitals (which have uniformly high occupancy rates); thus, the importance of physician surgical experience for these individuals indicates that differential patient management in high- and low-occupancy-rate hospitals was not responsible for the findings.

Readmissions Not Due to Complications

In the process of identifying complications, readmissions not due to complications were noted in the patient histories for comparison with the complications data. For all three procedures, individual patient health status (reflected in prior hospitalizations, chronic diagnoses, etc.) would be expected to be much more important for predicting the probability of a readmission *not* due to complications than for predicting the probability of a readmission due to complications. Moreover, if particular hospital and physician variables are causally related to subsequent complications, these variables should be more strongly associated with the "readmission due to complications" variable than with the "readmission not due to complications" variable. Table 8.6 presents results from the multiple logistic regression predicting readmission *not* due to complications in the 2 years after cholecystectomy. The importance of patient health status emerges in this analysis; similar results were found for the other two procedures. The higher hospital readmission rate for rural patients is also seen in Table 8.6; a relatively weak relationship with hospital experience in performing cholecystectomies also appears. The physician surgical experience variable was not predictive of readmissions for reasons other than complications for any of the three procedures.

Two additional analyses were performed. Because of the possibility of a physician's "propensity to readmit" affecting readmission for complications, an index of this propensity was calculated for each permanent physician performing 15 or more cholecystectomies over the 3-year period. The measure was generated by dividing the number of a physician's patients readmitted for reasons other than complications by the number of cholecystectomies performed by the physician and multiplying by 100. Adding this "rate of readmission for reasons other than complications" independent variable, the multiple logistic regression for readmission for complications after cholecystectomy was rerun. There was no change in the significant variables presented in Table 8.4; "physician propensity to readmit" did not enter into the regression. Finally, when each physician's "rate of readmission for postcholecystectomy complications" (per 100 surgical patients) was correlated with the "rate of readmission for reasons other than complications," the correlations were statistically and substantively insignificant (product moment $r = -0.08$, $N = 230$ permanent physicians).

Given the limitation of not conducting a randomized clinical trial, but rather using routinely collected, population-based data, findings appear to be quite strong. Six lines of evidence beyond the multiple logistic regression supported the importance of physician surgical experience as a predictor of readmission for complications after cholecystectomy:

1. successful cross-validation of the importance of physician surgical experience as a predictor,
2. the relative strength of the zero-order correlation between physician surgical experience and readmission for complications versus that for hospital location and readmission for complications,
3. the separate analyses for Winnipeg and rural patients and for Winnipeg and rural hospitals,
4. the logistic regression analyses of readmission for reasons other than complications,
5. the lack of importance of a physician's "rate of readmission for reasons other than complications" as a predictor of a patient's readmission for complications,
6. the lack of correlation between a physician's "rate of readmission for complications" and "rate of readmission for reasons other than complications."

Volume-Outcome Relationships

Luft[51] has forwarded an alternative explanation for the observed volume-outcome relationships. Perhaps physician experience with cholecystectomy is not a critical cause of outcome, but rather an existing referral system channels more patients to the more capable providers. Some readily available data bear on this possibility.

A previous study[52] has shown that a number of newly arrived rural general practitioners were able to generate substantial surgical workloads in a relatively short time (1 or 2 years). This occurred regardless of the existing overall or procedure-specific surgical rate, i.e., a recently arrived physician might do a number of cholecystectomies in an area where a considerable volume was already being performed. If such newcomers' capabilities were being assessed by other physicians, such assessment must take place rather quickly.

Except for new physicians, year-to-year correlations in the number of cholecystectomies performed by each physician are high (between .90 and .95) in both Winnipeg and rural areas; this suggests that information about "the more capable" providers becomes diffused and acted upon slowly. Since specialty is not a strong predictor of probability of patient readmission for complications, the more capable physicians cannot be identified on the basis of training alone.

However, changes in the mean number of cholecystectomies performed annually by long-term permanent physicians (1972–1978) provided some support for the referral hypothesis. Although analysis was complicated by an overall drop in the number of cholecystectomies, data from three time periods (1972–1973, 1974–1976, and 1977–1978) showed the smallest decline in the number of cholecystectomies performed by physicians with considerable ongoing experience (averaging 20 or more cholecystectomies annually in 1974–1976). Their "mean number performed" went from 59 in 1972 to 41 in 1978. Physicians averaging six or more such operations in 1974–1976 (N = 87) showed a drop in their "mean number performed" from 10.0 in 1972 to 4.8 in 1978. The decline was even greater proportionally for those operating occasionally (five or fewer annually in 1974–1976); the annual average went from 2.1 in 1972 to 0.4 in 1978 (N = 69). This smallest proportional drop in the cholecystectomies performed by experienced physicians might suggest operation of a referral system sensitive to physician experience.

DISCUSSION

The three procedures differ markedly in the ease of prediction of the probability of complications. A perusal of the rank order correlation coefficients[47] under Tables 8.3, 8.4, and 8.5 shows that the predictors worked quite well for cholecystectomy, somewhat less well for hysterectomy, and not well at all for prostatectomy. The three procedures also differ in the predictive importance of patient, hospital, and physician variables. After controlling for important patient variables, physician surgical experience was found to account for relatively large differences (almost two to one) in the probability of patient complications following cholecystectomy. Physician surgical experience was only a marginally significant predictor for hysterectomy; because of the intercorrelations among different predictors, no single variable or policy suggestion stands out. As noted earlier, a great majority of the physicians performing prostatectomy did more than 50 procedures annually; surgical volume was neither substantively nor statistically significant in predicting complications following prostatectomy. Various possible biases were brought up and eliminated.

This paper is innovative in using claims to provide detailed data on both covariates and outcomes. Approaching case mix in this way can be particularly persuasive when put into a substantive context. In this study, an inadequate adjustment for case mix would have confounded the overall results only if physicians with relatively few cases performed cholecystectomies on sicker patients.[53] The population-based Manitoba data and attention to reliability make it highly unlikely that these results are due to methodologic artifacts. Such data help improve researchers' ability to make interhospital comparisons, but the accuracy of routinely collected hospital data must be checked in other sites.[3]

Work has also been directed toward examining the results when less complete information is available. Because hospital claims are more accessible to researchers elsewhere, the Manitoba analysis has been duplicated using only hospital claims; results were very similar to those presented here using both hospital and medical claims. In similar fashion, because sensitivity, specificity, and predictive values have been shown to be high when readmissions for complications generated by computer algorithms were compared with those generated by physician panels,[5] results using these algorithm-based readmissions for complications after hysterectomy, cholecystectomy, and prostatectomy generated regression findings highly similar to those (based on physician panels) presented in this paper.

The frequencies of hysterectomy, cholecystectomy, and prostatectomy in North America are such that efforts to reduce associated complications are worthwhile. Because Manitoba's surgical rates are generally near the Canadian median, while overall readmission rates for complications for the three procedures compare favorably with those reported in the literature,[54-56] these findings suggest the appropriateness of parallel research in other political jurisdictions.

Such research is highly relevant to concerns about where procedures should be done, who should do them, and how they should be evaluated.[57] As recommended by Wennberg,[24] the paper adopts a procedure-by-procedure approach to looking at outcomes. At the same time, studying several operations simultaneously highlights where efforts at quality assurance might be directed. The importance of the individual physician's surgical experience in predicting complications after cholecystectomy, rather than surgical volume of the hospital, raises questions as to when centralization is an effective strategy for improving outcomes.

Cholecystectomy might be a candidate for certification because of the epidemiology of the operation: as of the mid-1970s, a substantial proportion of the cholecystectomies were being performed by physicians with comparatively little ongoing experience with this type of procedure. Thirty-six percent of the gallbladder operations were performed by Manitoba physicians averaging fewer than 20 such procedures annually; in contrast, only 13% of the prostatectomies were done by Manitoba physicians performing fewer than 50 such procedures. Another characteristic of biliary tract surgery calls attention to the operation. A procedure that starts out as a simple cholecystectomy may unexpectedly involve exploration of the common bile duct, adding considerable risk to the surgery and suggesting the need for an experienced surgeon.

The term certification usually refers to "board-certified," i.e., passing final specialty examinations. However, with regard to cholecystectomy, the variable using the dichotomy between board-certified specialist and general practitioner was not a significant predictor of readmission due to complications (crude odds ratio of 1.17, adjusted odds ratio of 0.79). Such findings suggest that, to be effective, certification would have to be directed toward strongly encouraging physicians without sufficient ongoing experience *not* to perform cholecystectomies. Such an extension of the certification concept would raise issues of access to surgery in some rural areas and necessitate considerable planning for allowing new practitioners to acquire the necessary experience.

Assessing the performance of individual hospitals raises a different set of issues. Direct monitoring has been proposed with regard to surgical rates,[58] and the computer technology to do this is becoming available. Monitoring would be complicated by any systematic biases in information reported across hospitals. Although comparisons of Manitoba hospital claims with hospital medical records have found little indication of inaccurate reporting, using these data explicitly for monitoring would increase this possibility. Encouraging overly long stays or placing administrative barriers in the way of readmission would obviously be perverse consequences of any strategy. Since length of stay is a measure widely monitored in current American systems based on diagnosis-related groups (DRGs), such changes could certainly be spotted.

Although the tactic of curtailing hospital admissions could be picked up in insurance systems that track ambulatory claims, application of the techniques described here should not be so heavy-handed as to force such behavior. Indeed, a focus on readmissions may well be a healthy counterbalance to DRG systems, which provide an incentive for doctors to increase the volume of hospitalization.[59] In the American context, Bunker and Fowles[3] have stressed that "if the goal of prospective payment is to provide incentives for cost-effective medical care—including fewer costly complications—the reimbursement per episode of care formula should logically include all complications, including readmissions."

This study has found that individual hospitals with particularly poor (and particularly good) records regarding postsurgical problems could be identified after controlling for a range of other variables. It is becoming increasingly possible to computerize the coding of complications and focus on individual hospitals that appear to have either superior or inferior outcomes.[5] Bunker and Fowles[3] have noted that American medical insurers might identify providers with particularly good outcomes and offer to their subscribers policies with economic incentives to patronize those "preferred providers." Such activity is highly relevant to the American Peer Review Organizations, which are oriented toward reducing readmissions, "unnecessary" admissions or invasive procedures, and "avoidable" mortality and morbidity.[60,61]

Somewhat different regulatory strategies are suggested by centralization, certification, and monitoring. Centralization and certification pose difficulties by imposing a uniform policy—even upon providers whose work is relatively problem-free—according to outcomes associated with the group to which they belong. These approaches may prove to be less palatable than a monitoring strategy that identifies particular hospitals for attention directed toward a specific problem. Monitoring could greatly improve the efficiency of standards committees by providing them with a focus and a list of cases for further investigation. Such an approach does concentrate on the larger hospitals, those performing enough procedures of a given type to meet the criteria for analysis at the individual hospital level. However, as Luft[11] has pointed out, many hospitals elsewhere in North America host more operations than do the larger Manitoba institutions; the research possibilities are substantial.

Use of a smaller N, aggregating more years, and adopting less stringent statistical criteria for identifying particular hospitals would all tend to "cast the net wider." Such approaches might well be justified in situations oriented specifically toward providing constructive input for standards committees. Along similar lines, in summarizing the National Halothane Study's findings of differences among hospitals in postoperative mortality rates, Moses and Mosteller[62] suggest that quiet, cooperatively-oriented efforts are required. More recent findings indicating substantial interinstitutional differences in mortality confirm the importance of paying attention to such differences.[33,63,64]

In Manitoba, the recent development of regional surgical centers has brought surgical specialists to several of the larger hospitals classified as "rural" (actually located in towns). These centers have tended to draw surgical activity away from smaller hospitals and, when compared with data from the mid-1970s, provide a "natural experiment" in regionalization. Over the next year we will be comparing data from the 1980s with those presented in this paper. This should permit better analysis of a number of questions recently raised regarding regionalization.[65]

Whatever the approach, discouraging certain physicians or hospitals from performing particular procedures is likely to be controversial if implemented by hospitals, insurers, or regulatory authorities. Although some notable successes have been reported,[66] educators disagree markedly as to the likely efficacy of efforts at feedback to individual institutions or providers.[24,67] Because of the overall frequency with which the common surgical procedures are performed, the choice of strategies for approaching quality-of-care issues has substantial implications for hospitals, physicians, and patients. Claims data from a well-defined population can help inform policy matters with regard to the three interrelated issues of centralization, certification, and monitoring.

Appendix 8.1a: Variables Assessed for Crude Association with Readmission for Complications following Hysterectomy

	Number of Operations	Number Readmitted for Complications	% Complications	Crude Odds	P
A. Patient Covariates					
Age: (20–39)	1222	55	4.5		
40–49	1818	76	4.2	0.93	0.670
50 +	1455	68	4.7	1.04	0.832
Residence: (Winnipeg)	2917	113	3.9		
Rural	1578	86	5.5	1.43	0.014
B. "Event" Variables					
Type of surgery:					
(Abdominal hysterectomy)	3203	128	4.0		
Vaginal hysterectomy	1155	67	5.8	1.48	0.011
Duration of operation—units of anesthetic: (<8)	2446	108	4.4		
8 +	2049	91	4.4	1.01	0.97
Multiple diagnoses: (No)	365	9	2.5		
Yes	4130	190	4.6	1.91	0.057
C. Medical History During 2 Years Prior to Surgery					
Hospital admissions: (No)	2750	104	3.8		
Yes	1745	95	5.4	1.46	0.008
Physician visits with					
a. Chronic diagnoses: (<10)	2262	84	3.7		
10 +	2233	115	5.2	1.41	0.019
b. Heart disease: (No)	4321	186	4.3		
Yes	174	13	7.5	1.80	0.047

Continued

Appendix 8.1a: Continued

	Number of Operations	Number Readmitted for Complications	% Complications	Crude Odds	P
D. Hospital Characteristics					
Type of hospital:					
(Winnipeg teaching)	1905	75	3.9		
Winnipeg nonteaching	1650	70	4.2	1.08	0.646
Rural	940	54	5.7	1.49	0.029
Number of hysterectomies at hospital per year: (100+)	3709	153	4.1		
<100	786	46	5.9	1.44	0.033
E. Surgeon Characteristics					
Specialty: (Gynecologist)	3505	144	4.1		
General surgeon	482	28	5.8	1.44	0.085
G.P.	465	26	5.6	1.38	0.138
Number of hysterectomies performed per year: (20+)	3082	123	4.0		
<20	1413	76	5.4	1.37	0.036

Appendix 8.1b: Variables Assessed for Crude Association with Readmission for Complications following Cholecystectomy

	Number of Operations	Number Readmitted for Complications	% Complications	Crude Odds	P
A. Patient Covariates					
Age: (20–44)	2452	46	1.9		
45–59	2427	71	2.9	1.57	0.017
60+	2277	106	4.7	2.55	0.0001
Sex: (Female)	5079	126	2.5		
Male	2077	97	4.7	1.93	0.0001
Residence: (Winnipeg)	4388	116	2.6		
Rural	2768	107	3.9	1.48	0.004
B. "Event" Variables					
Type of surgery:					
(Simple cholecystectomy)	6232	142	2.3		
More complex surgery	791	66	8.3	3.90	0.0001
Duration of operation—units of anesthetic: (<7)	3985	87	2.2		
7+	3065	131	4.3	2.00	0.0001
Multiple diagnoses: (No)	4696	128	2.7		
Yes	2460	95	3.9	1.43	0.009
C. Medical History During 2 Years Prior to Surgery					
Hospital admissions: (No)	4184	102	2.4		
Yes	2972	121	4.1	1.70	0.0001
Physician visits with					
a. Chronic diagnoses: (<8)	3512	96	2.7		
8+	3644	127	3.5	1.28	0.067
b. Heart disease: (No)	6358	190	3.0		
Yes	798	33	4.1	1.61	0.079

Continued

Appendix 8.1b: Continued

	Number of Operations	Number Readmitted for Complications	% Complications	Crude Odds	P
D. Hospital Characteristics Type of hospital:					
(Winnipeg teaching)	1885	58	3.1		
Winnipeg nonteaching	3321	89	2.7	0.87	0.406
Rural	1950	76	3.9	1.28	0.167
Number of cholecystectomies at hospital per year: (100+)	5722	170	3.0		
<100	1434	53	3.7	1.25	0.158
E. Surgeon Characteristics Specialty: (Non-G.P.)	5846	177	3.0		
G.P.	1310	46	3.5	1.17	0.362
Number of cholecystectomies performed per year: (20+)	5292	138	2.6		
<20	1864	85	4.6	1.78	0.0001

Appendix 8.1c: Variables Assessed for Crude Association with Readmission for Complications following Prostatectomy

	Number of Operations	Number Readmitted for Complications	% Complications	Crude Odds	P
A. Patient Covariates					
Age: (<65)	754	72	9.6		
65–74	1118	106	9.5	0.99	0.961
75+	938	90	9.6	1.01	0.975
Residence: (Winnipeg)	1675	156	9.3		
Rural	1135	112	9.9	1.07	0.623
B. "Event" Variables					
Type of surgery:					
(TUR)	1767	195	11.0		
Open prostatectomy	990	69	7.0	0.60	0.0005
Duration of operation—units of anesthetic: (<6)	1620	161	9.9		
6+	1151	59	8.6	0.85	0.234
Multiple diagnoses: (No)	889	80	9.0		
Yes	1921	188	9.8	1.10	0.509
C. Medical History During 2 Years Prior to Surgery					
Hospital admissions: (No)	1684	155	9.2		
Yes	1126	113	10.0	1.10	0.462
Physician visits with					
a. Chronic diagnoses: (<9)	1440	121	8.4		
9+	1370	147	10.7	1.31	0.036
b. Heart disease: (No)	1920	170	8.9		
Yes	890	98	11.0	1.27	0.070

Continued

Appendix 8.1c: Continued

	Number of Operations	Number Readmitted for Complications	% Complications	Crude Odds	P
D. Hospital Characteristics					
Type of hospital:					
(Winnipeg teaching)	1188	108	9.1		
Winnipeg nonteaching	1230	125	10.2	1.13	0.372
Rural	392	35	8.9	0.98	0.923
Number of prostatectomies at hospital per year: (100+)	2320	224	9.7		
<100	490	44	9.0	0.92	0.644
E. Surgeon Characteristics					
Specialty: (Urologist)	2713	263	9.7		
Other	97	5	5.2	0.51	0.135
Number of prostatectomies performed per year: (50+)	2450	236	9.6		
<50	360	32	8.9	0.92	0.654

APPENDIX 8.2: MEASURES USED

Identifying Complications

For each surgical procedure, a large number of readmissions that might possibly be complications were identified from the MHSC hospital claims on the basis of ICD-8-coded discharge diagnoses and operative procedures (if any) performed; for example, 158 readmissions that might have represented complications were noted following 1973 hysterectomies. These "possibles" represented approximately 80% more cases than were eventually chosen. These "possibles" were identified on the basis of liberally interpreted guidelines from the literature and consensus conferences.[68-70]

Abbreviated histories based on these claims data were presented to two specialists who independently judged whether or not the readmissions were due to complications. These specialists did not know which physician performed the surgery or where the operation was done. When more information was requested by the physicians, admission/separation forms filed by the hospitals with the Manitoba Health Services Commission were obtained to provide these data. The physicians then met to resolve the differences and decide on those readmissions that could be categorized as definite complications. (With regard to hysterectomy, readmissions for psychologic problems and for such other problems as repair procedures associated with incontinence, rectocele, or cystocele following an abdominal hysterectomy were not considered complications of surgery by the physicians.)

We assessed the interphysician reliability in coding complications.[5] In general, reliability checks using the Manitoba data have approximated results obtained in clinical trials.[35] Comparing initial independent ratings as to whether or not a readmission was a complication characteristically generated kappa values between 0.4 and 0.6. This measure corrects for the possibility of chance agreement and kappas between 0.4 and 0.6 are generally seen as acceptable.[71] One physician coded the same set of cholecystectomy complications twice several months apart; this "test–retest" kappa was 0.74.

Disagreements concerning the coding of readmissions as complications following hysterectomy were most marked for adhesions, both with and without obstruction. One physician coded all such adhesions as complications, the other thought the majority of them should not be seen as complications. The most significant disagreements about complications after cholecystectomy concerned pancreatitis (both acute and chronic), recurrent ventral hernia, and postoperative wound infection. Questions of timing were significant for disagreements between physicians concerning complications following prostatectomy. The major disagreement was whether or not orchitis and epididymitis should be considered complications if they occurred more than a month after surgery.

After coding the complications independently, each pair of physicians met to resolve differences. When compared with the initial independent ratings, the final decisions by the two physicians produced kappas in the 0.7–0.8 range. Only complications finally agreed upon by both physicians were retained in our analysis.

Case-Mix Covariates

The availability of hospital and medical claims information for the 2 years before surgery permitted generating several diagnosis-related indices. The number of indices was reduced by choosing just one index when two or more were substantively intercorrelated. Various indicators of hospital utilization were substantially intercorrelated; the measure selected was simply "whether or not admitted to hospital in the two years previous." Two indices were derived from claims associated with ambulatory visits: a chronic disease index based on a list of conditions derived from the United States National Health Survey 1969– 1971;[72] diagnostic codes not classified on the survey were reviewed by a physician panel and classified as chronic or acute; the NAMCS index of seriousness developed from the matching of diagnosis and seriousness provided by physicians on the National Ambulatory Medical Care Survey.[36] Medical claims associated with hospital visits were not included because they, in large part, duplicate information on the hospital claim. The two indices were intercorrelated and the chronic disease index was selected. Finally, a measure taken off the hospital claim from the surgical admission—comorbidity as indicated by multiple diagnoses—was essentially uncorrelated with the variables derived from hospital and medical claims accumulated over the previous 2 years. Considerable experimentation with both bivariate and multivariate analyses showed little information to be lost by eliminating predictors that were substantially correlated with others included in the analysis.

APPENDIX 8.3: RELIABILITY AND VALIDITY OF CLAIMS DATA

Previous analysis of the Manitoba claims data compared hysterectomies billed for by surgeons with those recorded in the hospital file. Ninety-four percent of the records showed an identical match: e.g., when an abdominal hysterectomy was recorded in the hospital discharge, the surgeon billed for this procedure. Discrepancies were frequently due to minor differences in dates or to the surgeon billing for a more extensive procedure associated with an abdominal malignancy; in this latter case, the hysterectomy was secondary. In these cases, the more extensive procedure was also recorded in the hospital claim. Cholecystectomy and prostatectomy results were generally similar.

Diagnoses on the hospital claims have corresponded closely with those on the hospital medical record. A set of checks using MHSC data and records from on Winnipeg hospital found 95% (37 out of 39) of diagnoses for gallbladder patients to be identical. Similar high levels of agreement were noted for serious coronary problems diagnosed in four Winnipeg and four rural hospitals.[35]

The admission and separation forms submitted by the hospitals to the Manitoba Health Services Commission contain the written diagnostic data prior to ICDA coding. This was used to help resolve the more difficult cases and provide information requested by members of the physician panels. Coding error seems minimal. The work on cholecystectomies mentioned above found two coding errors (digits transposed) among the diagnoses. Analysis of admissions and separations forms used to resolve questions in the coding of complications after prostatectomy showed complete agreement between written diagnosis and those coded on 35 out of 36 forms. The 36th form indicated a minor discrepancy vis-a-vis one of the three diagnoses coded.

Although a previous study of medical record coding among patients with myocardial infarction indicated that a few secondary and tertiary diagnoses on the hospital claims may not agree completely with the medical records, several lines of evidence suggest that few complications are missed by the methods discussed in this paper. We independently coded admission/separation forms for 50 cholecystectomies. A number of these forms had multiple diagnoses (18 had two and 10 had three diagnoses). In two instances, a fourth diagnosis might have been added, but only three diagnoses were permitted on the hospital claim.

Few additional complications are produced from the second and third diagnoses of the 232 complications after hysterectomy identified by both the computerized algorithms and the physician panels; 214 (92%) were generated from primary diagnoses. Of the postcholecystectomy complications, 218 out of 238 were from the primary diagnoses. Equivalent figures for prostatectomy were 245 out of 266 (92%). Because relatively few complications are identified from the second and third diagnoses, possible differences among providers in the number of diagnoses reported are relatively unimportant.

Although the recording of diagnoses is generally most reliable when fine distinctions are not made,[35,73] a number of four-digit ICDA codes on the hospital file were used to identify appropriate diagnoses leading to readmissions. When only three-digit ICDA codes were used in the hysterectomy analysis, decisions were changed very slightly. A more detailed analysis comparing physician decisions as to complications with decisions using computerized algorithms is presented in Roos et al.[5]

ACKNOWLEDGMENTS

The authors gratefully acknowledge the help of the Manitoba Health Services Commission with this research. Drs. Marsha Cohen, Joel Kettner, Arthur Majury, John McBeath, James Mitchell, and Ernest Ramsey generously contributed their time to the coding of complications. Interpretations and viewpoints contained in this paper are the authors' own and do not necessarily represent the opinion of either the Manitoba Health Services Commission or Health and Welfare, Canada. Earlier versions of this paper benefited from comments made at the National Bureau of Economic Research "Conference of Productivity in Health," Stanford, California, August 1983, and at the Royal College of Physicians and Surgeons of Canada meetings, Calgary, Alberta, September 1983.

REFERENCES

1. Bunker JP, Barnes BA, Mosteller F, et al. Summary, conclusions, and recommendations. In: Bunker JP, Barnes BA, Mosteller F (eds): Costs, Risks, and Benefits of Surgery. New York: Oxford University Press, 1977.
2. Moore FD. Scientific salients in surgery. Can J Surg 1979; 22:339.
3. Bunker JP, Fowles J. Medical audit by claims data? Am J Pub Health 1985; 75:1261.
4. Lohr KN, Lohr WR, Brook RH. Understanding variations in the use of services: are there clinical explanations? Health Affairs 1984; 3(2):139.
5. Roos LL, Cageorge SM, Austen E. et al. Using computers to identify complications after surgery. Am J Pub Health 1985; 75:1288.
6. Adams DF, Fraser DB, Abrams HL. The complications of coronary arteriography. Circulation 1973; 48:609.
7. Luft HS, Bunker JP, Enthoven AC. Should operations be regionalized? The empirical relation between surgical volume and mortality. N Engl J Med 1979;301:1364.
8. Flood AB, Scott WR, Ewy W. Does practice make perfect? I. The relation between hospital volume and outcomes for selected diagnostic categories. Med Care 1984; 22:98.
9. Flood AB, Scott WR, Ewy, W. Does practice make perfect? II. The relation between volume and outcomes and other hospital characteristics. Med Care 1984;22:115.
10. Farber BF, Kaiser DL, Wenzel R. Relation between surgical volume and incidence of postoperative wound infection. N Engl J Med 1981;305:200.
11. Luft HS. Regionalization in medical care. Am J Pub Health 1985;75:125.
12. Crile G. How to keep down the risk and cost of surgery. Inquiry 1981;18:99.
13. Verjaal M, Leshot NJ, Treffers PE. Risk of amniocentesis and laboratory findings in a series of 1500 prenatal diagnoses. Prenatal Diagnosis 1981;1:173.
14. Nickerson RJ, Colton T, Peterson OL, et al. Doctors who perform operations: a study on inhospital surgery in four diverse geographic areas. N Engl J Med 1976;295:921, 982.
15. Couch NP, Tilney NL, Rayner AA, et al. The high cost of low-frequency events: the anatomy and economics of surgical mishaps. N Engl J Med 1981;304:634.
16. Moore FD, Nickerson RJ, Colton T, et al. National surgical work patterns as a basis for residency training plans. Arch Surg 1977;296:921.
17. Folse R, D'Elia G, Birtch AG, et al. Surgical manpower and practice patterns in a nonmetropolitan area. Surgery 1980;87:95.
18. Cageorge SM, Roos LL. When surgical rates change: workload and turnover in Manitoba, 1974–1978. Med Care 1984;22:890.
19. Cageorge, SM, Roos LL, Danzinger RG. Gallbladder operations: a population based analysis. Med Care 1981;19:510.
20. Scott WR, Forest WH, Brown BW, Hospital structure and postoperative mortality and morbidity. In: Shortell SM, Brown M (eds). Organizational Research in Hospitals, Chicago: Blue Cross Association, 1976.
21. Roos LL. Alternative designs to study outcomes: the tonsillectomy case. Med Care 1979;17:1069.
22. Gallbladder Survey Committee. Hysterectomies in Ohio: results of a survey in Ohio hospitals by the Gallbladder Committee, Ohio Chapter, American College of Surgeons. Am J Surg 1970;119:714.

23. Mainen NW. The surgical role of family physicians. Am J Pub Health 1982;72:1359.
24. Wennberg JE. Dealing with medical practice variations: a proposal for action. Health Affairs 1984;3(2):6.
25. Leventhal ML, Lazarus ML. Total abdominal and vaginal hysterectomy, a comparison. Am J Obstet Gynecol 1951;61:289.
26. Hall WL, Sobel IA, Jones CP, et al. Anaerobic postoperative pelvic infections. Obstet Gynecol 1967;30:1.
27. Shapiro M, Munoz A, Tager IB, et al. Risk factors for infection at the operative site after abdominal or vaginal hysterectomy. N Engl J Med 1982;307:1661.
28. Horn SD, Sharkey PD, Bertram DA. Measuring severity of illness: homogeneous case mix groups. Med Care 1983;21:14.
29. Avery AD, Leah T, Solomon NE, et al. Quality of medical care assessment using outcome measures: Eight disease specific applications. Santa Monica, CA:The Rand Corporation, 1976.
30. Ziffren SE. Comparison of mortality rates for various surgical operations according to age groups, 1951–1977. J Am Geriatr Soc 1979;27:433.
31. Chilton CP, Morgan RJ, England HR, et al. A critical evaluation of the results of transurethral resection of the prostate. Br J Urol 1978;50:542.
32. Melchior J, Valk WL, Foret JD, et al. Transurethral prostatectomy: computerized analysis of 2223 consecutive cases. J Urol 1974;112:634.
33. Wennberg JE, Roos NP, Sola L, et al. Use of claims data systems to evaluate health care outcomes: mortality and reoperation following prostatectomy. JAMA 1987; 257: 933–36.
34. Roos LL, Nicol JP, Johnson C, et al. Using administrative data banks for research and evaluation: a case study. Eval Q 1979;3:236.
35. Roos LL, Roos NP, Cageorge SM, et al. How good are the data? Reliability of one health care data bank. Med Care 1982;20:266.
36. Roos NP. Impact of the organization of practice on quality of care and physician productivity. Med Care 1980;18:347.
37. Webb EJ, Campbell DT, Schwartz RD, et al. Nonreactive Measures in the Social Sciences. Boston: Houghton Mifflin, 1981.
38. Keys A. Seven Countries: A Multivariate Analysis of Death and Coronary Heart Disease. Cambridge, MA: Harvard University Press, 1980.
39. Roos LL. Surgical rates and mortality: a correlational analysis. Med Care 1984;22:586.
40. Roos, LL, Nicol JP, Roos NP. Using large-scale data banks—productivity and quality control. In: Bennett EM, Trute B (eds). Mental Health Information Systems: Problems and Prospects. New York: Edwin Mellen Press, 1984;81–98.
41. Anderson, GF, Steinberg EP. Hospital readmissions in the Medicare population. N Engl J Med 1984;311:1349.
42. Mossey JM, Roos LL. Using claims to measure health status: the illness scale. J Chronic Dis 1987;40:415.
43. Shapiro E, Roos LL. Using health care: rural/urban differences among the Manitoba elderly. Gerontologist 1984;24:270.
44. McNeil BJ, Hanley JA. Statistical approaches to clinical predictions. N Engl J Med 1981;304:1292.
45. Flood AB, Scott WR. Professional power and professional effectiveness: the power of the surgical staff and the quality of surgical care in hospitals. J Health Soc Behav 1978;19:240.
46. Flood AB. Hospital organization and outcomes of care. In: Hirsh RA, Forrest WH, Orkin FK, et al. (eds). Health Care Delivery in Anesthesia. Philadelphia: George F. Stickley, 1980;105–118.

47. SAS Institute. SUGI Supplemental Library's User's Guide. Cary, NC: SAS Institute, 1983.
48. Roos NP, Danzinger RG. Assessing surgical risks in a population: patient histories before and after cholecystectomy. Soc Sci Med 1986;22:571.
49. Cox DR. Regression models and life tables (with discussion). J Stat Soc B 1972;34:187.
50. Mosteller F, Tukey JW. Data Analysis and Regression. Reading, MA: Addison-Wesley, 1977.
51. Luft HS. The relation between surgical volume and mortality: an exploration of causal factors and alternative models. Med Care 1980;18:940.
52. Roos LL. Supply, workload and utilization: a population-based analysis of surgery. Am J Pub Health 1983;73:414.
53. Bunker JP, Roos LL, Fowles J, et al. Information systems and routine monitoring in the United States and Canada—with examples from surgical practice. In: Holland WW, Detels R, Know G (eds). Oxford Textbook of Public Health, Volume 3: Investigative Methods in Public Health. New York: Oxford University Press, 1985;77–86.
54. Mindell WR, Vayda E, Cardillo B. Ten year trends in Canada for selected operations. Can Med Assoc J 1983;127:23.
55. Roos NP. Hysterectomies in one Canadian province: a new look at risks and benefits. Am J Public Health 1984;74:39.
56. Fitzpatrick G, Neutra R, Gilbert JP. Cost-effectiveness of cholecystectomy for silent gallstones. In: Bunker JP, Barnes BA, Mosteller F (eds): Costs, Risks, and Benefits or Surgery. New York: Oxford University Press, 1977;246–261.
57. Bunker JP, Luft HS, Enthoven AC. Should surgery be regionalized? Surg Clin North Am 1982;63:685.
58. Gleicher N. Cesarean section rates in the United States: the short-term failure of the National Consensus Development Conference in 1980. JAMA 1984;252:3273.
59. Stern RS, Epstein AM. Institutional responses to prospective payment based on diagnosis-related groups: implications for cost, quality, and access. N Engl J Med 1985;312:621.
60. Lohr KN, Brook RH. Quality assurance in medicine. Am Behav Scientist 1984;27:583.
61. Dans PE, Weiner JP, Otter SE. Peer review organizations: promises and potential pitfalls. N Engl J Med 1985;313:1131.
62. Moses LE, Mosteller F. Institutional differences in postoperative death rates: commentary on some of the findings of th National Halothane Study. JAMA 1968;203:492.
63. Kennedy JW, Kaiser GC, Fisher LD, et al. Multivariate discriminate analysis of the clinical and angiographic predictors of operative mortality from the Collaborative Study in Coronary Artery Surgery (CASS). J Thorac Cardiovasc Surg 1980;80:876.
64. Knaus WA, Draper EA, Wagoner DP, et al. An evaluation of outcome for intensive care from major medical centers. Ann Intern Med 1986;104:410.
65. Maerki SC, Luft HS, Hunt SS. Selecting categories of patients for regionalization: implications of the relationship between volume and outcome. Med Care 1986;24:148.
66. Dyck FJ, Murphy FA, Murphy JK, et al. Effect of surveillance on the number of hysterectomies in the province of Saskatchewan. N Engl J Med 1977;296:1326.
67. Schroeder SA. ReViews: a medical educator. Health Affairs 1984;3(2):55.
68. Levinson CJ. Hysterectomy complications. Clin Obstet Gynecol 1972;15:802.
69. Jenkins VR. Unnecessary—elective—indicated? Audit criteria of the American College of Obstetricians and Gynecologists to assess abdominal hysterectomy for uterine leiomyoma. Quality Rev Bull 1977;3:7.

70. Brook RH, Lohr KN, Chassin M, et al. Geographic variations in the use of services: do they have any clinical significance? Health Affairs 1984;3(2):63.
71. Fleiss JL. Statistical Methods for Rates and Proportions. New York: John Wiley & Sons, 1981.
72. US Department of Health, Education and Welfare. Prevalence of selected chronic respiratory conditions, United States—1970. Vital and Health Statistics, Series 10, No. 84, DHEW Publication No. (HRA) 74-1511. Rockville, MD: National Center for Health Statistics, 1973.
73. Demlo LK, Campbell PM. Improving hospital discharge data: lessons from the National Hospital Discharge Survey. Med Care 1981;19:1030.

Chapter 9

Nonmortality Outcomes

Farber, Kaiser, and Wenzel explored the use of a statewide infection-surveillance program to assess wound infection, a relatively common adverse outcome of surgery. Although the pathogenesis of wound infection is multifactorial, it is likely to be determined at least in part by surgical skill, technique, and postoperative management. Because postoperative infection is relatively common compared to death for most types of surgery, it may be a more sensitive indicator of quality of hospital care.

Fortunately, death is a relatively rare outcome of most surgical care. For certain elective operations, the risk of death is so small that its use as an outcome indicator is limited. It is also self-evident that some adverse outcomes of health care do not result in death: wound infection, nosocomial (hospital-acquired) infections, amputation, poorly fitting prostheses, or permanent disfigurement. Measurement of more common outcomes would increase the statistical sensitivity of any research and might provide a more useful indicator of hospital quality.

This study takes the most direct approach to assessment of nonmortality outcomes. A surveillance program designed specifically to detect hospital infections was used to count wound infections in selected surgical patients. Other researchers have used data from hospital discharge abstracts to assess nonmortality outcomes. Hughes, Hunt and Luft (1987) and Showstack and his colleagues (1987) identified patients with a hospital stay greater than the 90th percentile as poor-outcome patients.[1] Although it makes sense that patients who suffer from complications usually stay longer in the hospital, it is not known whether the converse is true (or whether the patients stayed for other reasons). Other factors, such as difficulty in obtaining a nursing home placement, may be more important in determining the length of hospital stay. Another approach, using readmissions or number of related visits per year as adverse outcomes, was taken by Roos and his colleagues (1986) using a comprehensive claims data base in Manitoba, Canada.[2]

The strength of Farber, Kaiser, and Wenzel's approach is that the outcome measure may be more directly attributable to a specific process of care. A higher wound-infection rate may result from inadequate sterile techniques and conditions in the operating room, which could be specifically addressed in programs to improve the quality of medical care. It is easy to see how this approach could be used to identify specific hospitals with worse-than-expected results; it could also identify patterns related to volume. For example, the nursing staff in high-volume hospitals may be more adept at detecting complications while they are still minor, thus helping to avoid the more serious ones.

There are two problems with this approach: differences in reporting, and sample size limitations. All the hospitals in this study used the same surveillance system with a standardized training program. The authors tested for bias in reporting rates with respect to hospital size and found that no differences existed. Similar tests should be done in other surveillance systems, including those relying on routinely collected data. The sample in this study was limited to 22 selected hospitals and thus is of limited generalizability. One usually faces a trade-off between obtaining relatively superficial data from many hospitals or in-depth data from fewer sites.

NOTES

1. See Hughes, Hunt, and Luft (1987), reprinted in Chapter 17 of this volume, and Showstack et al. (1987), reprinted in Chapter 11 of this volume.
2. See reprint of Roos et al. (1986) in Chapter 8 of this volume.

Relation between Surgical Volume and Incidence of Postoperative Wound Infection

Bruce F. Farber
Donald L. Kaiser
Richard P. Wenzel

Postoperative wound infections account for 20 percent of all nosocomial infections[1] and occur at a rate of 81 per 10,000 patients hospitalized.[2] Their presence adds additional morbidity and expense to those expected from otherwise uncomplicated operations.[3] Unfortunately, the pathogenesis of these infections is complex and poorly understood. Exogenous microbial contamination resulting in infection seems to occur in the immediate operative period and is likely to reflect general operating-room technique.[4] Thus, improvement in surgical skill with experience might result in a reduction in rates of postoperative wound infection.

Recently, Luft and his colleagues demonstrated an excess mortality in patients undergoing certain complex surgical procedures in hospitals with a low volume of surgery.[5] We sought to examine the relation between rates of postoperative wound infection and volume of surgery. Using data generated by the Virginia Statewide Infection Control Program,[6] we selected for study seven surgical procedures performed at 22 community hospitals, and the data generated are the subject of this report.

METHODS

Hospitals

Of the 22 community hospitals providing data for this study, 19 were in Virginia and three in nearby states primarily served patients from Virginia. They were selected because of the regularity of their reporting to the statewide surveillance system. The hospitals were widely distributed and were divided into the following categories: six hospitals with fewer than 100 beds, nine with 100 to 300 beds, and seven with more than 300 beds. The study period extended from January 1, 1977, through May 31, 1979.

Reprinted from *The New England Journal of Medicine* 305, no. 4 (1981): 200–204, with permission from the Massachusetts Medical Society.

Supported by a grant (5-30160) from the Virginia Statewide Nosocomial Infection Control Program and an Infectious Diseases Training Grant (1-T32 AI 07046) from the National Institutes of Health.

Surveillance

Infection rates were obtained prospectively by practitioners with standardized training in infection control. Each hospital had its own infection-control practitioner or practitioners. The surveillance system used has been described previously.[7] It began with a review of the nursing-care plan (Kardex) of every patient on the ward. Admission date, diagnoses, and dates of commonly performed procedures and all operations were noted by the practitioner. Charts of patients remaining in the hospital for more than 48 hours after surgery were reviewed. Monthly reports from participating hospitals were sent to the University of Virginia. With use of supplementary surveillance this system has been demonstrated to have a 69 percent sensitivity and 99 percent specificity in identifying infection.[6]

Wound infection was defined as the presence of pus at the incision site. The number of operations was obtained monthly from operating-room logbooks by the practitioners in infection control.

Reporting Frequency

There was a maximum period of 29 months during which any participating hospital could have reported its data. The overall reporting frequency (75 percent) was calculated by adding up all the monthly reports submitted and dividing this total by the total number of possible months. The latter was calculated for each hospital from the first month in the year when the hospital sent in a report until the end of the study period. It should be noted that not every hospital joined the program at the beginning of the study period. A maximum of 154 infection rates (22 hospitals times seven operations) could be studied; 147 of these rates were available for analysis and seven were unavailable, either because the operation was not performed at that hospital or because sufficient data were not available. Five of these seven rates were in the hospitals with fewer than 100 beds, and one each was in the 100 to 300-bed group and the more than 300-bed group. The seven operative procedures selected for study were appendectomy, cholecystectomy, herniorrhaphy, colon resection, laminectomy, total abdominal hysterectomy, and cesarean section.

Statistical Analysis

To study variations in the quality of the data from hospital to hospital (according to size), we examined overall infection rates at all sites during the study period. We also examined the frequency of reporting.

It was hypothesized that smaller hospitals might be more reliable in both surveillance activities and reporting frequency than larger hospitals. If so, larger hospitals could be expected to report less often, and their overall infection rates would be lower than those in smaller hospitals. The hypotheses were tested with a general linear model that used hospital size as the independent variable and reported infections as the dependent variable. Adjustment was made in the model for overall admissions by using total admissions reported as a covariate, with the size group (fewer than 100 beds, 100 to 300 beds, or more than 300 beds) as the independent variable of interest.

Logistic regression was used to examine the occurrence of postoperative infection and its association with the frequency of an operation.[8] Operative frequency was expressed as the base 10 logarithm of the number of operations performed (according to type and hospital) during the study period.

Frequency of a procedure, rather than hospital size, was used as a predictor since there was no logic to the idea that large size alone would affect a hospital's infection rate as much as experience in performing a procedure, which would be reflected in operative frequency. It was obvious, however, that higher frequencies were likely to be observed in larger hospitals.

RESULTS

A total of 2118 operations were performed at hospitals with fewer than 100 beds, 8664 were performed at hospitals with 100 to 300 beds, and 15,159 at hospitals with more than 300 beds (Table 9.1). These figures are based on a reporting frequency of 75 percent. For each of the procedures studied the mean number of operations performed per hospital during the 29-month study period was lower at smaller hospitals than at larger ones. Overall, mean infection rates were lowest for laminectomy (1 percent), herniorrhaphy (1 percent), and cholecystectomy (2 percent), and highest for cesarean section (5 percent), appendectomy (5 percent), hysterectomy (7 percent), and colon resection (10 percent). The hospitals in the

Table 9.1:   Number of Operations Performed per Hospital for Selected Surgical Procedures, According to Hospital Size

Procedure	No. of Operations (By Hospital Size)*			Total
	<100 Beds (6)	100–300 Beds (9)	>300 Beds (7)	
Abdominal hysterectomy	369	1,532	3,216	5,117
Colon resection	58	294	979	1,331
Herniorrhaphy	498	1,875	3,059	5,432
Cholecystectomy	429	1,397	2,330	4,156
Appendectomy	469	1,134	2,068	3,671
Laminectomy	77	1,021	1,658	2,756
Cesarean section	218	1,411	1,849	3,478
Totals	2,118	8,664	15,159	25,941

*Figures in parentheses denote number of hospitals in size group.

Table 9.2:   Relation between Frequency of Procedures and Occurrence of Postoperative Wound Infections in 22 Hospitals—1977–1979*

Procedure	Chi-Square	P Value
Abdominal hysterectomy	203.45	<0.0001
Colon resection	16.56	<0.0001
Herniorrhaphy	13.95	0.0002
Cholecystectomy	11.48	0.0007
Appendectomy	4.95	0.0261
Laminectomy	3.68	0.0551
Cesarean section	0.52	0.4689

*Results were obtained from logistic regression with frequency of performance of a procedure by a hospital as the independent variable.

three size groups did not differ in frequency of reporting (fewer than 100 beds, 8.1 times per year; 100 to 300 beds, 8.8 times per year; and more than 300 beds, 8.9 times per year; P = 0.76). After adjustment for overall admissions, there was no difference according to size group in the overall occurrence of infection (adjusted means, less than 100 beds, 165 per year; 100 to 300 beds, 184 per year; more than 300 beds, 143 per year; P = 0.33).

The frequency of performance of a procedure was found to be a significant predictor of postoperative infection after appendectomy, cholecystectomy, herniorrhaphy, colon resection, and hysterectomy (Table 9.2 and Fig. 9.1). For laminectomy the relation was borderline (P = 0.055), and for cesarean section no significant relation was demonstrated.

DISCUSSION

Despite the widespread use of prophylactic antibiotics and other efforts at infection control, there is little evidence that rates of postoperative infection have changed over the past 20 years.[9] The Centers for Disease Control estimates that over 300,000 postoperative wound infections occur annually in the United States.[1] Nationally, over 10 percent of all surgery is performed in community hospitals with fewer than 100 beds, and over 50 percent is performed in hospitals with fewer than 300 beds.[10] Presumably, many of these operations are being performed in hospitals with a relatively low volume of surgery.

Contamination of an operative wound site can occur from a variety of sources[9] and should be suspected in the presence of high infection rates after "clean" procedures. The distinction between endogenous and exogenous contamination is important in comparing rates, since many infections from endogenous sources are not easily preventable. In contrast, data presented by Cruse suggest not only that a majority of wound infections after sterile procedures are

Figure 9.1:   Infection Rates after Selected Surgical Procedures

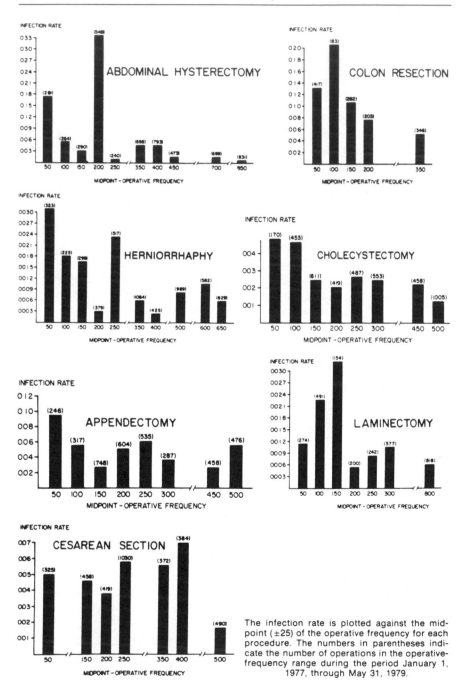

The infection rate is plotted against the midpoint (±25) of the operative frequency for each procedure. The numbers in parentheses indicate the number of operations in the operative-frequency range during the period January 1, 1977, through May 31, 1979.

preventable, but also that high infection rates after such procedures result from poor surgical technique.[11]

Our study demonstrated a significant inverse relation between the rate of infection and the number of procedures performed for appendectomy, cholecystectomy, herniorrhaphy, total abdominal hysterectomy, and colon resection. The relation was borderline for laminectomy and not significant for cesarean section.

There are several possible explanations for these relations. Physicians in hospitals with lower numbers of procedures may be operating on a population of patients at higher risk, perhaps with more emergencies. This explanation seems unlikely, however, in view of the fact that most hysterectomies and herniorrhaphies are elective.

It is possible that smaller hospitals (with fewer operations) have more mandatory and more accurate surveillance than that in larger hospitals. If so, the inverse relation between infection rates and the number of procedures performed could be an artifact of systematic surveillance. However, when we examined overall infections (all sites) in the same hospitals, no such relation was observed. In addition, there was no higher frequency of reporting in smaller hospitals. Thus, a surveillance artifact seems most unlikely. Furthermore, in smaller hospitals the practitioners performing surveillance usually work only part-time in hospital-infection control and do not have more hours of surveillance time per hospital bed.

Another possible explanation is that operating teams with more experience have better technique. With improved technique there may be a decreased risk of exogenous contamination and therefore of infection. The logarithmic relation suggests that the value of added experience is most important at hospitals with a very low volume of surgery. Thus, experience may be the most important factor in determining outcome when very little surgery is performed. As the number of operations performed increases, other factors assume more importance in influencing the risk of infection.

The lack of a significant relation for cesarean section may reflect the nature of the operation, since the degree of exogenous contamination may be less important than other factors (e.g., an indication for surgery or premature rupture of membranes).

Recently, Luft and his colleagues demonstrated an inverse relation between the frequency of surgery and mortality after certain complex operations (i.e., open heart surgery).[5] Another group of operations, including colectomy and cholecystectomy with duct exploration, also conformed to this relation, but death rates flattened out at the level of 10 to 50 procedures per year. A third group, which included cholecystectomy, did not demonstrate such a correlation. We are unaware of previous studies that have examined this relation with reference to morbidity. The volume-dependent nature of less complicated operations (cholecystectomy) with respect to morbidity but not to mortality suggests that the former is a more sensitive monitor of technique.

It should be emphasized that many questions about this relation need to be resolved. The relative contributions of the attending surgeon, house staff, anesthesiologist, and nursing personnel need to be explored. Examination of infection rates associated with individual surgeons might uncover a group of surgeons whose patients have high rates of postoperative infection that are hidden in overall rates at institutions with greater volumes. Finally, there are exceptions to this relation. In some hospitals where few procedures are performed, there were no infections or very low infection rates. Although this finding may be related to inaccuracies in surveillance, it should be noted that the reporting frequencies of these hospitals were similar to those of other institutions. Further study of these hospitals might disclose practices that are important in infection control and that could be extended to similar hospitals with higher rates.

Regionalization of open-heart surgery has been suggested as one mechanism to improve the quality of surgical care.[12,13] Objective data recently presented suggest that ensuring a minimum volume of surgery may lower mortality.[5] Our study evaluated relatively uncomplicated, commonly performed operations at 22 community hospitals with respect to morbidity (wound infection). Certainly, the potential effectiveness of regionalization of commonly performed surgery is a complex issue. Its effect on accessibility to medical care and to emergency procedures that cannot be regionalized has not been studied. Our study cannot answer the question of whether regionalization for surgical procedures is a valid concept, but it provides additional data clearly demonstrating that morbidity is higher in hospitals performing very little surgery. Further examination of the causes for this relation is needed.

We are indebted to Dr. J. M. Gwaltney, Jr., for his critical review of the manuscript.

REFERENCES

1. Dixon RE. Effect of infections on hospital care. Ann Intern Med. 1978;89:749–53.
2. Centers for Disease Control. National Nosocomial Infections Study report. Washington, D.C.: Government Printing Office, 1976:7. (DHEW publication no. (CDC)78-8257).
3. Green JW, Wenzel RP. Postoperative wound infection: a controlled study of the increased duration of hospital stay and direct cost of hospitalization. Ann Surg. 1977; 185:264–8.
4. Cruse PJE, Foord R. A five-year prospective study of 23,649 surgical wounds. Arch Surg. 1973; 107:206–10.
5. Luft HS, Bunker JP, Enthoven AC. Should operations be regionalized?: the empirical relationship between surgical volume and mortality. N Engl J Med. 1979; 301:1364–9.
6. Wenzel RP, Osterman CA, Townsend TR, et al. Development of a statewide program for surveillance and reporting of hospital-acquired infections. J Infect Dis. 1979; 140:741–6.
7. Wenzel RP, Osterman CA, Hunting KJ, Gwaltney JM Jr. Hospital-acquired infections. I. Surveillance in a university hospital. Am J Epidemiol. 1976; 103:251–60.

8. Harrell F. The logist procedure: SAS supplemental library user's guide. Cary, N.C.: SAS Institute, 1980:83–102.
9. Altemeier WA. Surgical infections: incisional wounds. In: Bennett JV, Brachman PS, eds. Hospital infections. Boston: Little, Brown, 1979:287–306.
10. Hospital statistics: AHA 1977 annual survey. Chicago: American Hospital Association, 1978:20.
11. Cruse PJE. Surgical wound sepsis. Can Med Assoc J. 1970; 102:251–8.
12. Scannell JG, Brown GE, Buckley MJ, et al. Report of the Inter-society Commission for Heart Disease Resources: optimal resources for cardiac surgery: guidelines for program planning and evaluation. Circulation. 1975; 52:A23–37.
13. Cardiovascular Committee of the American College of Surgeons. Guidelines for minimal standards in cardiovascular surgery. Ann Thorac Surg. 1973; 15:243–8.

Chapter 10

Case-Mix and Severity Scores

Kelly and Hellinger explored the association between hospital volume, physician volume, and patient outcomes for four selected groups of surgical patients. This is one of the few studies to assess physician volume, and it provides a good example of a unique system of adjusting for severity of illness. The whole issue of case-mix adjustment is complex and has been under intensive scrutiny as a result of hospital mortality rates released by the Health Care Financing Administration. Not surprisingly, the HCFA analysis showed that many of the hospitals with higher-than-expected mortality rates claimed that their patient mix was sicker than average, even after the study controlled for diagnosis-related groups (DRGs) and other factors.

Although better measures of case-mix adjustment are always desirable, their importance may differ depending on whether one is measuring patterns of outcomes across a large number of hospitals with different patient volumes or attempting to identify individual hospitals with particularly high mortality rates. Identifying high or low outliers among individual hospitals is difficult because there are only small numbers of each type of patient. When there are relatively few patients, the confidence intervals become very broad, so wide-ranging outcome rates are still not statistically different from the expected rate.[1] As a consequence, hospital mortality rates have generally been released as case-mix–adjusted rates for heterogeneous combinations of admissions. (The procedure-specific hospital mortality rates released by the *Los Angeles Times* constitute an exception [Steinbrook 1988].) The aggregated data on outcomes provide little information about a hospital's quality in delivering different types of services, which may be poorly correlated with each other. More important, the aggregation of various types of cases highlights the necessity of adjusting for severity.

Case-mix adjustment in volume studies is usually a more finely tuned process because a certain degree of homogeneity among patients is already achieved by the initial criteria for selecting the diagnosis or procedure under study. In part, this type of selectivity is possible because the volume-outcome studies are designed for research, rather than for administrative or public information purposes. Thus it is reasonable for researchers to exclude various types of cases within a diagnosis or procedure category in order to achieve a more homogeneous patient mix. Such exclusions are less reasonable in the evaluation of individual hospitals because they end up excluding a significant fraction of the patients, thereby reducing the usefulness of the information. The smaller sample size results in even larger confidence intervals around the results for individual hospitals. In volume-outcome studies, however, one is not interested in the results for specific hospitals. Instead, attention is focused on the relationship between volume and outcome. Although the estimates for individual hospitals are not very precise, this imprecision does not affect the estimation of patterns across large numbers of hospitals.

The predominance of volume-outcome studies of surgical patients, rather than medical patients, partly reflects an attempt to control for differences in case-mix severity among hospitals. For surgical patients, a minimal degree of fitness is usually required to undergo an operation, especially for procedures that can be postponed. Variables such as age and gender are available from most data sets and are clinically plausible adjustors for patient risk. Variables that account for the variation in the patient's severity or acuity of illness and general fitness are more complex, and several systems are currently under study.

Kelly and Hellinger used a system known as "disease staging" to control for the severity of illness of the principal diagnosis (Gonnella, Hornbrook, and Louis 1984). A computer algorithm classifies patients into different stages of illness based on the diagnoses listed in the data set. Two important principles in judging whether such a system plausibly assesses hospital quality are (1) whether there is a reasonable association with the patient's short-term outcome, and (2) whether it focuses on the patient's status at admission rather than subsequent status. In this study, it is clinically plausible that the stages defined for peptic ulcer and abdominal aneurysm strongly determine the short-term outcome for these patients, but it is less plausible for cancer of the stomach and colon, where the cancer stage largely determines the patient's long-term prognosis rather than in-hospital mortality. For cancer and other chronic diseases, it is plausible that the stages defined were present on admission to the hospital (less convincingly so for aneurysm and ulcer).

A case-mix system should not adjust for variation in illness caused by the hospitalization. All systems relying on data currently coded in the discharge abstract, such as disease staging, are unable to discriminate between problems present on admission and those occurring after admission, perhaps even as a result of treatment.[2] However, none of the newer systems, which account only for admission status is widely available for a large number of hospitals.

The patient's general fitness and other medical conditions are also important risk factors. Kelly and Hellinger used the number of diagnoses listed on the discharge abstract in addition to the severity of the "target" condition to assign patients to risk categories. However, these other diagnoses (e.g., shock) are sometimes used to determine severity in the disease-staging system. Other researchers have used approaches ranging from a simple distinction between whether the patient had one diagnosis or several (Luft, Bunker, and Enthoven 1979), the presence of specific comorbidities (Showstack et al. 1987), or prior hospitalizations (Roos et al. 1986).[3] A possible source of error is that the diagnoses may not have been present on admission and could represent complications of treatment rather than comorbidities. For example, Showstack and his colleagues used acute myocardial infarction, which can increase the risk of coronary artery bypass graft surgery, or may be a complication of the surgery. Most data sets cannot distinguish between these two cases. The HCFA mortality data released in December, 1988, used selected chronic conditions as comorbidities, thereby undercounting acute conditions present on admission that may present increased risk of poor outcome.

NOTES

1. For further discussion, see Luft and Hunt (1986), reprinted in Chapter 19.
2. For a discussion of some alternative methods of measuring severity, see Aronow (1988).
3. See Luft, Bunker, and Enthoven (1979), reprinted in Chapter 12; Showstack et al. (1987), reprinted in Chapter 11; and Roos et al. (1986), reprinted in Chapter 8.

Heart Disease and Hospital Deaths

An Empirical Study

Joyce V. Kelly
Fred J. Hellinger

Heart disease is the leading cause of death and the second most common reason for hospitalizations in the United States. Nonetheless, mortality due to the disease decreased by 21 percent between 1968 and 1976 after increasing steadily for 30 years. A recent study attributes 40 percent of this decline to new surgical and medical techniques and the remaining 60 percent to lifestyle changes [1].

Heart procedures that have become prevalent include direct heart revascularization or coronary artery bypass graft (CABG), cardiac catheterization, valve replacement or repair, and correction of congenital anomalies of the heart. Of these, CABG and cardiac catheterization are the most common and the fastest growing. CABG, a procedure in which a vein from a patient's thigh or abdomen is used to bypass an obstructed artery, is the standard treatment for patients with left main artery disease and/or intractable angina. Cardiac catheterization, a diagnostic procedure used to determine the extent and location of blockages in the coronary arteries, has become a standard tool for diagnosing heart disease.

The purpose of this study is to determine whether patients with diagnosed heart disease who survive their first day in the hospital are more likely to be discharged alive when they are treated by physicians and hospitals with particular characteristics. Separate analyses are conducted for three groups: (1) patients with a principal diagnosis of atherosclerosis who undergo a CABG operation; (2) patients with a principal diagnosis of atherosclerosis who undergo a cardiac catheterization and do not undergo a CABG operation during the same hospital stay; and (3) patients with a principal diagnosis of acute myocardial infarction (AMI) who do not undergo any surgical procedure during the stay. Relevant physician characteristics include board certification status and the volume of similar patients treated. Relevant hospital characteristics include the presence of a coronary care unit, teaching status, size, and the volume of similar patients treated.

Reprinted from *Health Services Research* 22, no. 3 (1987): 369–95, with permission from The Hospital Research and Educational Trust.

The views expressed in this article are those of the authors and no official endorsement by the National Center for Health Services Research or the Department of Health and Human Services is intended or should be inferred.

Previous studies indicate that heart patients are more likely to survive when they are hospitalized in facilities that provide greater volumes of services to similar patients. For example, Luft, Bunker, and Enthoven found that in-hospital mortality decreased with an increasing number of operations performed for open-heart surgery, vascular surgery, transurethral resection of the prostate, and coronary bypass patients [2]. Investigators also have determined that the presence of coronary care units in hospitals increases inpatient survival of coronary patients [3]. However, investigators have not had data that relate patient characteristics to specific characteristics of their attending physicians, such as their board certification status or the volume of similar patients that they treat. Since our analysis files do link physician and patient data, we can distinguish whether the characteristics of physicians or the characteristics of the hospitals themselves account for better inpatient outcomes in high-volume hospitals.

The first section of this article describes the empirical model and the data that are employed in this study. Then, each of the three groups of hospitalized heart patients is discussed separately. The findings of previous research are summarized and the results of our empirical analyses are presented in the three sections on CABG, cardiac catheterization, and AMI patients. The article concludes with a summary of findings, a discussion of methodological issues pertaining to the three analyses, and a discussion of policy implications.

EMPIRICAL SPECIFICATION AND DATA SOURCES

We analyze the determinants of variation in hospital mortality by regressing patient-specific outcome (discharged alive or dead) on hypothesized determinants of variation in patient death rates. Separate multivariate regression equations are estimated for three groups of heart patients—CABG, cardiac catheterization, and acute myocardial infarction (see Table 10.1)[1] The number of patients in each group treated by specific physicians and the number treated in specific hospitals are employed as explanatory variables. These variables measure the effects on patient outcome of the experience of physicians and hospitals in treating similar patients. Other hypothesized determinants of in-hospital mortality include: (1) patient severity of illness, age, sex, and the number of diagnoses; (2) hospital ownership, size, location, teaching status, resources expended, and the presence of a coronary care unit; and (3) board certification status of the attending physician or surgeon who operated.

This analysis used Hospital Cost and Utilization Project (HCUP) sample data collected by the Hospital Studies Program of the National Center for Health Services Research and Health Care Technology Assessment (NCHSR). The HCUP sample contains patient discharge abstract and other data for 373 short-term, general nonfederal hospitals across the nation for 1977. Discharge abstract data include patients' discharge status (alive or dead), principal and secondary discharge diagnoses, procedures, age, sex, principal expected source of pay-

Table 10.1: Staged Disease Condition, Principal Diagnoses, and Principal Surgical Procedures of Patients Included in Each Study Group (1977 HCUP Sample)

Study Group	Staged Disease Condition	Principal Diagnoses (HICDA-2 Codes)	Principal Surgical Procedures (HICDA-2 Codes)
Direct heart revascularization with atherosclerosis	Atherosclerosis of coronary arteries	Chronic ischemic heart disease (412.0, 412.9), angina pectoris (413), other acute and subacute forms of ischemic heart disease (411), heart failure (427), etc.	Direct heart revascularization (CABG) (36.1)
Cardiac catheterization with atherosclerosis	Atherosclerosis of coronary arteries	Chronic ischemic heart disease (412.0, 412.9), angina pectoris (413), other acute and subacute forms of ischemic heart disease (411), heart failure (427), etc.	Cardiac catheterization (93.3)
Acute myocardial infarction	Acute myocardial infarction	Acute myocardial infarction (410), cardiac arrest (415.8), and postmyocardial infarction syndrome (420.2)	None

Source: Hospital Studies Program, National Center for Health Services Research and Health Care Technology Assessment.

ment, a hospital-specific code number for the attending physician, similar codes for up to two surgeons, and other variables.

This analysis also used a physician file that contains biographical information on physicians with 15 or more patient encounters for 1977. Of 373 HCUP sample hospitals, 160 hospitals agreed to participate in this phase of data collection. The American Medical Association provided information on these physicians from its 1984 Physician Master-file. We assume that physicians possessed these same characteristics in 1977. The HCUP physician file contains data on approximately 10,000 physicians and can be linked directly to patient discharge abstract records.

In order to account for differences in the likelihood of dying among hospitalized patients, we include variables measuring patient age, disease stage, sex, number of diagnoses, and Medicaid or no insurance coverage. Seven age groups are defined for CABG and cardiac catheterization patients, and nine age groups are defined for patients with AMI. All patients above the age of 99 and below the age of 18 years are deleted from the study.

Disease staging is used to control for variation in patient severity of illness within principal diagnostic categories. This technique was designed by a panel of physicians to describe the progression of disease for nearly 400 diagnoses [5]. Disease staging used diagnostic information from patient discharge abstracts to classify patients along an ordinal scale within a single disease condition, according to the stated extent of medical complications. Generally, stage 1 of a disease consists of conditions with no complications or with problems of minimal severity; stage 2 conditions are limited to an organ or system and have significantly increased risks of complications; stage 3 conditions affect multiple sites or present generalized systemic involvement; and stage 4 is death.

Disease stages are determined solely by patients' medical conditions; unlike Diagnosis Related Groups, disease staging was not designed to reflect utilization of resources by patients [6]. We have applied the disease-staging algorithm to our data, omitting the death stage, because we seek to examine the relationship between the pre-death stage of illness and the probability of dying in the hospital. Table 10.2 illustrates the stages within the two staged disease conditions used in this study. Patients are included who have a principal diagnosis of atherosclerosis of the coronary arteries and undergo a CABG or a cardiac catheterization procedure. Patients are also included who have a principal diagnosis of acute myocardial infarction and do not undergo any surgical procedure.

It is likely that certain hospital characteristics are correlated with in-hospital mortality. We include two variables to adjust for teaching status: COTH and MSA (NONCOTH). COTH hospitals are members of the Council of Teaching Hospitals of the Association of American Medical Colleges,[2] and MSA (NONCOTH) hospitals are affiliated with medical schools but are not members of COTH. We also include regional variables to account for regional variations in practice patterns. Prior studies have shown that patients in Western U.S. hospitals are less likely to die in the hospital, possibly because their lengths of stay are shorter [8]. We include variables denoting public hospitals, and Medicaid or no insurance coverage (LOCOV), because patients in public hospitals and patients with Medicaid or no insurance coverage may be different from other patients in ways that are not accounted for by age, sex, or disease stage. For example, such patients may have fewer alternative sources of care and, therefore, would be more likely to die in the hospital.

In addition, we include variables measuring the number of hospital inpatient admissions because prior studies have shown that larger hospitals (that is, hospitals with larger than average numbers of beds or admissions as opposed to higher volumes of patients who receive a specific service) have higher mortality rates when other factors are held constant [8–10]. In-hospital mortality rates of

Table 10.2: Description of Stages within Disease Conditions Studied

Stage	Label*	Atherosclerosis of Coronary Arteries Description	Stage	Label*	Acute Myocardial Infarction Description
1.0	A	Angina pectoris induced by prolonged exertion, or hill-climbing, or hurrying, or emotional stress, or variant angina	1.1	A	Myocardial infarction manifested by chest pains and/or electrocardiographic or enyzmatic changes consistent with diagnosis
2.1	A†	Angina pectoris produced by any one of the following: walking more than one or two blocks on the level or climbing one flight of stairs	1.2	B	Myocardial infarction plus heart block or supraventricular arrhythmia or ventricular arrhythmia other than fibrillation or pericarditis
2.2	B	Physical evidence of minimal congestive heart failure (i.e., pulmonary rales, or peripheral edema secondary to ischemic heart disease)	2.1	C	Myocardial infarction plus emboli to other organ systems leading to a peripheral vascular occlusion, or infarction of GI tract or infarction of kidney
2.3	C	Physical evidence of moderate congestive heart failure (i.e., one or more of the following: pulmonary rales, positive hepatojugular reflux, ascites, sacral edema, plus pitting, peripheral edema)	2.2	D	Myocardial infarction manifested by chest pains and/or electrocardiographic or enzymatic changes consistent with the diagnosis plus congestive heart failure
3.1	C†	Angina or symptoms of cardiac insufficiency present during the performance of any of the activities of daily living beyond the personal toilet	2.3 2.4 2.5	E F G	Cerebral vascular accident Papillary muscle rupture Ventricular aneurysm
3.2	C†	Angina or symptoms of cardiac insufficiency present at rest	3.1	H	Evidence of shock (hypotension, oliguria, obtundation, signs of peripheral vascular collapse) or ventricular fibrillation or pulmonary edema
3.3	D	Acute myocardial infarction or pulmonary edema	3.2	I	Cardiac arrest
4.0	—‡	Death	4.0	—‡	Death

*Stages are labeled as A–I in Table 10.4 and 10.6.

†A separate stage is defined, but patients cannot be classified in this stage because discharge abstract data are not sufficiently detailed. Therefore, patients are classified in the labeled stage.

‡Ordinarily, patients who die in the hospital are placed in the "death" stage. To examine the relationship between the predeath stage of illness and the probability of dying, we omit the death stage as an option of the staging algorithm and we classify patients in the predeath stage of illness.

Source: Joseph S. Gonnella, M.D. (ed.). *Clinical Criteria for Disease Staging.* Santa Barbara, CA: SysteMetrics, Inc., 1983.

medical patients also may be related to the characteristics of their attending physicians, while characteristics of the surgeons who operate may help explain in-hospital mortality rates of surgical patients. We include board certification variables to measure the qualifications of individual practitioners. Other things being equal, we expect patients of board-certified physicians to experience better inpatient outcomes per admission.

We created three patient files specifically for this analysis. Each file contains data for all patients discharged from sample hospitals in 1977 with one of the three conditions described in Table 10.1. These data are linked to hospital information obtained from the American Hospital Association Annual Survey for 1977 and to the physician data described above. Characteristics of attending physicians are linked to data for AMI patients and characteristics of surgeons who operate are linked to data for CABG and cardiac catheterization patients. Table 10.3 and Table 10.4 present means and standard deviations for all variables used in these analyses. Comparison of these data with data from the universe of short-term, general nonprofit hospitals in 1977[3] indicates that the hospitals included in this analysis are disproportionately large, urban, medical school affiliated, and private nonprofit. Included hospitals have these characteristics for two reasons: among HCUP sample hospitals, such hospitals were more likely to provide physician data, and such hospitals are more likely to perform CABG and cardiac catheterization procedures.

The individual patient is the unit of analysis and the dependent variable is set equal to one if the patient is discharged dead and equal to zero if the patient is discharged alive. Logistic regression is used to obtain efficient least squares estimators.[4] Special computer software is used to protect the identity of individual patients, physicians, and hospitals.

Data are not available to distinguish patient admission type (urgent, emergent, or elective) or the stage (severity) of AMI upon admission. In order to examine correlates of the quality of inpatient care, however, interhospital differences in the severity of patients upon admission must be controlled. Patients with one-day lengths of stay are deleted from the analysis because death so soon after admission may reflect the patient's medical condition upon admission as well as the skills of emergency department personnel rather than the quality of inpatient services in the hospital. One-day stay AMI patients represented 9.6 percent of all AMI patients admitted to HCUP sample hospitals in 1977.

Patients who were discharged during the first day of their stay after receiving either a cardiac catheterization or a coronary artery bypass procedure also are deleted. Discharge during the first day was unusual in 1977; only 3.1 percent of cardiac catheterization and .15 percent of CABG patients were discharged within 24 hours of admission. Performance of these procedures followed by discharge (alive or dead) so early in the stay may reflect patient characteristics that are not otherwise controlled for in regression analyses, such as type of admission or stage of the principal diagnosis upon admission.

Table 10.3: Variable Definitions and Descriptive Statistics for Hospital and Physician Characteristics (1977 HCUP Hospital Sample)

		Direct Heart Revascularization with Atherosclerosis		Cardiac Catheterization with Atherosclerosis		Acute Myocardial Infarction	
Number of Hospitals		26		39		146	
Number of Physicians		99		145		926	
Number of Patients		3,883		4,835		11,033	
Number Who Died		107		38		1,511	
*Definition**	*Acronym*	*Mean†*	*(Std. Dev.)*	*Mean†*	*(Std. Dev.)*	*Mean†*	*(Std. Dev.)*
Coronary care unit	CCU	.923	(.266)	.903	(.296)	.703	(.457)
Volume of specific procedure							
In hospital	HOSPVOL	355.999	(319.453)	398.554	(401.153)	146.163	(96.142)
By physician	MDVOL	109.220	(64.789)	96.669	(70.053)	29.630	(25.683)
Board certified							
Family practice	BCFP	NI‡		NI		.129	(.336)
Internal medicine	BCIM	NI		.864	(.343)	.447	(.497)
Any other specialty	BCOTH	NI		NI		.020	(.140)
Council of Teaching Hospitals	COTH	.267	(.442)	.295	(.456)	.164	(.370)
Medical school affiliation	MSA (NONCOTH)	.477	(.500)	.611	(.488)	.449	(.497)
Geographical location							
	NOREAST	.071	(.256)	.152	(.359)	.301	(.459)
	NORCENT	.557	(.497)	.557	(.497)	.406	(.491)
	SOUTH	.230	(.421)	.206	(.404)	.238	(.426)
Public hospital	PUBLIC	.044	(.205)	.036	(.187)	.152	(.360)

*The reference group for categorical (dummy) variables consists of patients with disease stage A in the 18–45 years of age group, and non-board-certified physicians and hospitals that are Western, private nonprofit, and not medical school affiliated. Other variables included in regression analyses but not displayed here are: sex of the patient, presence of a cardiac catheterization procedure (CABG patients only), urban or rural location of the hospital, total hospital admissions, and total hospital expenses per day.

†All statistics are calculated from patient-level data.

‡NI: This category is not included.

Source: Hospital Studies Program, National Center for Health Services Research and Health Care Technology Assessment.

Table 10.4: Variable Definitions and Descriptive Statistics for Patient Characteristics (1977 HCUP Hospital Sample)

		Direct Heart Revascularization with Atherosclerosis		Cardiac Catheterization with Atherosclerosis		Acute Myocardial Infarction	
	Number of Hospitals	26		39		146	
	Number of Physicians	99		145		926	
	Number of Patients	3,883		4,835		11,033	
	Number Who Died	107		38		1,511	
*Definition**	*Acronym*	*Mean†*	*(Std. Dev.)*	*Mean†*	*(Std. Dev.)*	*Mean†*	*(Std. Dev.)*
Mortality rate	MORTALITY	.028	(.164)	.008	(.088)	.137	(.344)
Stage of disease	Stage B	.025	(.157)	.049	(.216)	.084	(.278)
	Stage C	ND§		ND		.010	(.102)
	Stage D	.037	(.188)	.019	(.136)	.121	(.326)
	Stage E	NI‡		NI		.027	(.162)
	Stage F	NI		NI		.003	(.053)
	Stage G	NI		NI		.006	(.078)
	Stage H	NI		NI		.040	(.196)
(Most severe)	Stage I	NI		NI		.059	(.235)

Number of diagnoses	NUMDX	2.240	(1.444)	2.060	(1.275)	2.991	(1.709)
Patient age	46–50 years	.142	(.349)	.155	(.362)	.072	(.259)
	51–55 years	.216	(.411)	.211	(.408)	.113	(.316)
	56–60 years	.232	(.422)	.218	(.413)	.137	(.344)
	61–65 years	.172	(.377)	.155	(.362)	.140	(.347)
	66–70 years	.096	(.295)	.072	(.259)	.141	(.348)
	71–75 years	NI		NI		.127	(.333)
	76–80 years	NI		NI		.103	(.304)
	81–85 years	NI		NI		.060	(.238)
	86–99 years	NI		NI		.038	(.190)
	71–99 years					NI	
	LOCOV	.026	(.158)	.032	(.177)	.084	(.278)
No insurance/Medicaid		.050	(.217)	.061	(.240)	NI	

*The reference group for categorical (dummy) variables consists of patients with disease stage A in the 18–45 years of age group, and non-board-certified physicians and hospitals that are Western, private nonprofit, and not medical school affiliated. Other variables included in regression analyses but not displayed here are: sex of the patient, presence of a cardiac catheterization procedure (CABG patients only), urban or rural location of the hospital, total hospital admissions, and total hospital expenses per day.

†All statistics are calculated from patient-level data.

‡NI: This category is not included.

§ND: No deaths. No patients in this stage died in the hospital; therefore, the maximum likelihood estimates would have been unbounded.

Source: Hospital Studies Program, National Center for Health Services Research and Health Care Technology Assessment.

CORONARY ARTERY BYPASS GRAFT SURGERY
(DIRECT HEART REVASCULARIZATION)

Ten years ago, the average operative mortality of CABG patients ranged between 6 and 7 percent [12, 13]. Now, fewer than 3 percent of CABG patients die within 30 days after surgery, on average [14, 15]. The determinants of in-hospital mortality for CABG patients have been examined in studies by Luft et al. and Sloan et al. [2, 10]. These analysts found a significant negative relationship between hospital volume and in-hospital mortality. However, analysts did not have data on the number of procedures performed by surgeons who operate and they did not use staging to adjust for severity-of-illness differences.

Within the 160 HCUP hospitals with physician data for 1977, 99 physicians in 26 hospitals conduct CABG operations on 3,883 patients with a principal diagnosis of atherosclerosis (Table 10.3). On average, 356 procedures are performed in those hospitals offering CABG; surgeons perform an average of 109 procedures per year. One hundred seven (or 2.8 percent) of these 3,883 CABG patients died during their hospital stay. Their mortality rate and age distribution are comparable to that reported for patients included in the Coronary Artery Surgery Study (CASS, 1975–present), sponsored by the National Heart, Lung, and Blood Institute. About 12 percent of patients are older than 65 years of age and about 1 percent also underwent cardiac catheterization during their hospital stay (Table 10.4). Approximately 80 percent are male and 5 percent have Medicaid or no insurance coverage. Since virtually all surgeons conducting CABG are board-certified surgeons and all hospitals are located in urban areas, both of these variables are omitted from the regression equation.

Of the characteristics of the hospital in which the patient undergoes CABG, three variables included in multivariate regression analyses are significantly different from zero—the total volume of CABG procedures performed in the hospital, the presence of a coronary care unit (CCU), and Southern U.S. location (Table 10.5). Our analysis demonstrates that the number of CABG procedures performed in the hospital in which the patient undergoes CABG is negatively related to in-hospital mortality. We reject the hypothesis of no hospital-volume effect at a significance level of .05. The coefficient indicates that CABG patient mortality would decrease by 1 percent in hospitals that added 200 CABG procedures.[5] Since the average hospital serves 356 CABG patients annually with a mean mortality rate of 2.8 percent, this finding suggest that a 56 percent increase in the number of CABG patients served in the average hospital (200/356) would result in a 36 percent decrease in mortality (.01/.028).[6]

The number of CABG procedures performed by individual surgeons is not related to in-hospital mortality. This findings suggest that the inverse relationship found in this and previous studies between hospital volume and in-hospital mortality is not a manifestation of an underlying relationship between physician volume and in-hospital mortality. Thus, patients in hospitals where relatively

Table 10.5: Probability of In-Hospital Mortality Based on Logistic Regression Analyses, Hospital and Physician Variables (1977 HCUP Sample)

Definition†	Acronym	Direct Heart Revascularization with Atherosclerosis		Cardiac Catheterization with Atherosclerosis		Acute Myocardial Infarction	
		Coefficient††	(t-Ratio)	Coefficient††	(t-Ratio)	Coefficient††	(t-Ratio)
Intercept		-.154**	(5.464)	-.075**	(4.546)	-.410**	(10.793)
Coronary care unit	CCU	-.032**	(2.528)	-.006	(1.229)	-.004	(0.361)
Volume of specific procedure							
In hospital	HOSPVOL (00's)	-.005**	(2.640)	-.001*	(1.931)	-.0003	(0.000)
By physician	MDVOL (00's)	.007	(1.245)	-.001	(0.361)	-.049**	(2.977)
Board certified							
Family practice	BCFP	NI‡		NI		-.042**	(3.245)
Internal medicine	BCIM	NI		-.002	(0.374)	-.031**	(3.479)
Any other specialty	BCOTH	NI		NI		.037	(1.526)
Council of Teaching Hospitals	COTH	.009	(0.678)	-.004	(0.566)	-.027*	(1.778)
Medical school affiliation	MSA (NONCOTH)	.015	(1.510)	.008	(1.400)	-.025**	(2.138)
Geographical location							
	NOREAST	.011	(0.616)	.008	(0.812)	.040*	(1.884)
	NORCENT	.023	(1.559)	.008	(0.954)	.024	(1.204)
	SOUTH	.028*	(1.658)	-.001	(0.100)	.036*	(1.720)
Public hospital	PUBLIC	-.031	(1.378)	.001	(0.173)	.022*	(1.876)

*Statistically significant at the .10 level, using a two-tailed t-test.

**Statistically significant at the .05 level, using a two-tailed t-test.

†The reference group for categorical (dummy) variables consists of patients with disease stage A in the 18–45 years of age group, and non–board–certified physicians and hospitals that are Western, private nonprofit, and not medical school affiliated. Other variables included in regression analyses but not displayed here are: sex of the patient, presence of a cardiac catheterization procedure (CABG patients only), urban or rural location of the hospital, total hospital admissions, and total hospital expenses per day.

††All statistics are calculated from patient–level data. Probabilities were calculated by multiplying logistic coefficients by [P·(1–P)] where P is the average observed probability of dying in the hospital for all patients in each study group. Thus, coefficients were evaluated at the mean mortality value for each study group.

‡NI: This category is not included.

Source: Hospital Studies Program, National Center for Health Services Research and Health Care Technology Assessment.

large numbers of CABG procedures are performed are less likely to die as inpatients regardless of the volumes of procedures performed by their own surgeons. Our findings may be explained by the presence of more skilled surgeons, better protocols, more skilled professional help (for example, better nurses and surgical assistants), and more opportunities for sharing knowledge in high-volume hospitals. In the discussion section below, we describe the tests that we conducted to rule out multicollinearity as a reason for our findings.

Patients who undergo coronary bypass surgery in hospitals with coronary care units are considerably less likely to die in the hospital than are patients who undergo CABG in hospitals without coronary care units. The presence of a CCU decreases in-hospital mortality rates by 3.2 percent. We reject the hypothesis of no CCU effect at a significance level of .05. Hospitals with coronary care units may be better equipped to handle patient complications that develop during and after surgery; also, hospitals with such units may have more up-to-date equipment. We expected regional variables to be positive because the Western United States is the omitted region and has the shortest length of stay. The variable representing the South is positive and significant.

The disease-staging variables perform quite well. The omitted or reference stage is the least severe—those atherosclerosis patients with mild to moderate angina pectoris induced by such activities as hill-climbing or climbing one flight of stairs (stage A in Table 10.2). A comparison of patients in the omitted stage with patients who have physical evidence of minimal congestive heart failure (stage B in Table 10.6) indicates that the latter are 5 percent more likely to die in the hospital following CABG. Similarly, compared to patients in the omitted stage, patients who suffer an acute myocardial infarction or pulmonary edema (stage D) are 5 percent more likely to die. The presence of additional diagnoses also increases the chance of dying in the hospital. Each additional diagnosis beyond atherosclerosis increases the likelihood of being discharged dead by nearly 1 percent. For these coefficients, we reject the hypothesis of no effect at a significance level of .05.

The relationship between patient age and mortality is interesting. Up to age 60, CABG patients are no more likely to die in the hospital than patients in the omitted age group (18–45 years of age). Beyond the age of 60, however, patients are considerably more likely to die. CABG patients between the ages of 61 and 65 or 66 and 70 years of age are 3.6 percent and 3.2 percent, respectively, more likely to die in the hospital. After age 70, the chance of dying in the hospital increases dramatically, with patients in the 71–99 years of age group being 5.7 percent more likely to die following CABG than patients aged 18–45.

CARDIAC CATHETERIZATION

Coronary angiography, the standard test for diagnosing coronary artery disease, is performed during cardiac catheterization. Other procedures performed during

Table 10.6: Probability of In-Hospital Mortality Based on Logistic Regression Analyses, Patient Variables (1977 HCUP Hospital Sample)

Definition[+]	Acronym	Direct Health Revascularization with Atherosclerosis		Cardiac Catheterization with Atherosclerosis		Acute Myocardial Infarction	
		Coefficient[††]	(t-Ratio)	Coefficient[††]	(t-Ratio)	Coefficient[††]	(t-Ratio)
Stage of disease	Stage B	.051**	(5.675)	.029**	(6.925)	−.045**	(2.433)
	Stage C	ND‡‡		ND		.104**	(3.302)
	Stage D	.051**	(6.331)	.036**	(7.479)	.040**	(4.942)
	Stage E	NI*‡		NI		.121**	(6.694)
	Stage F	NI		NI		.308**	(6.719)
	Stage G	NI		NI		.041	(0.735)
	Stage H	NI		NI		.237**	(16.266)
	Stage I	NI		NI		.399**	(30.200)
Number of diagnoses	NUMDX	.009**	(5.123)	.002	(1.507)	−.004	(1.446)
Patient age	46–50 years	.008	(0.510)	.008	(0.831)	−.015	(0.424)
	51–55 years	.019	(1.389)	.007	(0.800)	.040	(1.342)
	56–60 years	.011	(0.825)	.013	(1.435)	.076**	(2.722)
	61–65 years	.036**	(2.814)	.013	(1.425)	.127**	(4.730)
	66–70 years	.032**	(2.265)	.012	(1.261)	.170**	(6.414)
	71–75 years	NI		NI		.221**	(8.356)
	76–80 years	NI		NI		.249**	(9.389)
	81–85 years	NI		NI		.273**	(9.895)
	86–99 years	NI		NI		.357**	(12.588)
	71–99 years	.057**	(3.587)	.027**	(3.00)	NI	

Continued

Table 10.6: Continued

Definition†	Acronym	Direct Health Revascularization with Atherosclerosis		Cardiac Catheterization with Atherosclerosis		Acute Myocardial Infarction	
		Coefficient††	(t-Ratio)	Coefficient††	(t-Ratio)	Coefficient††	(t-Ratio)
No insurance/Medicaid	LOCOV	.005	(0.412)	.004	(0.648)	.028*	(1.664)
-2 Ln (likelihood ratio)		800.21		237.60		6,523.6	
Model Chi-Square (degrees of freedom)		179.40***(23)		206.40***(23)		2,289.41***(35)	
Sample size		3,883		4,835		11,033	

*Statistically significant at the .10 level, using a two-tailed *t*-test.
**Statistically significant at the .05 level, using a two-tailed *t*-test.
***Statistically significant at the .01 level, using a one-sided Chi-square test.
†The reference group for categorical (dummy) variables consists of patients with disease stage A in the 18–45 years of age group, and non-board-certified physicians and hospitals that are Western, private nonprofit, and not medical school affiliated. Other variables included in regression analyses but not displayed here are: sex of the patient, presence of a cardiac catheterization procedure (CABG patients only), urban or rural location of the hospital, total hospital admissions, and total hospital expenses per day.
††All statistics are calculated from patient-level data. Probabilities were obtained by multiplying logistic coefficients by [P · (1 − P)] where P is the average observed probability of dying in the hospital for all patients in each study group. Thus coefficients were evaluated at the mean mortality value for each study group.
‡NI: This category is not included.
‡‡ND: No deaths. No patients in this stage died in the hospital; therefore, the maximum likelihood estimates would have been unbounded.
Source: Hospital Studies Program, National Center for Health Services Research and Health Care Technology Assessment.

cardiac catheterizations include right ventriculograms (x-rays of the right ventricle of the heart) and other physiologic tests. Coronary angiography is an invasive procedure involving the injection of iodinated dye or contrast medium into the left ventricle of the heart. After the left ventriculogram is completed, the contrast medium is injected in the coronary arteries, as the catheter is guided through. The procedure is recorded on cine film and enables the cardiologist to determine the extent and location of coronary artery disease.

The National Health Guidelines recommend that cardiac catheterization laboratories perform at least 300 procedures each year, since there is evidence that patients in high-volume laboratories experience lower mortality and morbidity rates.[7] One study showed that institutions performing ten or fewer procedures were five times more likely to experience an untoward event than were institutions performing 400 or more procedures [16]. Such results prompted Levin to ask whether "the performance of coronary arteriography (should) be consolidated or centralized in a relatively small number of hospitals throughout the country."[18]

Our study examines the relationship between in-hospital mortality and hospital volume, taking into account the effect of patient and hospital factors that were not considered in the studies described above. In our sample of 1977 data, 4,835 patients with a principal diagnosis of atherosclerosis undergo cardiac catheterizations conducted by 145 physicians in 39 hospitals (Tables 10.3 and 10.4). On average, 399 procedures are performed in those hospitals offering cardiac catheterization and surgeons perform an average of 97 procedures annually. Nearly 86 percent of the surgeons who operate are board certified in internal medicine, reflecting the diagnostic nature of the cardiac catheterization procedure. The reference class, non-board-certified physicians, comprises 14 percent of surgeons who operate (the few physicians who are board certified in other specialties are deleted from the analysis).

Our analysis of in-hospital mortality for cardiac catheterization patients who do not undergo CABG surgery confirms studies described above. Mortality associated with cardiac catheterization is low. Approximately .8 percent of cardiac catheterization patients in our sample die in the hospital while .2 percent of CASS patients die [18]. The mortality rate in our sample is higher for two reasons: the CASS study excludes patients with severe angina or significant occlusion in the left main artery, and our data are from an earlier year. More importantly, the number of procedures performed and in-hospital mortality are inversely related. The coefficient indicates that, in order to decrease mortality by .5 percent, the average hospital must add 500 procedures ($-.005 \div -.00001$, see Note 5). Since the average hospital treats 399 cardiac catheterization patients annually with a mean mortality rate of .8 percent, this finding implies that a 125 percent increase in patients (500/399) would decrease mortality by 63 percent (.5/.8). Note that this assumes a relatively constant relationship between the number of patients treated and mortality.

The number of procedures performed by individual physicians is not related to in-hospital mortality, nor does physician board certification in internal medicine (compared to no board certification) improve patient outcome. Just as with CABG surgery, these findings suggest that the effect of hospital volume overwhelms any learning-by-doing effect attributable to individual physicians. High-volume hospitals either attract more skillful physicians and support personnel, or they exhibit a learning-by-doing effect that is not specific to physicians (for instance, support personnel may become more skillful as they assist with more procedures and monitor more postoperative patients).

The disease-staging variables perform as expected. Patients with physical evidence of minimal congestive heart failure (stage B in Table 10.6) are 2.9 percent more likely to die following a cardiac catheterization compared to patients with mild to moderate angina pectoris (stage A, the omitted stage). Similarly, patients with an acute myocardial infarction or pulmonary edema (stage D) are 3.6 percent more likely to die compared to patients in the omitted stage. Also, compared to patients in the reference age group (18–45 years), cardiac catheterization patients in the 71–99 years of age group are 2.7 percent more likely to die in the hospital. For these coefficients, we reject the hypothesis of no effect at a significance level of .05. However, coefficients for the other age categories and for the number of diagnoses are not significantly different from zero, suggesting that age up to 70 years and the presence of additional diagnoses do not increase the probability of death in the hospital following a cardiac catheterization.

ACUTE MYOCARDIAL INFARCTION

About 60 percent of those who die from an acute myocardial infarction (AMI) die before they reach the hospital. The remaining 40 percent die in the hospital. We examine factors that affect in-hospital mortality rates for the approximately 500,000 people hospitalized each year with AMI.

Treatment in coronary care units (CCUs) is the only aspect of hospital treatment of AMIs that has been the subject of clinical trails. The purpose of such units is to lessen early hospital mortality among AMI patients. Their effectiveness in this regard, however, is still in question. The major randomized clinical trails involving CCUs show no significant impact on mortality for AMI patients when compared to home care [19, 20]. Goldman argues that the sample sizes of these trials were too small to detect an impact of the expected magnitude; he argues that CCUs reduce the hospital mortality rate of AMI patients by about 4 percent [21].

Statistical studies (as opposed to clinical trails), by Shortell and LoGerfo, and Stross, examined factors associated with in-hospital mortality of AMI patients. Shortell and LoGerfo found that the presence of CCUs decreased in-hospital mortality rates of AMI patients [3]. They concluded that in-hospital mortality is inversely related to the average number of AMI patients treated per family practitioner or internist on a hospital's staff. However, because investigators could not link physician and patient data, they had to assume that each physician on a hospital's medical staff treated the average number of patients. Clearly, individual physicians are likely to treat more or fewer patients than average. Nonetheless, they found a statistically significant relationship between case volume per physician and in-hospital mortality. They also found that physician board certification is not related to the mortality of AMI patients, when board certification status is measured by the percent of family practitioners and internists on staff who are board certified.

Stross et al. conducted an empirical study that compares in-hospital mortality rates and the volume of cases treated in a hospital CCU [22]. They found that CCUs treating fewer than 60 AMI patients experienced twice the mortality of CCUs treating more than 60 AMI patients. However, the impact on in-hospital mortality of factors other than the volume of patients treated in CCUs was not taken into account in the study.

We are studying 11,033 patients, admitted to the sample of HCUP hospitals in 1977 with a principal diagnosis of AMI, who do not undergo surgery and who survive their first day in the hospital. Of these patients, 1,511 (13.7 percent) die sometime during their stay (Table 10.4). AMI patients are considerably older than patients who undergo cardiac catheterization or CABG surgery. Almost half of the AMI patients are 65 years of age or older. The average number of AMI patients treated per hospital is 146, and the average number of AMI patients treated per physician is 30. Far more hospitals serve AMI patients than provide either CABG or cardiac catherterization services. Further, compared to HCUP hospitals providing CABG or cardiac catheterization services, hospitals serving AMI patients are smaller, less likely to be affiliated with COTH or to have a coronary care unit, less likely to be located in urban areas, and more likely to be public. Nearly 45 percent of AMI patients are attended by physicians who are board-certified internists, 13 percent are attended by physicians who are board certified in family practice, and 2 percent are attended by physicians who are board certified in other specialties. The omitted class of non-board-certified physicians attends the remaining 40 percent of AMI patients.

Regression results indicate different relationships between physician and hospital volume and in-hospital mortality for AMI patients than was found for CABG or cardiac catheterization patients (Table 10.5). There is a negative relationship between in-hospital mortality and the number of AMI patients treated by individual physicians; yet there is no relationship between mortality and physician volume for CABG or cardiac catheterization patients. Further, there is no statistically significant relationship between mortality and the number of AMI patients treated in hospitals, while equations discussed previously indicate a negative and significant relationship between in-hospital mortality and the number of patients treated by hospitals for CABG or cardiac catheterization patients. Thus, our findings for AMI patients lend support to prior research studies which show that the inverse relationship between hospital volume and in-hospital mortality is stronger for surgical patients than for medical patients.[8]

These results suggest that the skill of the support staff, the availability of equipment, and other characteristics of high-volume hospitals are determinants of outcome of CABG and cardiac catheterization patients. However, the experience of physicians in treating similar types of patients helps determine outcomes of AMI patients. This reasoning is supported by the negative and significant coefficients in the AMI equation for board certification in family practice or internal medicine. (Board certification was not a significant factor in the cardiac catheterization equation; board certification was not included in the CABG equation because all surgeons in this group were board certified in surgery.)

Other significant variables in the AMI equation include teaching status, geographical location, ownership, and expenses per day. Patients in COTH, or in medical school-affiliated but non-COTH hospitals, are 2.7 percent and 2.5 percent, respectively, less likely to die in the hospital. Hospitals outside the Western United States have higher in-hospital mortality rates, as do public hospitals. Further, AMI patients with attending physicians who are board certified in family practice or internal medicine are 4.2 percent and 3.1 percent, respectively, less likely to die in the hospital.

Seventy percent of AMI patients are admitted to hospitals with coronary care units (Table 10.3). The regression coefficient on the presence of a CCU indicates a negative, but quite small and insignificant, relationship between the presence of a CCU and the mortality of AMI patients. This result may reflect the fact that AMI patients who died during their first day in the hospital were deleted from this study. If such patients disproportionately died in hospitals without CCUs, then the negative coefficient may have achieved statistical significance. However, this hypothesis cannot be tested with available data.

The staging variables perform as expected (Table 10.6). With a single exception, patients in higher stages of AMI are more likely to be discharged dead, compared to patients in the omitted or reference stage. In general, the stages increase monotonically, with patients in higher stages being more likely to die in the hospital, compared to patients in lower stages. The age variables perform similarly—they monotonically increase, showing that older patients are considerably more likely to die in the hospital compared to younger patients.

DISCUSSION AND CONCLUSIONS

This study examines the effects of selected physician and hospital characteristics on the in-hospital mortality of three groups of heart patients who survive their first day in the hospital. The number of patients in each group treated by specific physicians (MDVOL), and the number treated in specific hospitals (HOSPVOL), measure provider experience with similar patients. Other hypothesized determinants of in-hospital mortality include: (1) patient severity of illness, age, sex, and the presence of comorbidities; (2) hospital ownership, size, location, teaching status, resources expended, and the presence of a coronary care unit; and (3) board-certification status of the attending physician or surgeon who operated. Empirical results are described in Tables 10.5 and 10.6. The Chi-square test statistic, an overall measure of model fit, is highly significant for all three specifications.

Our findings indicate that heart patients who undergo a CABG or a cardiac catheterization procedure are more likely to survive when their procedures are performed in high-volume hospitals. However, there is no statistical relationship between patient outcome and the volume of similar procedures performed by surgeons (MDVOL). The dominant effect of the volume of similar surgical cases treated by hospitals may reflect the importance of a learning-by-doing effect for operative and postoperative staff, the reliance on complex medical equipment during surgical procedures, or other characteristics of high-volume hospitals. The most appropriate entity for measuring the effect of experience on treating surgical patients may be the experience of the operating room staff in performing similar types of procedures.

AMI patients are more likely to survive when their attending physicians treat high volumes of AMI patients, or are board certified in family practice or internal medicine (compared to non-board-certified physicians). Outcomes of medical heart patients do no depend on operating room staff and are less dependent on complex medical equipment. They depend on the ability of physicians to diagnose illness correctly and to prescribe appropriate treatment.

The relatively high average values of MDVOL for CABG and cardiac catheterization procedures may account for our failure to observe a downward-sloped "learning curve" for physician volume. The average values of MDVOL for CABG and cardiac catheterization patients are considerably higher than is true for AMI (109, 97, and 30, respectively; see Table 10.3). Further, for CABG and cardiac catheterization patients, possible values of MDVOL range from 1 to 248 and 1 to 252, respectively, with values rather evenly located throughout the ranges. In contrast, possible values of MDVOL for AMI patients range from 1 to 122, with considerable clustering at the low end of the range. The higher surgical volumes may reflect the presence of formal or informal guidelines. For example, the *National Guidelines for Health Planning* published in 1978 recommended a minimum of 200 cardiac procedures [17]. No such recommendations exist for treatment of AMI patients. If physicians and hospital teams learn by doing, then it may be that surgeons who perform CABG or cardiac catheterization procedures are on the flat portion of the learning curve, having passed the threshold beyond which additional experience is not related to improved patient outcome. Finally, it is important to note that the findings reported here hold only for the range of values included in this study.

Other variables in these equations perform as expected. With a single exception, patients who are more severely ill, as measured by disease staging, are significantly more likely to die in the hospital. The age variables also perform as expected. The results are particularly dramatic for AMI patients, where coefficients increase monotonically. The presence of a coronary care unit decreases the chance that heart patients will die in the hospital, but this variable is only significant for CABG patients. Similarly, AMI patients who are hospitalized in teaching facilities are less likely to die, compared to AMI patients in hospitals not affiliated with medical schools.

Recognizing that collinearity may confound these results, we tested for it in several ways. First, we tested the sensitivity of regression results to collinearity between hospital volume and physician volume, between these two volume measures and patient severity of illness, and between these two volume measures and physician board certification. To conduct these sensitivity analyses, we estimated many different versions of the basic regression equations, deleting a single variable (for example, HOSPVOL or MDVOL) or a set of variables (for example, the staging variables). The magnitude and statistical significance of HOSPVOL or MDVOL did not change appreciably in any specification. Then, we re-estimated equations using a two-stage approach proposed by Flood and Scott [24]. In the first stage, we regressed mortality on patient characteristics in order to attribute to the patient variables any variation resulting from collinearity between them and other variables. We used residuals from this stage as dependent variables and all other hypothesized determinants of mortality as independent variables in a second-stage regression equation. Again, the signs and levels of significance of variables remained about the same. Finally, we examined correlation coefficients between HOSPVOL and MDVOL. They were below .40 for the three patient groups.

These findings suggest that policies concerned with in-hospital mortality should consider discriminating on a service basis. For medical procedures such as AMI, the choice of hospital as a regional center may not be as important as ensuring that each physician treats an appropriately high number of patients. For surgical procedures such as CABG, the choice of regional center may be quite important. In any case, further research on the differential effect of physician experience on in-hospital mortality rates for medical and surgical patients is needed to formulate a sound policy for the regionalization of hospital services.

ACKNOWLEDGMENTS

The authors are grateful for programming assistance provided by Ed Hoke and Danita Holt of Social and Scientific Systems, Incorporated, under the direction of Sophie Nemirovsky; and by Ben Kamhi of SysteMetrics, under the direction of Craig Spirka. For their helpful suggestions, we thank John Burkhardt, Rosanna Coffey, Ernest Feigenbaum, Donald Goldstone, Nancy Lemrow, Ira Raskin, and Lawrence Rose. We also thank Erika Polomeskey for her skilled typing.

NOTES

1. See Kelly and Hellinger [4] for an analysis of four groups of surgical patients.
2. Hospitals that are members of the Council of Teaching Hospitals (COTH) must participate in at least four approved active residency programs, in addition to other requirements. See [7] for details.
3. Patients in investor-owned hospitals were omitted from the study because they comprise fewer than 2 percent of patients in the analysis files. Logistic regression coefficients are unreliable for classes that contain fewer than 2 percent of patients.
4. The dependent variable in the logistic model is defined as the log of the odds of dying in the hospital, i.e., $\log P/(1 - P)$. See [11].
5. The additional number of hospital (or physician) procedures necessary to obtain a target reduction in mortality (such as 1 percent) is obtained by dividing the target reduction by the coefficient on the relevant variable. In this case, $-.01 \div -.00005 = 200$.
6. This ratio is not a true elasticity because the calculation includes the actual probability of dying in the sample, rather than the expected probability. In the limit, the actual and expected values are equal.
7. See [16, p. 89] for a discussion of economies of scale in cardiac laboratories. The National Health Guidelines recommendation on cardiac laboratories appeared in [17].
8. See [23, p. 113] for a discussion of this point.

REFERENCES

1. Goldman, L., and E. F. Cook. The decline in ischemic heart disease mortality rates: An analysis of the comparative effects of medical interventions and changes in lifestyle. *Annals of Internal Medicine* 101(6):825–36, 1984.
2. Luft, H. S., J. P. Bunker, and A. S. Enthoven. Should operations be regionalized? The empirical relation between surgical volume and mortality. *New England Journal of Medicine* 301(25):1364–69, December 20, 1979.
3. Shortell, S. M., and J. P. LoGerfo. Hospital medical staff organization and quality of care: Results for myocardial infarction and appendectomy. *Medical Care* 19(10):1041-55, October 1981.
4. Kelly, J. V., and F. Hellinger. Physician and hospital factors associated with mortality of surgical patients. *Medical Care* 24(9):785–800, September 1986.
5. Gonella, J. S., M. C. Hornbrook, and D. Z. Louis. Staging of disease: A case-mix measurement. *Journal of the American Medical Association* 251:637–44, February 3, 1984.
6. Coffey, R., and M. Goldfarb. DRGs and disease staging for reimbursing Medicare patients. *Medical Care* 24(9):814–29, September 1986.
7. Council of Teaching Hospitals. *Committee Structure and Membership Directory, 1983.* Washington, DC: American Association of Medical Colleges, 1983.
8. Luft, H. S. The relation between surgical volume and mortality: An exploration of causal factors and alternative models. *Medical Care* 18(9):940–59, September 1980.
9. Flood, A. B., W. R. Scott, and W. Ewy. Does practice make perfect? Part II: The relation between volume and outcomes and other hospital characteristics. *Medical Care* 22(2):115–24, February 1984.
10. Sloan, F., J. Perrin, and J. Valvona. In-hospital mortality of surgical patients: Is there an empiric basis for standard setting? *Surgery* 99(4): 446–53, 1986.
11. Kmenta, J. *Elements of Econometrics.* New York: Macmillan Publishing Co., Inc., 1971.

12. Cannom, D. S., et al. Long-term follow-up of patients undergoing saphenous vein bypass surgery. *Circulation* 49(1):77–85, 1974.
13. Hall, R., et al. Coronary artery bypass. *Circulation* 47–48(Suppl. 3):III-146–III-150, 1973.
14. CASS Principal Investigators and Their Associates. Coronary Artery Surgery Study (CASS): A randomized trial of coronary artery bypass surgery—Survival data. *Circulation* 68(5):939–50, November 1983.
15. Cosgrove, D., F. Loop, and W. Sheldon. Results of myocardial revascularization: A 12-year experience. *Circulation* 65(Suppl. 2):II-37–II-43, 1982.
16. Adams, D. F., and H. L. Abrams. Complications of coronary arteriography: A follow-up report. *Cardiovascular Radiology* 2(1):89–93, 1979.
17. *National Guidelines on Health Planning*. Department of Health, Education and Welfare, Publication No. (HRA)78– 643. Washington, DC: U.S. Government Printing Office, 1978.
18. Levin, D. Invasive evaluation (coronary arteriography) of the coronary artery disease patient: Clinical, economic, and social issues. *Circulation* 66(Suppl. 3):III-77–III-79, 1982.
19. Hill, J. D., J. R. Hampton, and J. R. Mitchell. A randomized trail of home versus hospital management for patients with suspected myocardial infarction. *Lancet* 1(8069):837–41, 1978.
20. Mather, R. M., S. G. Blount, and E. Genton. Acute myocardial infarction: Influence of a coronary care unit. *Archives of Internal Medicine* 122(3):473–75, 1968.
21. Goldman, L. Coronary care units: A perspective on their epidemiologic impact. *International Journal of Cardiology* 2(2):284-87, 1982.
22. Stross, J. K., et al. Effectiveness of coronary care units in small community hospitals. *Annals of Internal Medicine* 85(6):709–13, 1976.
23. Flood, A. B., W. R. Scott, and W. Ewy. Does practice make perfect? Part I: The relation between hospital volume and outcome for selected diagnostic categories. *Medical Care* 22(5):98–114, May 1984.
24. Flood, A. B., and W. R. Scott, *Hospital Structure and Performance*. Baltimore: Johns Hopkins University Press, 1987.

Chapter 11

Defining Patient Categories

The study by Showstack and his associates demonstrates the importance of analyzing a well-defined group of patients. In particular, the volume-outcome relationship may be different for patients who undergo emergency surgery. Consider, for example, the entire set of patients undergoing coronary artery bypass graft (CABG) surgery. Some patients also undergo valve surgery, others receive emergency surgery after a complication of coronary angiography or an acute myocardial infarction, and still others have a chronic cardiac condition and are scheduled for surgery. We would expect different outcomes for these different groups of patients because those whose surgery is not scheduled are likely to be more acutely ill. Furthermore, if the operation is performed on an emergency basis, the regular open-heart surgery team may not be on hand and prepared to operate. A less skilled surgical team may not be able to save as many critically ill patients.

Acute episodes and the need for emergency surgery may occur at random among patients with heart disease, but these different subgroups of patients may not be randomly distributed among hospitals. A hospital with a cardiac angiography program or a large emergency room would see a disproportionate share of emergency cases with poorer expected outcomes. Therefore, a failure to take account of such differences in case mix might lead to incorrect interpretations with respect to volume. For example, Showstack's data indicate that low-volume hospitals tend to have a disproportionate share of emergency cases that have a higher expected death rate. If one did not account for this difference, low-volume hospitals would appear to have relatively worse outcomes than they actually do. Showstack and his colleagues used two approaches to deal with the problem of defining homogeneous groups of patients for analysis. First, they excluded patients with concurrent mitral valve and CABG surgery from the outcome analysis (although those patients were included in the hospital volume of CABG surgery). Second, they estimated separate regression equations for scheduled and nonscheduled CABG surgery and found that the association between higher volume and survival was stronger for nonscheduled patients; that is, the reductions in mortality in high-volume hospitals relative to low-volume hospitals were greater for the high-risk (nonscheduled) patients than for the lower-risk (scheduled) patients.

Defining admissions as emergency, nonelective, or nonscheduled, and selecting the proper terminology are difficult tasks. Without access to medical records, it is not possible to know if an admission is a true medical emergency. Although the hospital discharge abstract designates the reason for admission (as elective, urgent, or emergency), it may be biased. For example, medical records coders may be more likely to record an "urgent" or "emergency" designation when a patient dies. Admission to the hospital through the emergency room also can vary according to the hospital's routine procedures. Therefore, Showstack and his associates inferred the status of the admission from the number of days after admission that the operation took place. They categorized as "nonscheduled" those patients whose operations took place on the day of admission or three or more days after admission. The latter group primarily comprises those who were admitted for another condition or who deteriorated to the point of needing CABG surgery. Those patients who were operated on the day after or second day after admission are likely to have been scheduled for the surgery.

It is important to be careful with such approaches. Showstack felt that in 1983, the year from which his data were drawn, same-day surgery was rare for scheduled CABG patients. One could not make the same assumption about data from 1987 or 1988, because many scheduled admissions now enter the hospital on the day of their surgery.

Riley and Lubitz (1985) also used both approaches, exclusion of patients and statistical control for patients' risk factors, in a regression equation.[1] For their analyses of hip arthroplasty, femur fracture reduction, inguinal hernia repair, cholecystectomy, and CABG surgery, they excluded cases with a principal diagnosis of cancer for the hospital stay during which the patient underwent surgery. Although fewer than 1.2 percent of the patients undergoing each of these operations had cancer, their mortality experience was considerably different than that of the noncancer patients. For transurethral prostatectomy and resection of the intestine, cancer patients were retained in the analyses and controlled for in the mortality regression equations. The rationale for this difference in approach is that although many prostatectomy specimens contain cancerous cells, prostate cancer is unlikely to cause death in the immediate postoperative period, and most intestinal surgery is done for cancer.

Kelly and Hellinger (1987), who also studied heart disease, omitted patients with a length of stay of one day from their analysis of CABG surgery, cardiac catheterization, and acute myocardial infarction.[2] Because these patients have mortality rates that are much higher than average, they were classified as emergency patients. Since Showstack showed a stronger volume-outcome relationship for nonscheduled patients, Kelly and Hellinger might have shown larger coefficients for volume if they had included patients with a one-day length of stay.

Both careful selection of patients and separate analysis of scheduled and nonscheduled admissions were important in Showstack's work, but the approach may not be necessary for all diagnoses or procedures. For example, nonscheduled cases of mastectomy, hysterectomy, or transurethral prostatectomy are extremely rare. In contrast, common bile duct exploration and cholecystectomy are sometimes analyzed together, even though common bile duct surgery poses considerably more risk to the patient. Therefore, the researcher must consider carefully whether there may be a subset of patients whose outcomes might be worse or better than average for reasons that will not be captured by variables used to adjust for case mix. Reasons might include emergency surgery, a diagnosis of cancer, another concurrent procedure, or trauma.

Whether it is better to handle such risk factors by including variables in a combined regression, by estimating separate regressions for subsets of patients, or by excluding certain groups from the analysis depends on several factors. If there is reason to believe that a patient subgroup exhibits a particular relationship with respect to key variables, then interaction terms or separate regressions are necessary. If, however, there is merely a greater risk of a poor outcome, then simpler controls for the risk factors are appropriate. When subgroups represent a small portion of the total sample, separate analyses are impossible and exclusion becomes a reasonable alternative.

NOTES

1. Riley and Lubitz (1985) is reprinted in Chapter 15 of this volume.
2. Kelly and Hellinger (1987) is reprinted in Chapter 10 of this volume.

Association of Volume with Outcome of Coronary Artery Bypass Graft Surgery

Scheduled vs. Nonscheduled Operations

Jonathan A. Showstack
Kenneth E. Rosenfeld
Deborah W. Garnick
Harold S. Luft
Ralph W. Schaffarzick
Jinnet Fowles

Empirical evidence suggests that, for many surgical procedures, mortality rates are lower in hospitals performing a higher volume of a given procedure.[1-5] This association between volume of surgery at a hospital and outcome has received increasing attention both because it is measurable and because it may be amenable to policy intervention. Luft et al[1] reported substantially higher procedure-specific death rates in hospitals performing fewer than 200 coronary artery bypass graft (CABG) operations annually compared with hospitals that performed 200 or more procedures (5.7% mortality vs 3.4% for 1974 to 1975). If higher volume is associated with lower mortality and, potentially, lower costs because of shorter lengths of stay, then directing patients to higher-volume hospitals may lead to both better clinical outcomes and lower per-case costs. Recognizing the need for open heart surgery teams to perform a minimum number of operations, the American College of Surgeons has recommended that each team perform at least 150 operations per year.[6]

A variety of patient and hospital characteristics (other than the volume of surgery at the operative hospital) may be associated with the outcome of surgery. For CABG surgery, a significant association between volume and outcome remains when patient characteristics such as age, single or multiple diagnoses, and sex are accounted for, as well as when hospital-specific characteristics (eg, hospital size, teaching status, and geographic location) are considered. Advancing age and female sex are almost uniformly associated with increased risk of mortality for patients undergoing CABG. [1,3,7-10] Clinical risk factors found to be associated with poor surgical outcome include the presence and severity of angina[7,10] and the presence of heart failure,[7,10] although diabetes,[7] hypertension,[7] and previous

Journal of the American Medical Association 257, no. 6 (1987): 785–89. Copyright 1987, American Medical Association. Reprinted with permission.

acute myocardial infarction[7,9,10] have not been found to be significantly associated with in-hospital death.[7,9,10] Priority of surgery (emergency or urgent rather than elective)[7,9] and additional surgical procedures (eg, valve replacement)[7] are associated with higher mortality, while the number of coronary artery grafts inserted appears to be unrelated to outcome.[9]

In recent years, criteria for CABG surgery appear to have been expanded to allow more severely ill patients to undergo surgery. Previously reported empiric evidence of the association between the volume of CABG surgery and outcome, however, was generally drawn from the experience of patients who had surgery in the 1970s, and these studies accounted for relatively few patient characteristics. Previous studies also were limited to self-selected hospitals or samples of Medicare patients and, thus, may not be generalizable.

This study extends previous empiric work by addressing two key questions: First, has the volume-outcome relationship for CABG surgery continued to exist in recent years, particularly when data are drawn from hospitals and patients in a broad geographic area? Second, is the relationship between volume and outcome similar for all types of patients, or does it vary according to clinical and other patient characteristics, such as the emergency nature of the procedure?

MATERIALS AND METHODS

Data Sources

The source of data for this analysis was individual patient discharge abstracts for 1983 obtained from the California Health Facilities Commission (CHFC). Each discharge abstract contained a variety of demographic, clinical, and hospitalization data that characterized a specific hospitalization. The patient's principal and secondary diagnoses, and the principal and secondary procedures performed on the patient during the hospital stay, were classified according to the *International Classification of Diseases, Ninth Revision, Clinical Modification (ICD-9-CM)*.[11] All discharges with a primary or secondary *ICD-9-CM* procedure code of 36.1 through 36.19 ("bypass anastomosis for heart revascularization") were separated into a data file that included 20,093 cases.

Frequency distributions were computed for each variable in the data set. Several factors that were thought to be important to the subsequent data analysis were noted in these frequency distributions. Of the patients who had CABG surgery, 1077 also had a heart valve replacement during the same hospitalization. Because of the likely different outcome of these patients, we decided to exclude them from subsequent analyses. In addition, 15 hospitals that reported only one CABG operation during 1983, one hospital that reported only five operations, and two hospitals that had not yet reported their data to the CHFC at the time of this analysis were excluded. This left a total of 18,996 patients with CABG surgery (and no valve replacement) from 77 hospitals.

Scheduled vs. Nonscheduled Operations

Previous studies of the relation between volume of CABG surgery and in-hospital outcome did not distinguish between outcomes for different types of patients. Because of recent studies showing that new categories of patients may now be receiving CABG surgery, we hypothesized that the volume-outcome relationship might be different for higher-risk patients, such as patients admitted for an acute myocardial infarction.[12] There could be a variety of reasons for a different volume-outcome effect for "scheduled" compared with "nonscheduled" operations. For example, a patient who receives a nonscheduled CABG operation may be sicker and more acutely ill than one who receives a scheduled operation. Also, a hospital's open heart surgery team is much more likely to be on hand and prepared for a scheduled operation than for a nonscheduled operation.

The CHFC data did not list whether an operation was scheduled, and we were unable to go directly to a patient's medical record to determine the reason for the operative admission. There were, however, data available that allowed inference about the emergency nature of the CABG procedure. For example, the number of days after the admission that the operation took place was recorded. It might be hypothesized that "scheduled" operations are likely to take place on the first or second day after admission, with emergency CABG operations taking place on the day of admission. Patients who have a CABG operation on the third or subsequent day after admission also seem likely to be those who are at high risk, because they were likely admitted for another condition and/or deteriorated to the point of needing a CABG operation. Also recorded was the "reason for admission," which was coded according to whether the admission was "emergency," "urgent," or "elective." While the reason for admission might seem to be a good characterization of the concept that we were trying to assess, it is potentially biased: a medical record coder might be more likely to record "emergency" or "urgent" on the discharge abstract if there was a poor outcome. Because the day of surgery is an objective measure, the results reported below are from analyses that used day of surgery as the criterion for defining scheduled or nonscheduled surgery. (Other analyses that used a variety of other characterizations of the nature of the admission, including whether the admission was emergency, urgent, or elective, produced results entirely consistent with the results of the analyses reported below that used day of surgery as the criterion.)

Data Analysis

The methods used to analyze the data consisted of computing frequency distributions, simple bivariate correlation analyses to determine the relationships between individual independent variables, and regression equations to assess the independent associations of patient and hospital characteristics with the primary outcomes of interest: survival at the time of discharge and postoperative length of stay. Two units of analysis, patients and hospitals, are possible with this data set.

Data reported below are from analyses in which the patient was the unit of analysis; when the hospital was defined as the unit of analysis, results were similar to results of analyses of patient-level data. With the patient as the unit of analysis, the final regression equations consisted of 18,986 cases (ten cases were omitted because individual data items were missing).

Two primary *dependent variables* were analyzed: (1) discharge status (in-hospital death vs other type of discharge), and (2) "poor outcome" (the total of in-hospital death and long post-operative length of stay [for survivors only, postoperative length of stay beyond the 90th percentile for all patients undergoing CABG surgery in the state]). In-hospital mortality is a limited, although easily measured, indicator of poor quality. While objective measures of complications would be desirable, discharge abstracts did not indicate whether specific listed diagnoses were present on admission or developed after the procedure. Therefore, postoperative length of stay was used as a proxy for complications that developed subsequent to the operation. It can be argued that, after adjusting for case mix, any hospital with a high rate of patients staying longer than 15 days after the day of operation (the 90th percentile postoperative length of stay) has an unusually high rate of complications.

The *independent variables* included in the analyses were the volume of CABG surgery at the operating hospital, sex, age group, ethnic group (white vs other), presence of primary or secondary diagnostic codes of current acute myocardial infarction, congestive heart failure, and/or angina, and presence of primary or secondary *ICD-9-CM* procedure codes of coronary catheterization, and/or coronary angioplasty. The volume of surgery at the hospital was coded to include all CABG surgery, whether a valve replacement was performed or not (although *patients* who had a concurrent valve replacement were *excluded* from the analysis). For purposes of interpretation, and because of a potential nonlinear relationship between age and the dependent variables, age was entered into the regression equations as three dichotomous variables plus one reference group: age less than 50 years, age 50 to 64 years, and age over 74 years, with age 65 to 74 years as the reference group. A variable was also included to characterize whether a patient was discharged to another facility, thus not having the "chance" to die in that hospitalization.

Adjusted means were calculated from regression equations that included all of the independent variables. An adjusted mean is an estimate based on the hypothetical situation that all (hospital volume) groups had the same values on each of the independent variables that were entered into the regression equation. (A complete description of the process of adjustment was provided by Cohen and Cohen.[13] The regression equations for discharge status are shown in Table 11.1.) Analyses of the volume-outcome relationship that did not include any covariates, ie, that were analyses of variance with the volume groups as the only independent variables, produced results similar to, although slightly less sensitive statistically than, the results produced in the full regression equations that included the entire set of covariates.

Table 11.1:   Association of Patient Characteristics and Hospital Surgical Volume with In-Hospital Death Rate for Coronary Artery Bypass Graft Surgery, California, 1983

	$\beta \pm SE$		
	Total Group	*Scheduled**	*Nonscheduled†*
Patient characteristics			
Sex (male-1)	-0.0207 ± 0.0032‡	-0.0207 ± 0.0037‡	-0.0182 ± 0.0058§
Age, y			
<50	-0.0378 ± 0.0046‡	-0.0267 ± 0.0049‡	-0.0504 ± 0.0090‡
50–64	-0.0227 ± 0.0031‡	-0.0110 ± 0.0034§	-0.0365 ± 0.0058‡
≥75	0.0301 ± 0.0055‡	0.0292 ± 0.0067‡	0.0265 ± 0.0092‡
Ethnic group (white -1)	-0.0120 ± 0.0040§	$-0.0100 \pm 0.0043\|$	-0.0129 ± 0.0076
Presence of			
Acute myocardial			
infarction (yes -1)	0.0602 ± 0.0039‡	0.0611 ± 0.0051‡	0.0536 ± 0.0062‡
Congestive heart failure			
(yes -1)	0.0964 ± 0.0071‡	0.0891 ± 0.0097‡	0.0937 ± 0.0110‡
Angina (yes -1)	-0.0123 ± 0.0030‡	$-0.0079 \pm 0.0032\|$	-0.0161 ± 0.0059§
Cardiac catheterization			
(yes -1)	-0.0088 ± 0.0028§	0.0005 ± 0.0035	-0.0407 ± 0.0057‡
Coronary angioplasty			
(yes -1)	0.0252 ± 0.0069‡	0.0119 ± 0.0075	0.0429 ± 0.0133§
Other discharge (yes -1)	-0.0495 ± 0.0052‡	-0.0346 ± 0.0055‡	-0.0768 ± 0.0104‡
Hospital surgical volume			
20–100 (yes -1)	0.0207 ± 0.0069§	0.0076 ± 0.0082	0.0304 ± 0.0117§
101–200 (yes -1)	0.0077 ± 0.0039	0.0052 ± 0.0045	0.0077 ± 0.0070
201–350 (yes -1)	0.0096 ± 0.0030§	$0.0073 \pm 0.0032\|$	$0.0125 \pm 0.0059\|$
Constant	0.0686 ± 0.0053‡	0.0515 ± 0.0058‡	0.1094 ± 0.0104‡
Adjusted R^2	0.042	0.033	0.048
N	18,986	11,497	7,489

*Surgery on first or second day after admission.
†Surgery on day of admission or three or more days after admission.
‡$P<.001$.
§$P<.01$.
‖$P<.05$.

The use of secondary data to address clinical questions presents certain potential problems, such as possible miscoding of subjective data. In this study, data were derived from hospital discharge abstracts, which are coded after the fact by nonclinicians who are usually trained in abstracting medical records. The primary questions of interest addressed in this study, however, depend on the accurate coding of data elements that are relatively objective, such as day of surgery, length of stay, and discharge status. The addition of more subjective data elements to the analyses, such as presence of angina, made the results somewhat more sensitive statistically but did not alter the inferences that one might have drawn from unadjusted results. Also, there is little reason to believe that any of the data elements studied was recorded systematically in one way at higher-volume hospitals and in another way at lower-volume hospitals. Therefore, it seems reasonable to assume that the results of this study would be confirmed if detailed primary data were collected directly from patients' clinical records.

Reported below are analyses of the total group of patients, and subgroups divided according to the day after admission that their operation took place (one or two days ["scheduled"] vs any other day ["nonscheduled"]). The central questions addressed by this analysis are whether the volume of CABG surgery at a hospital is associated with in-hospital death and postoperative length of stay and how this relationship differs for scheduled surgery compared with nonscheduled surgery.

RESULTS

The 22% of hospitals with over 350 operations in 1983 accounted for 44% of all CABG surgery, while the 16% of hospitals with 100 or fewer operations accounted for only 4% of all CABG surgery (Table 11.2). Almost half (44%) of the hospitals studied had fewer than 200 operations, accounting for one fifth of all surgeries.

Table 11.3 shows the characteristics of the total group of patients studied and of patients whose operations were scheduled or nonscheduled. Most of the operations were performed on men, although there was a relatively high number of women in the nonscheduled group. Almost 90% of patients were white. Approximately one of seven patients had a current acute myocardial infarction, one of 25 patients had congestive heart failure, one of four patients had angina, slightly fewer than half of all patients had a coronary catheterization during the operative hospitalization, and approximately one of 25 patients had a coronary angioplasty performed during the study hospitalization (Table 11.3).

Patients undergoing nonscheduled surgery were much more likely to have had a current acute myocardial infarction (22% vs 9%; $P < .001$) and/or congestive heart failure (6% vs 2%; $P < .001$) and/or a cardiac catheterization during the study hospitalization 72% vs 23%; $P < .001$). Thus, these data suggest that the characterization of scheduled vs nonscheduled is capturing a real effect;

Table 11.2:   Distribution of Patients and Hospitals
According to Hospital Volume of Coronary Artery Bypass
Graft Surgery, California, 1983

No. of Operations	% of Hospitals	% of Patients
20–100	16	4
101–200	28	16
201–350	34	36
>350	22	44

Table 11.3:   Characteristics of Patient Population*

	Total Group	Scheduled Operations†	Nonscheduled Operations‡
Sex, % M	77.2	80.4	72.3
Mean age, y	61.2	60.4	62.5
Ethnicity, % W	86.7	86.6	87.0
% With diagnosis			
Acute myocardial infarction	14.2	9.1	21.8
Congestive heart failure	3.7	2.3	5.8
Angina	27.8	29.7	24.8
% With procedure (during operative hospitalization)			
Cardiac catheterization	42.4	22.9	72.4
Angioplasty	3.9	3.9	3.8
No. of patients	18,986	11,505	7,491

*On all characteristics, except the percentage of patients who received angioplasty, scheduled patients were significantly different from nonscheduled patients ($P < .001$).
†Surgery on first or second day after admission.
‡Surgery on day of admission or three or more days after admission.

patients with scheduled operations are much more likely to have had their cardiac catheterization prior to the operative admission, implying earlier preparation for the procedure, and are less likely to have other current serious medical conditions. All of the characteristics listed in Table 11.3, except ethnic group, were found in subsequent analyses to be significantly associated with the outcomes of interest.

The association of volume of surgery with in-hospital death rates, adjusted for patient characteristics, is shown in Table 11.4 and the Figure [11.1]. For the entire group of patients there was a fairly strong association of volume with adjusted death rate. For patients who received CABG surgery in hospitals performing 20 to 100 operations per year, the adjusted death rate was 0.052, falling to 0.039, 0.041, and 0.031 for patients who had surgery in hospitals with volumes of 101 to 200 operations, 201 to 350 operations, and 351 or more operations, respectively. When patients were divided according to whether they received scheduled or nonscheduled operations (as defined by their day of operation), there was a trend toward an association of volume with outcome in the group that was admitted for scheduled surgery, with a much stronger association of volume with outcome occurring for patients who were admitted for nonscheduled surgery (Table 11.4). Similar effects were seen when this effect was modeled using other categorizations of scheduled vs nonscheduled operations. For example, a substantial association of volume with adjusted in-hospital death rate was found for patients with an "emergency/urgent" admission compared with a much lower volume-outcome association for patients with an "elective" admission.

To assess total "poor outcome," patients were defined as having a poor

Table 11.4: Adjusted* In-Hospital Deaths and Poor Outcomes According to Hospital Volume of Coronary Artery Bypass Graft Surgery, California, 1983

No. of Operations	Mean %		
	Total Group (N = 18,986)	Scheduled† (N = 11,497)	Nonscheduled‡ (N = 7,489)
In-hospital deaths			
20–100	5.2§	3.0	7.7§
101–200	3.9	2.7	5.5
201–350	4.1§	2.9‖	5.9‖
>350	3.1	2.2	4.6
Poor outcomes¶			
20–100	21.7#	16.1#	27.9#
101–200	15.5#	11.5§	20.6#
201–350	11.8	8.9	16.3
>350	12.0	9.3	16.3

*Adjusted for sex, age, ethnic group, and presence of acute myocardial infarction, congestive heart failure, angina, cardiac catheterization, and coronary angioplasty.
†Surgery on first or second day after admission.
‡Surgery on day of admission or three or more days after admission.
§$P<.01$ vs. highest-volume group.
‖$P<.05$ vs. highest-volume group.
¶"Poor outcome" is the sum of the in-hospital death rate and the percentage of patients discharged alive who had a postoperative length of stay beyond the 90th percentile (15 days).
#$P<.001$ vs. highest-volume group.

outcome if they either died in the hospital or stayed beyond 15 days (the 90th percentile postoperative length of stay). A strong volume-outcome association was apparent, with the likelihood of poor outcome in the highest-volume hospitals approximately two thirds of that in the lowest-volume hospitals (Table 11.4). The magnitude of the volume-outcome effect is by far largest in the non-scheduled group, with 28% of nonscheduled patients in the lowest-volume group having a poor outcome.

To understand better the implications of these data, several estimates were derived based on the *hypothetical* situation that patients in the lowest-volume hospitals could be treated with the same efficacy and efficiency as patients in higher-volume hospitals. Of the 18,986 patients studied who received CABG surgery in California in 1983, 789 (approximately 4%) were operated on in hospitals providing *100 or fewer* operations. Their adjusted death rate was 0.053 compared with an adjusted death rate of 0.035 in hospitals with volumes above 200 CABG operations a year. Hypothetically, if the death rate for the 789 patients was similar to the case mix–adjusted death rate for patients who received their surgery in hospitals with volumes above 200 CABG operations a year, 12 lives might be saved (28% of deaths in the low-volume hospitals), 85% of which would

Figure 11.1:   Adjusted Death Rate According to Hospital Surgical Volume

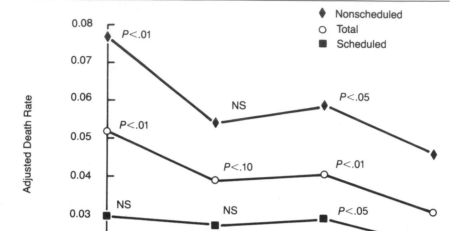

P values shown are for difference between lower-volume group and highest-volume group.
NS indicates not significant.

be in the nonscheduled group (Table 11.5). If the group of patients from the lower-volume hospitals is broadened to include patients who had surgery in hospitals with *200 or fewer* operations (approximately 20% of total patients), the total number of lives saved might increase to 18 (about 11% of deaths in hospitals with 200 or fewer operations), with 74% in the nonscheduled group. Thus, over half of the potential lives saved would be in nonscheduled operations in the lowest-volume hospitals.

COMMENT

The results of this study suggest that the association of volume of CABG surgery with in-hospital survival found by other investigators occurs for both scheduled and nonscheduled procedures, while the lifesaving potential of regionalization may be concentrated in patients who are sicker and need surgery on an emergency basis. These results imply that the greater skills of surgical teams at higher-volume hospitals may be particularly necessary to care for patients undergoing nonscheduled CABG surgery. In particular, recent evidence suggests that mem-

Table 11.5: Estimated Lives Saved if Patients at Lower-Volume Hospitals Had Outcomes Similar to Those of Patients at Higher-Volume Hospitals

Comparison Group	Estimated Lives Saved*		
	Scheduled†	Nonscheduled‡	Total
Volume≤100	1.7	9.9	11.6
Volume 101–200	2.9	3.1	6.0
Total (volume≤200)	4.6	13.0	17.6

*Compared with hospitals with a volume of more than 200 operations per year.
†Surgery on first or second day after admission.
‡Surgery on day of admission or three or more days after admission.

bers of the team in addition to the primary surgeon, in particular the anesthesiologist, may be equally important in determining outcome.[14] Empiric support is also provided for the recommendation by the American College of Surgeons that at least 150 open heart procedures be performed by a surgical team each year.[?] The volume of surgery at a hospital was also found to be positively associated with outcomes other than survival; average postoperative length of stay and the percentage of patients who had long stays were significantly lower for patients who received surgery in higher-volume hospitals.

The hypothetical savings that might result from performing all operations at higher-volume hospitals are based on several assumptions that might not prove to be true if patients were actually diverted to higher-volume hospitals. In particular, most of the lifesaving potential is seen in patients having nonscheduled surgery. Thus, the availability of a *nearby* higher-volume hospital performing CABG surgery is an essential assumption. On the other hand, the comparison group for this hypothetical analysis is the 80% of patients in hospitals with volumes greater than 200 operations. If the comparison group had been, for example, patients who received surgery in hospitals with yearly volumes of greater than 350 CABG operations, the savings might be even larger, although a focus of concern would then shift increasingly to issues such as access. These hypothetical projections should be viewed with some caution, but they may be regarded as rough approximations of the savings in lives that might occur if CABG surgery were provided to patients only in higher-volume hospitals.

The elimination of nonscheduled surgery at lower-volume hospitals would result in even lower volumes, and possibly poorer outcomes for the remaining scheduled patients. A more attractive strategy might be to shift all CABG surgery to medium- and higher-volume facilities. This shift could be accomplished in a variety of ways, such as by making hospital and/or specialty accreditation dependent on the volume of surgery performed, or by selective contracting by health insurers. Given the poor outcomes at lower-volume hospitals reported in this and other studies, the likelihood of increased numbers of malpractice suits at lower-volume hospitals might also have the effect of forcing the closure of lower-volume surgery units.

The implications of this study for regionalization and other policies related to selective use of certain hospitals will depend, to some extent, on future studies of the reasons for the differential outcomes of CABG surgery and on the location of hospitals in a particular geographic area. The fact that, in this study, most of the low-volume hospitals with poor outcomes were located within 40 miles of a high-volume hospital implies that, at least in California, further regionalization of CABG surgery may be possible without major access problems. Outcomes have to be linked closely to the clinical conditions of patients and the medical appropriateness of referral prior to admission or transferring a severely ill patient in need of surgery to another (higher-volume) hospital. Because a perforated coronary artery during coronary angioplasty necessitates immediate CABG surgery, the results of this study also suggest that coronary angioplasty should be performed only in facilities with a readily available, experienced, high-volume CABG surgery team.

The question of which specific hospitals should perform CABG surgery cannot be answered directly by this study. Despite the overall results that show a positive effect for volume, it is always possible that a particular lower-volume hospital may have good outcomes, while an individual high-volume hospital may have poor outcomes.[15] In the aggregate, however, the data suggest strongly that average outcomes would be improved if patients who require CABG surgery, particularly nonscheduled surgery, have this procedure in higher-volume hospitals.

This study was supported by a contract with the Blue Shield of California Education and Research Foundation. This study involved efforts by a number of persons who were instrumental in its inception and conduct, including Tom Purvis and Paul Gottlober from the Office of Analysis and Inspections, Office of the Inspector General, US Department of Health and Human Services, San Francisco; Amos Carey from Blue Shield of California, San Francisco; John Bunker, MD, and Byron W. Brown, PhD, from Stanford (Calif) University; and Stephen J. McPhee, MD, Benson B. Roe, MD, Cary Fox, Jan Tetreault, Deborah Peltzman, and Elizabeth Afshari from the University of California, San Francisco. Without the help and insights of these and other persons, this project would not have been possible.

REFERENCES

1. Luft HS, Bunker J, Enthoven A: Should operations be regionalized? The empirical relation between surgical volume and mortality. *N Engl J Med* 1979;301:1364–1369.
2. Luft HS: The relation between surgical volume and mortality: An exploration of causal factors and alternative models. *Med Care* 1980;18:940–959.
3. Flood AB, Scott WR, Ewy W: Does practice make perfect? I. The relation between hospital volume and outcomes for selected diagnostic categories. *Med Care* 1984;22:98–114.
4. Flood AB, Scott WR, Ewy W: Does practice make perfect? II. The relation between volume and outcomes and other hospital characteristics. *Med Care* 1984;22:115–125.
5. McGregor M, Pelletier G: Planning of specialized health facilities: Size vs. cost and effectiveness in heart surgery. *N Engl J Med* 1978;299:179–181.

6. Guidelines for minimal standards in cardiac surgery. *Am Coll Surgeons Bull* January 1984, pp 67-69.
7. Kennedy JW, Kaiser GC, Fisher LD, et al: Clinical and angiographic predictors of operative mortality from the collaborative study in coronary artery surgery (CASS). *Circulation* 1981;64:793–801.
8. Hammermeister KE, Kennedy JW: Predictors of surgical mortality in patients undergoing direct myocardial revascularization. *Circulation* 1974;49-50(suppl 2):112–115.
9. Campeau L, Lespérance J, Crochet D, et al: Clinical and angiographic determinants of early mortality related to autocoronary bypass surgery. *Can J Surg* 1979; 22:221–224.
10. Chaitman BR, Rogers WJ, Davis K, et al: Operative risk factors in patients with left main coronary-artery disease. *N Engl J MEd* 1980;303:953–957.
11. *International Classification of Diseases, Ninth Revision, Clinical Modification,* ed 2, publication (PHS) 80– 1260. US Dept of Health and Human Services, Public Health Service, Health Care Financing Administration, September 1980, vol 1–3.
12. Showstack JA, Hughes Stone M, Schroeder SA: The role of changing clinical practices in the rising costs of hospital care. *N Engl J. Med* 1985;313:1201–1207.
13. Cohen J, Cohen P: *Applied Multiple Regression/Correlation Analysis for the Behavioral Sciences,* ed 2. Hillsdale, NJ, Lawrence Erlbaum Associates Inc, 1983.
14. Slogoff S, Keats AS: Does perioperative myocardial ischemia lead to postoperative myocardial infarction? *Anesthesiology* 1985;62:107–114.
15. Luft HS, Hunt SS: Evaluating individual hospital quality through outcome statistics. *JAMA* 1986;225:2780–2784.

Chapter 12

Graphic Display of Information

The authors of the study that follows explored the relation between surgical volume and mortality for several types of surgical procedures in a relatively simple, direct fashion with the results displayed in graphical form. The use of volume categories allowed a visual display of the range of relationships between volume and outcome, without the restraint of a specific functional form. Other authors, including Farber, Kaiser, and Wenzel, (1981) and Showstack and his colleagues (1987) also visually displayed the "shape" of the relationship.[1] The plot of actual hospital death rates gives the most powerful picture of the relationship—the reader can control for case mix by direct comparison with the plot of expected death rates. Researchers often prefer to present standardized mortality ratios, which are the actual death rates divided by the expected death rates. One advantage of Luft, Bunker, and Enthoven's approach is that it could demonstrate that the expected death rate did not rise with volume, thereby providing some evidence against the argument that high-volume centers attract the sickest patients.

This was the first study to examine surgical outcomes for multiple procedures. After demonstrating that patterns may vary among procedures, the authors discussed a range of policy options. Regionalization was discussed with reference to the potential benefits of concentrating certain procedures, weighed against the need for adequate access to services and the need for emergency provision of certain services. In a later paper, Maerki, Luft, and Hunt (1986) explored the trade-off between the proportion of patients who would have to be shifted to higher-volume centers and the potential lives saved. Luft, Bunker, and Enthoven also pointed out the possibility that the observed relationship may be due to selective referrals to better surgeons and hospitals. If so, then any policy encouraging regionalization would have to refer patients to the better settings.

The study did not address the role of several potentially confounding issues, such as the importance of teaching status and hospital size. A discussion of these issues is found in Luft's analysis of the same data using regression techniques (Luft 1980).[2] By today's standards, Luft's method of adjusting for case severity was primitive. Currently, patient data are commonly available to researchers, and there is a plethora of case-mix adjustment systems from which to choose. However, even though such adjustments are crucial for the more accurate identification of individual hospital performance, they seem to add little to the interpretation of broad trends among large groups of hospitals. The authors recognized the crudeness of their approach when they began the study and chose to use broad volume categories as a way to reduce the sensitivity of their results to errors in adjusting for case mix. They seem to have been fortunate in their assumption that aggregation would reduce the potential influence of omitted variables.

NOTES

1. See Farber, Kaiser, and Wenzel (1981), reprinted in Chapter 9 of this volume, and Showstack et al. (1987), reprinted in Chapter 11.
2. See Luft (1980), reprinted in Chapter 16 of this volume.

Should Operations Be Regionalized?

The Empirical Relation between Surgical Volume and Mortality

Harold S. Luft
John P. Bunker
Alain C. Enthoven

There is a wide acceptance of the hypothesis that, other things being equal, the quality of care improves with the experience of those providing it. If true, surgical mortality rates should be lower in hospitals performing higher volumes of a given procedure. Also, the "experience effect" should be more pronounced in more complex procedures. The "experience curve," or "learning curve," describing a logarithmic decline in unit costs as a function of cumulative production experience, has been widely recognized and well documented in industrial economics.[1-3] The experience hypothesis—if true—would have important implications for the organization of medical care:[4] optimal quality as well as cost savings from economies of scale and experience could potentially be realized through "regionalization." Our search of the medical literature has yielded little statistical documentation for the hypothesis,[5-7] and no broadly based empirical evidence of what volumes are required to obtain these benefits for specific procedures. To meet this need, we have examined the relation between volume and mortality for 12 operations or operation groups from nearly 1500 hospitals.

METHODS

Basic data for use in this study were supplied by the Commission on Professional and Hospital Activities (CPHA), Ann Arbor. In these data the identities of individual hospitals are not revealed in any way. Any analysis, interpretation, or conclusion based on these data is solely our own, and CPHA specifically disclaims responsibility for any such analysis, interpretation, or conclusion. All United States short-term general hospitals participating in the Professional Activity Study during 1974 and 1975 were eligible for inclusion in the study. To test the hypothesis, surgical procedures and diagnoses of differing degrees of com-

Reprinted from *The New England Journal of Medicine* 301, no. 25 (1979): 1364–69, with permission from the Massachusetts Medical Society.

Supported by a grant from the Henry J. Kaiser Family Foundation.

plexity and anticipated mortality were chosen. Table 12.1 lists the procedures chosen for the study.

A total of 33,336 patients were excluded because they were transferred, discharged against medical advice, or had missing data on age or sex. This resulted in 420,538 patients in 1974 and 437,147 in 1975. Patients were then classified by five age categories (0 to 19, 20 to 34, 35 to 49, 50 to 64, and 65 +), sex, and whether there were single or multiple diagnoses; the latter are known to have substantially higher mortality rates.[8] Classifying by age, sex, and diagnosis (5 × 2 × 2) yielded 20 cells. For each of the resulting 20 cells for each operation or operation group, the mortality rate was computed as the number of in-hospital deaths divided by the number of patients in the cell. This set of mortality rates used the largest possible sample of patients and hospitals in order to increase the reliability of the figures. Subsequently, an additional 15,063 patients were ex-

Table 12.1: Operations and Diagnosis Groups in the Study

Group	No. of Patients Included in the Estimation of Mortality Rates, 1974–75	Operation Code Number*
1	55,397	Operations on heart, pericardium, and heart vessels (35.0–37.6)
1a	34,505	Direct heart revascularization (36.1)
2	91,343	Operations on blood vessels, except ligation and bypass (38.0–38.3, 38.5–38.7, 39.3–39.5, 39.7–39.9)
2a	9,613	Resection of vessel with graft (38.3) and abdominal aortic aneurysm (441.0, 441.3, 441.4, 441.9, 093.0)
3	17,932	Vagotomy (44.0)
3a	9,090	Vagotomy (44.0) and/or pyloroplasty (44.1) and/ or bypass gastroenterostomy (44.2) and ulcer of duodenum without hemorrhage or perforation (532.0)
4	73,427	Colectomy (45.5–45.6)†
5	330,473	Cholecystectomy (51.5)
5a	8,085	Cholecystectomy and incision of bile ducts (51.1 and 51.3)
6	18,408	Operations on biliary tract and gallbladder except cholecystectomy (51.0, 51.2–51.9)
7	176,337	Transurethral prostatectomy (60.2)
8	33,075	Total hip replacement (81.5)

*The numbers in parentheses are the surgical procedure codes (XX.X) or diagnosis codes (YYY.Y) from the *Hospital Adaptation of the ICDA* (Second edition).

†A search for patients with complete colectomy and primary diagnosis of "malignant neoplasm of large intestine except appendix and rectum" yielded only 505 cases for the two-year sample and thus was not pursued.

cluded because they were in 35 hospitals that were missing certain data or were not on the Master Facility Index of the National Center for Health Statistics. Thus, the hospital-based mortality data presented here are drawn from 842,622 patients operated on during 1974 and 1975 in 1498 hospitals.

To correct for differences in the severity of their patients' illnesses, each hospital's expected death rates were calculated using the specific death rates for the whole sample, weighted by the proportion of each hospital's patients who were classified in each of the 20 age-sex-single/multiple-diagnosis cells. The actual number of deaths for each hospital was also computed. Hospitals were categorized by the number of procedures performed in each year (1, 2 to 4, 5 to 10, 11 to 20, 21 to 50, 51 to 100, 101 to 200, and 201 +), and the average number of actual and expected deaths was computed for all hospitals in each volume category. Within each size category, average death rates were computed from the sum of deaths in all hospitals divided by the sum of patients in all hospitals, rather than the average of each hospital's death rate. (Our technique is less sensitive to the problem of small denominators.) The actual and expected death rates for each volume level and each operation or operation group appear in Figure 12.1.

The data presented in this paper are the average results for the years 1974 and 1975. For example, in Table 12.2 the first entry in column 1 (11,997) represents the average annual number of open-heart operations in hospitals doing 200 or fewer such procedures in either 1974 or 1975, with each year counted as a separate observation. The hospital figures (column 2) indicate the average number of hospitals with that volume each year. The expected death rate in those hospitals (column 4) is derived from the expected deaths in 1974 by using the 1974 mortality rates, and the expected deaths in 1975 by using the 1975 mortality rates.

By visual examination of the plots in Figure 12.1 and consideration of the number of hospitals that each point represents, we estimated the range of volumes for which the actual death rate ceased falling relative to the expected death rate. We call this the "flat of the curve." For some procedures, the relative death rate continues its decline throughout the observed range. In such cases, 200 + operations per year is taken arbitrarily as the flat of the curve, although it might be at a substantially higher volume. In selecting the point at which the curve flattens, care was taken to exclude death rates based on small numbers of hospitals, because such estimates are statistically unstable.

As indicated above, each point in Figure 12.1 represents the results for all patients treated in hospitals with the indicated volumes; as a result, there are no standard deviations. We also did a regression analysis in which each hospital is an observation.[9] This allowed us to perform the conventional statistical analysis. According to a two-tailed t-test, the coefficients for the log of patient volume are significant for open-heart surgery, coronary-artery bypass, vascular surgery, resection and graft for abdominal aortic aneurysm, colectomy, transurethral resec-

Figure 12.1: Actual and Expected Death Rates for Selected Procedures by Annual Number of Procedures in Each Hospital

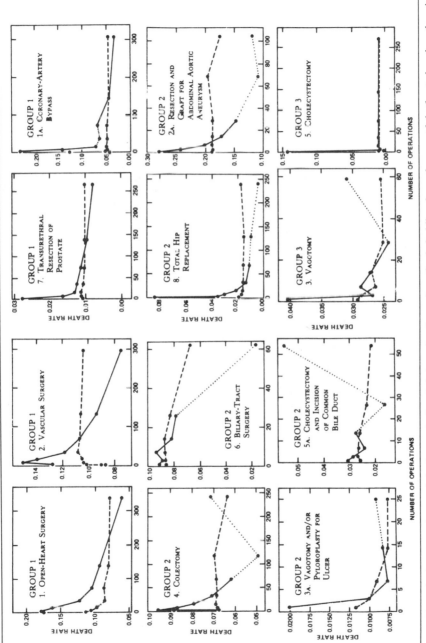

The solid line shows the actual death rates for hospitals in each volume class, the dashed line shows the expected death rate based on the mix of patients by age, sex, and single or multiple diagnosis, and the dotted line shows the death rate based on 15 or fewer hospitals. The procedures in Group 1 exhibit a falling death rate through the measured range of volumes; in Group 2, the actual death rate tends to flatten out at relatively low volumes, i.e., 10 to 50 procedures per year; Group 3 shows no consistent relation between volume and mortality.

Table 12.2: Actual and Expected Death Rates for Selected Procedures in High- and Low-Volume Hospitals and Estimates of Excess Mortality*

		Average Annual Experience, 1974–1975						Excess As:	
								The % of Deaths in Low-Volume Hospitals	The % of Deaths in All Hospitals
Group and Procedure	Volume Category	Number of Cases	Number of Hospitals	Actual Death Rate	Expected Death Rate	Projected Death Rate	Excess Deaths		
		1	2	3	4	5	6	7	8
Group 1									
1 Open-heart surgery	≤200	11,997	541	0.107	0.086	0.066	492	38	22
	>200	15,474	46	0.061	0.079	—	—	—	—
2 Vascular surgery	≤200	39,285	1,291	0.111	0.107	0.077	1,327	30	27
	>200	5,501	18	0.075	0.103	—	—	—	—
7 Transurethral resection	≤200	71,964	1,162	0.011	0.010	0.008	396	25	22
	>200	14,750	55	0.008	0.010	—	—	—	—
1a Coronary-artery bypass	≤200	9,549	157	0.057	0.047	0.034	224	41	28
	>200	7,616	25	0.034	0.047	—	—	—	—
Group 2									
4 Colectomy	≤50	21,523	1,191	0.074	0.068	0.061	291	18	12
	>50	14,560	199	0.061	0.069	—	—	—	—
6 Biliary-tract surgery	≤10	4,500	1,007	0.092	0.087	0.081	51	12	7
	>10	4,457	271	0.080	0.086	—	—	—	—
8 Total hip replacement	≤50	10,297	725	0.019	0.016	0.011	85	43	32
	>50	6,042	79	0.011	0.016	—	—	—	—

Procedure	Volume							
2a Resection and graft, abdominal aortic aneurysm	≤20	3,384	654	0.203	0.189	0.141	209	30	24
	>20	1,240	38	0.141	0.180	—	—	—	—
3a Vagotomy and/or pyloroplasty for duodenal ulcer	≤5	1,305	606	0.012	0.010	0.010	3	17	7
	>5	3,011	332	0.008	0.009	—	—	—	—
5a Cholecystectomy and incision of common bile duct	≤5	1,287	609	0.029	0.027	0.026	4	13	5
	>5	2,293	285	0.025	0.027	—	—	—	—
Group 3									
3 Vagotomy, all	≤1	161	161	0.040	0.027	0.029	2	27	1
	>1	8,543	947	0.027	0.027	—	—	—	—
5 Cholecystectomy	≤1	3	3	0.143	0.007	0.007	<1	95	0.02
	>1	162,569	1,478	0.010	0.010	—	—	—	—

*The two volume categories for each procedure represent annual volumes below and above those identified by the "flat of the curve." Actual death rates are based on the total procedure-specific deaths in the volume category divided by the number of cases (column 1). Expected death rates are based on the total death rates for each age-sex-single/multiple-diagnosis cell weighted by the case mix of patients in all hospitals within the volume category. Projected death rates are computed by multiplying the expected death rate for low-volume hospitals by the ratio of the actual to expected death rates for high-volume hospitals, e.g., 0.066 = 0.086 (0.061/0.079). The number of excess deaths is derived by multiplying the number of patients in low-volume hospitals by the difference between the actual and projected death rates. Figures in columns 5–8 may not add owing to rounding.

tion of the prostate, and total hip replacement (P<0.001) and cholecystectomy with incision of the common duct (P<0.05). Results were not statistically significant for the other procedures.

The influence of additional variables such as hospital size, total surgical volume, region, expenditures, and teaching status was examined by use of multiple regressions.[9] These regressions used the hospital as a unit of observation, and the dependent variable was the difference between actual and expected death rate. Independent variables included the logarithm of the number of patients with the procedure (to capture the nonlinear effect), the number of beds in the hospital, the number of surgical procedures of all kinds, the house-staff-to-bed ratio, whether or not the hospital was located in a Standard Metropolitan Statistical Area, its geographic region, and expenses per patient-day. Although a number of these variables are intrinsically interesting, the crucial point for this discussion is that in no case did their inclusion in the equation cause a statistically significant reduction in the coefficient for the volume measure (log of patients with procedures). In most cases, the inclusion of other factors increased the significance of the volume effect, as measured by the t-ratio.

The data are summarized in Table 12.2. The table shows the experience of hospitals with volumes above and below the flattening point for each procedure. The column headed "projected death rate" provides projections of what would occur if those patients treated in hospitals with volumes below the flat of the curve had the same experience as patients in the high-volume hospitals. Ideally, we would like to use a new set of expected death rates based only on the experience of the high-volume hospitals. These data, however, are not readily available, so we have approximated them in the following manner. Recognizing that case mix, and therefore expected death rates, may differ in high-volume and low-volume hospitals, we applied the observed proportionate reduction in deaths in high-volume hospitals to the expected deaths in low-volume hospitals. For example, in Table 12.2, for open-heart surgery the actual death rate in high-volume hospitals was only 77 percent (0.061/0.079) of that which was expected on the basis of their case mix. Low-volume hospitals had a greater proportion of patients in those age-sex-single/multiple-diagnosis cells having higher risk, yielding an expected death rate of 0.086. Multiplying this figure by 0.77 yields a projected death rate of 0.066. This projected death rate may then be compared to the actual death rate in those hospitals and the difference between the two, 0.107−0.066, when applied to the number of operations, yields an estimate of number of excess deaths.

RESULTS

The data provide clear evidence of the relation between volume and surgical mortality rates for several procedures. As seen in Figure 12.1, there are three major patterns of mortality rates. In the first group are those procedures that exhibit a falling death rate throughout the measured range, whereas the expected death rate is relatively invariant with respect to volume. Open-heart surgery, coronary-artery bypass, vascular surgery, and transurethral resection of prostate are in this category. Not only does the actual death rate continue to fall throughout the range, but the average death rates in hospitals doing only a small number of procedures are often several times that which would be expected after controlling for their mix of patients on the basis of age, sex, and multiple diagnoses.

The second group of procedures shows the importance of volume, but the death rate tends to flatten out at a relatively low volume, 10 to 50 procedures per year. Included in this category are colectomy, biliary-tract surgery without cholecystectomy, total hip replacement, resection and graft for abdominal aortic aneurysm, vagotomy and/or pyloroplasty for ulcer of duodenum, and cholecystectomy and incision of bile ducts.

The third group of procedures shows essentially no influence of volume on mortality (with the exception of those hospitals doing only one such procedure a year). Vagotomy for any diagnosis and cholecystectomy are in this third category.

For the four procedures in Group 1, substantial excess mortality occurs, assuming that all such operations could be done with outcomes similar to those of hospitals currently performing 200 or more procedures per year. For instance, outcomes such as those obtained in "flat of the curve" hospitals would avert 492, or 38 percent, of deaths after open-heart procedures in low-volume hospitals, and 1327, or 30 percent, of the deaths among patients undergoing vascular surgery. The excess deaths represent 22 to 28 percent of all deaths among patients with those procedures in all hospitals.

Some of the operations in the second group show similarly substantial savings if procedures were done in hospitals having the same outcomes as those in the flat range of the curve rather than at the low-volume, high-death-rate end. For instance, if all total hip replacements were performed with the results found in hospitals doing 50 or more procedures a year, 32 percent of all in-hospital deaths of patients with that procedure could be averted. For some of the procedures in this category, the flat of the curve is reached with very low volumes (five to 10 patients per year), and the potential mortality savings are small. For cholecystectomy and vagotomy, as long as hospitals perform more than one such procedure a year, there is no measurable difference between expected and actual mortality regardless of volume of those procedures.

It is often asserted that large hospitals receive the more complex cases whereas small hospitals treat the easier patients. Such an allocation of patients makes intuitive sense. The expected death rates in our analysis include the influence of age, sex, and presence of multiple diagnoses, three factors found to be highly correlated with more sensitive measures of disease severity and American Society of Anesthesiologists ratings of preoperative condition.[10-12] For most of the procedures examined, the expected death-rate curves are either flat or downward sloping, suggesting that hospitals with higher volumes are not treating a disproportionate share of patients in the higher risk categories. In fact, in the case of open-heart operations and vagotomy alone or in combination with pyloroplasty for ulcer, hospitals with relatively fewer patients a year have a mix of patients that is substantially riskier in terms of their expected death rates.

DISCUSSION

We report herein clear evidence of a relation between surgical volume and surgical mortality in hospitals participating in the Professional Activities Study (PAS) data system. Can the results be generalized to all hospitals? In 1974–75, 29 percent of all nonfederal, short-term hospitals in the United States were in the PAS system, and they accounted for 40 percent of all nonfederal, short-term discharges.[13] Thus, the PAS system is weighted towards larger hospitals. Given the correlation we found between hospital size and number of procedures, this suggests that hospitals not in the PAS system include a greater proportion of hospitals with small surgical volumes. If these hospitals have a mortality experience similar to that of PAS hospitals of comparable patient volumes, the proportion of excess deaths for the country as a whole is greater than the one we estimated.

This study provides evidence of a strong negative correlation, for some operations, between the number of surgical procedures done in a hospital and the in-hospital mortality rate for those patients. Can we explain its cause? Patient selection is an obvious and important candidate. Hospitals operating on sicker patients will predictably experience poorer outcomes. There is some evidence that, for some operations, this was the case. For example, the expected death rate for hospitals undertaking fewer than 20 open-heart operations per year was 0.11, indicating a patient mix disproportionately weighted toward riskier categories, whereas the expected death rate for hospitals undertaking more than 200 open-heart operations per year was 0.08, almost one-third lower. For most of the operations studied, the expected death rate shows no relation to volume or is greater than average only for hospitals undertaking a very small number of procedures (fewer than five per year), perhaps reflecting the occasional patient requiring emergency surgery who is too ill to refer elsewhere. This might, for example, be the case for resection and graft for ruptured abdominal aortic aneurysm.

A higher proportion of emergency cases in smaller hospitals cannot, however, explain the steady decrease in death rates observed over the full range of procedure rates for open-heart surgery, coronary-artery bypass graft, vascular surgery, and transurethral resection, since only a very small proportion of any of these procedures is undertaken on an emergency basis. To explain this steady decline on the basis of patient selection, one might postulate that hospitals that only occasionally undertake a given operation are reluctant to operate except when the indications are very strong, whereas hospitals with larger experience, and lower mortality, may be more willing to operate on low-risk patients with fewer indications. Concerning how large the effect of patient selection is, and for how many of the operations, we can say relatively little from the data on which risk is estimated in the present study. These data include age, sex, and multiple diagnoses, three factors that correlate highly with more sensitive measures of physical status,[12] but they may not reflect subtle variations in the severity or diagnosis of surgical disease. For instance, patients in high-volume hospitals may, because of the more experienced staff, have more diagnoses identified and thus fall in a higher risk category. We should note, however, that our measures do not support the hypothesis that the lower mortality rates in high-volume hospitals can be easily explained away by a mix of patients with lower than average risk of death.

A second potential explanation for the observed effect, and the hypothesis on which this study was based, is that higher volumes or greater experience or both lead to improved results. There is substantial evidence from industry that the cost of producing an item falls as the work team gains experience with that specific process.[1,2] Learning by doing is commonly observed and is the basis for much of medical education. Accordingly, the relation should be between mortality and experience, rather than volume, but the two are difficult to separate. More importantly, our data do not allow an investigation of whether the relevant experience is that of specific surgeons, the operating-room team, or perhaps the whole hospital staff.

A third alternative is that the observed correlations are the results of referral patterns: that larger surgical volumes are the result of better results, rather than the cause. Some hospitals have more skillful surgeons (operating-room teams, nurses, etc.), and as a result may attract a larger share of the patients suffering from a particular condition. That this may be the case is suggested by the fact that for some procedures, such as open-heart and coronary-artery bypass, there is already a substantial concentration of patients in hospitals with low mortality rates. For instance, 56 percent of open-heart operations are performed in 8 percent of the hospitals doing open-heart surgery (Table 12.2). Policy statements[14-16] by various professional groups recommending regionalization of heart surgery may well have contributed to this concentration.

CONCLUSIONS AND RECOMMENDATIONS

The data in this study establish, for some operations, a negative correlation between the annual number done in a hospital and postoperative mortality, after controlling for patients' age, sex, and single or multiple diagnoses. These results may be explained by the effect of volume or experience on mortality, or by the referral of a larger volume of patients to those institutions or surgeons known to have better outcomes. The results may also reflect, in part, differences in patient mix not measured by our statistical controls; for example, institutions with better outcomes may be able to justify operating on patients with less severe disease. The case for regionalization does not depend on the relative importance of these determinants, however. Accordingly, we should not postpone developing policies to encourage the regionalization of those procedures whose outcomes are markedly less satisfactory in low-volume hospitals.

The first step in such a policy should be to implement comprehensive, regional surgical-outcome data systems in order to confirm the results presented here, to include many of the operations we have not examined, and to provide information for each hospital and operation as a basis for policy decisions. A second step would seek to extend this study below the hospital level and test for comparable effects for the individual surgeon, anesthesiologist, or support team. Outcome data should include morbidity as well as mortality. (We call attention to the fact that morbidity was not examined in the present study and that important differences may have been missed. For example, although there was no measurable relation between volume and mortality after simple cholecystectomy, the possibility that complications such as injury to the common bile duct occur more often in less experienced hospitals was not tested.)

Those operations that are confirmed as having important relation between volume and mortality should be considered for regionalization. For instance, among the procedures examined in this paper, candidates for early regionalization would be open-heart surgery, major vascular surgery, and total hip replacement. The guiding principle should be: the greater the excess risk of low-volume surgery, the greater the distance one should be willing to travel to a hospital or surgeon with high volumes and good outcomes. Moreover, specific regionalization decisions should reflect local geographic resources and preferences and should be carried out with a minimum of disruption of services.

Previous recommendations for the regionalization of open-heart surgery, including minimum numbers of procedures for a given institution, have relied on the opinions of experts.[14-16] The data presented here provide an objective basis on which to formulate such recommendations. The data presented do not, however, allow precise definition of the optimal volume for each operation. For example, the "true" flat of the curve for hip replacements might start at 30, 75, or even 100 procedures per year. Although we may not be able to identify an appropriate minimum with precision, it does not appear appropriate for such procedures to be performed in hospitals only one to four times a year, as in 209 hospitals in the PAS data system in 1975. Nor does it seem appropriate to perform on an occasional basis any procedures for which the risk is substantially higher in low-volume hospitals, except in the case of emergency surgery—for example, resection and graft of ruptured aortic aneurysm.

We should emphasize that operations are performed and patients are cared for not by hospitals but by surgeons, anesthesiologists, operating-room teams, and nursing staffs. The poor outcomes in a specific hospital may be the result of the good outcomes of one well qualified surgeon being swamped by the poor outcomes of several "occasional" surgeons.[17] Similarly, a high-volume institution may harbor some "occasional" surgeons, but their failures can be more readily masked in aggregate statistics. We do not propose that statistics of this type can substitute for careful quality review by the hospital staff. Instead, such statistical analyses may serve as starting points for more detailed examinations by hospital staffs, by local professional standards review organizations, and by other review bodies.

Not all procedures will need to be regionalized. There are no apparent mortality savings in regionalizing relatively simple procedures such as cholecystectomies and vagotomies. Even with vagotomies and/or pyloroplasty done for ulcer of the duodenum, which show some sensitivity to volume, the mortality rate stabilizes at five patients per year. It may be that many operations performed in short-term general hospitals are in the category in which volume does not markedly affect performance. Moreover, after the volume of the specific procedure has been controlled for, hospital size or total surgical load have relatively little correlation with outcomes.[9] Rather than by concentrating all surgery in a few large, all-purpose medical centers, regionalization may be achieved with moderate-sized hospitals doing a full range of safer, volume-insensitive procedures, and a high volume of a selected number of riskier, volume-sensitive procedures in which they specialize. Thus, although regionalization may require a substantial improvement in the referral patterns for certain, more complex procedures, it is possible that large segments of surgical practice may not require change.

We are indebted to Wayne Ewy, Byron Wm. Brown, and William Forrest for assistance in the early design of this study, to Walter Wood, for management of data-processing activities at CPHA, to Luke Froeb for able research assistance, and to members of the UCSF Health Policy Program and Stanford Health Services Research Seminar for valuable comments on earlier drafts.

REFERENCES

1. Perspectives on Experience. Boston, Boston Consulting Group, 1972
2. Wright TP: Factors affecting the cost of airplanes. J Aeronaut Sci 3:122, 1936
3. Asher H: Cost-Quantity Relationships in the Airframe Industry, Santa Monica, California, Rand Corporation, 1956
4. McGregor M, Pelletier G: Planning of specialized health facilities; size vs. cost and effectiveness in heart surgery. N Engl J Med 299:179-181, 1978
5. Adams DF, Fraser DB, Abrams HL: The complications of coronary arteriography. Circulation 48:609–618, 1973
6. Iber FL, Cooper M: Jejunoileal bypass for the treatment of massive obesity: prevalence, morbidity, and short- and long-term consequences. Am J Clin Nutr 30:4–14, 1977
7. Chalmers TC: Randomization and coronary artery surgery. Ann Thorac Surg 14:323–327, 1972

8. Hospital Mortality: PAS hospitals, United States, 1972–73. Ann Arbor, Michigan, Commission on Professional and Hospital Activities, 1975

9. Luft HS: The relationship between surgical volume and mortality: an exploration of causal factors and alternative models. Presented at the 54th annual meeting of the Western Economic Association, Las Vegas, Nevada, June 17–21, 1979

10. The National Halothane Study: A study of the possible association between halothane anesthesia and postoperative hepatic necrosis. Edited by JP Bunker, WH Forrest Jr, F Mosteller, et al. Bethesda, Maryland, National Institute of General Medical Sciences, 1969

11. Staff of the Stanford Center for Health Care Research: Comparison of hospitals with regard to outcomes of surgery. Health Serv Res 11:112–127, 1976

12. The Staff of the Stanford Center for Health Care Research: Study of the Institutional Differences in Postoperative Mortality (PB 250 940/LK). Springfield, Virginia, National Technical Information Service, 1976

13. Hospital Mortality: PAS hospitals, United States, 1974–75. Ann Arbor, Michigan, Commission on Professional and Hospital Activities, 1977

14. Scannell JG, Brown GE, Buckley MJ: Report of the Inter-society Commission for Heart Disease Resources: optimal resources for cardiac surgery: guideline for program planning and evaluation. Circulation 52:A23–A37, 1975

15. Cardiovascular Committee of the American College of Surgeons: Guidelines for minimal standards in cardiovascular surgery. Ann Thorac Surg 15:243–248, 1973

16. U.S. President's Commission on Heart Disease, Cancer and Stroke: Report to the President: A national program to conquer heart disease, cancer and stroke. Volume 2. Washington, DC, Government Printing Office, 1965

17. Hotchkiss WS: Patent ductus arteriosus and the occasional cardiac surgeon. JAMA 173:244–247, 1960

Chapter 13

Comparisons of Volume Categories or Regression Analyses?

The study by Sloan, Perrin, and Valvona provides an example of how authors can examine a question using both fairly simple methods categorizing observations by a crucial variable, such as volumes or outcomes, and a more sophisticated approach using multiple regression analysis. The first approach allows the reader to compare the findings with common perceptions of the world. (Few of us are able to "hold everything else constant" in our heads.) This is often important when one is addressing policymakers and clinicians, rather than health services researchers. The second approach allows the analyst and researcher to explore *why* certain results are observed.

Sloan, Perrin, and Valvona asked an important health policy question: Does the empirical evidence provide a sufficient basis for establishing minimum volume standards for certain surgical procedures? They also asked three research-oriented questions: Does the evidence support a conclusion that volume of a procedure in a hospital affects inpatient mortality? What is the mortality experience of hospitals beginning or discontinuing certain procedures? Do mortality rates within hospitals vary substantially among procedures?

A policymaker might interpret the first question as the following: If one were to classify hospitals as having low, medium, or high mortality rates, would these categories be associated with such markedly different volume levels that clear minimums could be established? After classifying hospitals on the basis of their procedure-specific mortality rates, Sloan, Perrin, and Valvona found that both low- and high-mortality hospitals performed fewer procedures, on average, than medium-mortality hospitals. An analysis of year-to-year groupings by mortality rate demonstrated substantial movement by hospitals from one group to another, and there was essentially no correlation in mortality rates among procedures within hospitals. Although these findings may be due, in part, to the inherent instability of mortality rates based on small numbers of patients, this very instability is a crucial political problem for the policymaker.[1] It may be quite difficult for a regulatory authority or state legislature to resist the arguments that some low-volume hospitals have no deaths and some high-volume hospitals have high death rates.

Sloan, Perrin, and Valvona were also able to show that their multiple regression results were consistent with those of other researchers who found decreasing mortality rates associated with increased volume, at least up to a point. A quadratic equation with volume and volume-squared was estimated; it implied a minimum mortality rate at some level. With the exception of the estimates for coronary artery bypass graft surgery, these findings indicated that only a small percentage of hospitals (0.4 percent to 5.6 percent) have volumes above that associated with the estimated minimum. As is the case for all the other studies estimating regression models, Sloan, Perrin, and Valvona did not report on alternative functional forms, so there is no way of knowing whether the quadratic model is the best.

The role played by regressions and comparisons among categories varies among studies. Sloan, Perrin, and Valvona gave about equal weight to both sets of analyses in their presentation of findings. Their regressions are consistent with those of other researchers, thus increasing confidence in the analysis. The specific findings of the regressions and comparisons among categories were not contrasted, but both can be interpreted as lending support to the notion that volume may not be a good enough predictor of low mortality to be valid as a regulatory measure.

Farber, Kaiser, and Wenzel (1981) and Showstack and his colleagues (1987) also reported results using both volume categories and regressions.[2] They found that the same patterns observed using categories are generally found even after controlling for other variables. In contrast, Roos and his colleagues (1986) and Flood, Scott, and Ewy (1984a) began with simple bivariate results and found that the influence of hospital volume was lessened when other variables were held constant.[3] One potential explanation for the differences in the two sets of studies is in the number of categories used. The latter two studies each used a simple classification of high versus low volume, but the first three studies used between three and eight categories. If much of the "action" is concentrated in hospitals with very low volumes or in those with very high mortality rates, then the use of more categories helps prevent the effect of these important, but infrequent, observations from being swamped by other, more normal observations. Sloan, Perrin, and Valvona noted a similar problem and pointed out that their regression results tended to hide the good outcomes of some hospitals with very low volume.

This discussion of presentation techniques brings us back to the goals of the authors with respect to policy and research. Multiple regression models are important tools in the attempt to hold other variables constant and to rule out the potential influence of confounding factors. Policymakers, however, generally do not understand regression models. More important, few regulations are established to account for multiple factors. More frequently, they are relatively simple rules, such as "a hospital must have at least x procedures a year." If the qualitative results of a study are the same using both a simple classification and a more scientifically correct model holding other factors constant, then it is far easier to make policy recommendations.

NOTES

1. See, for example, Luft and Hunt (1986), reprinted in Chapter 19 of this volume.
2. See Chapter 9 for reprint of Farber, Kaiser, and Wenzel (1981), and Chapter 11 for reprint of Showstack et al. (1987).
3. The study by Roos et al. (1986) is reprinted in Chapter 8 of this volume; Part I of Flood, Scott, and Ewy (1984a) is reprinted in Chapter 14.

In-Hospital Mortality of Surgical Patients

Is There an Empiric Basis for Standard Setting?

Frank A. Sloan
James M. Perrin
Joseph Valvona

Mainly because of cost-containment concerns, insurers and planners are increasingly under pressure to develop standards to guide both payment decisions and the review of facilities and services. A prominent example of such standards is the federal health planning guidelines promulgated in 1978.[1] These guidelines establish specific standards for states to follow in regulating certain types of hospital facilities and services under certificate of need programs. Several private bodies (e.g., professional organizations) have developed numerical criteria for certain services, such as obstetric units.[2] These standards reflect both quality and cost concerns. However, unlike the federal guidelines, they lack the force of law. Like most "structure" criteria, relatively few have been shown to relate to better outcomes.

Proponents of standard setting emphasize the need for external intervention to regulate cost and quality and the responsibility of the payer and planner to intervene on behalf of the patient and premium payer or taxpayer.[3] Those opposed to standard setting question the scientific base underlying the criteria, the value issues inherent in standard setting, and the anticompetitive or franchising effects that may follow from excluding certain providers. Further, they note that variations among both patients and providers around any measure of central tendency make difficult the application of specific guidelines.[4,5]

A relationship often discussed in standard setting is the one between the frequency with which a given procedure is performed at a hospital and the associated in-hospital mortality rate. This study asks four questions. First, does the empiric evidence support a conclusion that the frequency of performing a procedure affects the likelihood that a patient will be discharged from the hospital alive? Second, what is the mortality experience of hospitals that decide to begin

Reprinted from *Surgery* 99, no. 4 (1986): 446–53, with permission from The C. V. Mosby Company.

Supported in part by a grant from the National Center for Health Services Research entitled "Diffusion of Surgical Technology" (No. 1 R01 HS04762-01) to the Institute for Public Policy Studies, Vanderbilt University.

or discontinue certain surgical procedures? Third, do mortality rates for different procedures vary within hospitals or are they more likely to be characteristic of hospitals? Fourth, does the empiric evidence provide a sufficient basis for establishing minimum volume standards? We explored these issues by analyzing variations in in-hospital mortality rates associated with patients who underwent any of seven surgical procedures during their hospital stays in a national cohort of more than 500 hospitals.

METHODS

Sample and Data Base

The basic data for this study were drawn from discharge abstracts on 521 hospitals that subscribed to the Commission on Professional and Hospital Activities (CPHA) discharge abstracting service continuously between 1972 and 1981. The CPHA constructed a file for purposes of this study containing annual measurements by hospital for 1972 to 1981 on the frequency that each of several surgical procedures was performed in each hospital. For each procedure, data were assembled on in-hospital mortality rates, length of stay, patient age and sex, procedure-specific indicators of patient severity of illness, and source of payment expected at time of discharge. For the purpose of this study, surgical mortality was defined as death during the same hospitalization in which the procedure was performed. Discharge summaries do not allow analysis of the direct relation between procedure and death, but we assumed that mortality as defined here would likely have been avoided in the very near term if the patient had not been hospitalized for surgery.

We confined the sample to short-term general (community) hospitals. Because we had to choose from CPHA-subscribing hospitals, the sample is not fully representative of community hospitals in the United States. Large, teaching, and midwestern hospitals are somewhat overrepresented and for-profit hospitals underrepresented.

The seven surgical procedures selected represent both high- and low-mortality procedures performed by a variety of surgical specialists. ICD-9-CM procedure codes were: hip arthroplasty (81.5–81.6), coronary artery bypass (36.0–36.9), morbid obesity surgery (44.3, 44.5, 45.6, 45.90–45.93 with diagnosis code 278.0), hysterectomy (68.3–68.8), mastectomy (85.4), nephrectomy (55.4–55.5), and spinal fusion (81.0).[6] Various coding schemes were applied before 1979, the year in which the ICD-9-CM system was initiated. We developed bridges among three coding systems (H-ICDA-1 and -2, and ICD-9-CM), which, for some procedures, necessitated minor compromises in definition.

At an early stage in the research, we found appreciable variation in hospital mortality rates, both cross sectionally and over time. To assess these differences, we established criteria for grouping hospitals by year into one of three categories according to the hospital's procedure-specific mortality rate in that year. We termed hospitals with no deaths during the year among patients undergoing the procedure as low mortality; the high-mortality classification applied when the hospital mortality rate for the procedure was at least 1 SD above the procedure mean for the year or in the top 10% of rates, whichever was less. We called the remaining hospitals medium mortality. For some procedures, more than 90% of hospitals had 0% mortality rates for the procedure. In such cases we combined the high and medium categories.

For six of the seven procedures with appreciable mortality (all except spinal fusion), we examined a number of hospital characteristics and patient- and procedure-specific variables using multiple regression analysis. The dependent variable was the hospital's mortality rate for a procedure in each year.

Several independent variables measured hospital characteristics, bed size, several indicators of teaching status, and ownership (government versus other). Variables describing characteristics of the hospital's medical staff, hospital region, and metropolitan status were initially studied but later excluded after we failed to detect an association with mortality.

Patient- and procedure-specific independent variables included, in addition to volume (number of times the procedure was performed at the hospital during the year) and volume squared (to measure nonlinear effects of volume on mortality), the percent of patients by age and sex, multiple versus single diagnosis, whether the operation was performed within 6 hours of admission or later, expected payment source at time of discharge, and the percent of patients with procedure-specific risk factors. (For example, for surgery for morbid obesity, such factors were diabetes and cardiac disease.) Choice of risk factors was in part determined by the information available from the discharge abstracts. For the classification of multiple diagnoses, we required that two or more organ systems be involved. In some regressions, we included variables to measure the influence of state mandatory hospital rate-setting programs on mortality. Main regression results are presented here, with further detail on the risk factors and additional analysis in Appendix A.[*]

RESULTS

Trends in operative mortality show a wide range of mortality rates for the seven procedures chosen, with a general trend toward lower mortality rates over time (Table 13.1). Mortality rates in 1981 varied from 5.9% for nephrectomy, 4.5% for coronary artery bypass, 4.3% for hip arthroplasty, and 1.7% for surgery for morbid obesity to less than 1% for the remaining procedures.

---

[*]Appendix A (*Results of Regression Analysis of In-Hospital Mortality*) filed with the National Auxiliary Publications Service (NAPS) (ASIS-NAPS, Microfiche Publications, P.O. Box 3513, Grand Central Station, New York, NY 10163, deposit XXXXX).

Table 13.1: Number of Hospitals in Low-, Medium-, and High-Mortality Categories

Surgical Procedure	Year	Mean (%)	Boundaries (%)		No. of Hospitals		
			Low to Medium Mortality	Medium to High Mortality*	Low	Medium	High
Hip arthroplasty	1972	6.0	0	15.4	167	181	39
	1981	4.3‡	0	9.1	168	227	48
Coronary artery bypass	1972	11.2	0	20.0	10	30	5
	1981	4.5‡	0	7.6	1	58	8
Morbid obesity surgery	1972	5.6	0	—	80	10	—
	1981	1.7§	0	—	101	9	—
Hysterectomy	1972	0.2	0	0.6	374	75	61
	1981	0.1‡	0	0.3	421	36	55
Mastectomy	1972	0.8	0	1.7	430	15	51
	1981	0.3†	0	—	461	40	41
Nephrectomy	1972	3.1	0	10.0	293	54	—
	1981	5.9†	0	16.1	244	109	45
Spinal fusion	1972	1.0	0	—	268	29	—
	1981	0.7	0	1.3	262	10	31

*Dashes indicate that there was no high category.
†Significant at the 1% level (t test for differences between 1972 and 1981 mean values).
‡Significant at the 5% level (t test for differences between 1972 and 1981 mean values).
§Significant at the 10% level (t test for differences between 1972 and 1981 mean values).

Mortality Rates and Frequency of Procedures

The boundary above which a hospital's mortality rate was classified as high varied greatly across procedures (Table 13.1). In 1972 hospitals performing hip arthroplasty operations had to have a death rate of at least 15.4% to be in the high group. By 1981 that classification had dropped to a death rate of 9.1% or greater. A mortality rate of 20% or greater for coronary artery bypass was high in 1972, and a mortality rate above 7.6% in 1981 was high. In some cases there were an insufficient number of non-0% rates to even define a high group.

With the exception of hip arthroplasty and coronary artery bypass, more than three fifths of hospitals performing a procedure had no deaths. For procedures with sizeable mortality rate, a consistent pattern was observed, with both high- and low-mortality hospitals performing fewer procedures than did hospitals with intermediate mortality rates (Table 13.2). The hospitals in the low-mortality group tended to have low volume and were smaller than hospitals in other groups. Most likely, a patient selection mechanism was present in the low-volume, low-mortality hospitals.

The 1981 figures for coronary artery bypass show that one hospital averaged only 19 procedures per year and had no deaths. Fifty-eight hospitals in the medium group performed an average of 329 procedures per year, with an average mortality rate of 3.7%. In contrast, eight hospitals, with a mean of 118 coronary bypass operations, had an average mortality rate of 11%.

Using the regression coefficients on the volume and volume square variables, we calculated the volumes for each of the procedures at which mortality reaches its minimum level (Table 13.3). The estimated minimums were relatively invariant regardless of whether hospitals with 0% mortality rates were excluded from the regression. However, we found substantial differences among procedures in the points of minimum mortality; they ranged from around 30 for nephrectomy to about 500 for coronary bypass surgery and about 1100 for hysterectomy. The vast majority of hospitals had volumes far below these minimums in 1981. Using the regression coefficients based on the full sample, we computed the rate of decline in in-hospital mortality rates for various increases in volume (Table 13.4). We found declines of a percentage point or more for a 50-unit increase in volume for two procedures, hip arthroplasty and coronary bypass surgery. Although the volume associated with minimum mortality was very high for hysterectomy (Table 13.3), the estimated rate of decrease in the mortality rate for a 50- or even 100-unit increase in volume was less than 0.1%.

We generally found a negative relationship between mortality rates and the number of procedures the hospital performed per annum. The volume figures show that as a hospital performs more operations of several types, its proficiency increases as measured by lower mortality rates. This so-called learning effect may result from the surgeon's skills being called on more often and a more cohesive nature to the entire surgical team because of greater experience together.

Table 13.2: Mortality, Volume, and Bed Size by Low-, Medium-, and High-Mortality Categories

Surgical Procedure	Year	Mortality (%)		Volume (Mean)			Bed Size (Mean)		
		Medium	High*	Low	Medium	High*	Low	Medium	High*
Hip arthroplasty	1972	6.6	29.1	12	41	12	194	335	213
	1981	4.0†	20.9‡	25	65	13	185	342	174
Coronary artery bypass	1972	9.6	43.3	6	70	10	319	482	466
	1981	3.7†	11.0†	19	329	118	539	494	300
Morbid obesity surgery	1972	50.3	—	5	14	—	342	372	—
	1981	20.6	—	18	36	—	353	453	—
Hysterectomy	1972	0.4	1.6	161	402	134	191	372	208
	1981	0.2†	1.2	139	506	193	209	499	304
Mastectomy	1972	1.3	7.1	25	83	31	213	486	253
	1981	4.1§	—	27	50	—	233	369	—
Nephrectomy	1972	5.9	21.7	8	24	10	232	399	300
	1981	8.8†	30.5‡	7	20	11	230	405	288
Spinal fusion	1972	9.9	—	19	50	—	283	442	—
	1981	0.9	7.0	20	156	43	306	491	412

*Dashes indicate that there was no high category.

*Significant at the 1% level (t test for differences between 1972 and 1981 mean values).

†Significant at the 5% level (t test for differences between 1972 and 1981 mean values).

‡Significant at the 10% level (t test for differences between 1972 and 1981 mean values).

Table 13.3:   Volume at Minimum Mortality

	Full Sample		Non-0% Sample	
Surgical Procedure	Volume at Minimum Mortality	% of Hospitals Exceeding Volume at Minimum Mortality (1981)	Volume at Minimum Mortality	% of Hospitals Exceeding Volume at Minimum Mortality (1981)
Hip arthroplasty	135	4.5	118	9.8
Coronary artery bypass	510	16.4	479	19.7
Morbid obesity surgery	192	0.9	105	11.1
Hysterectomy	1092	0.4	824	3.3
Mastectomy	101	2.2	90	10.0
Nephrectomy	30	5.6	33	7.7

Table 13.4:   Effects of Volume Changes on Mortality Rates*

	Volume Change (per 50 U)			
Surgical Procedure	5 to 50	50 to 100	100 to 200	200 to 350
Hip arthroplasty	−1.7	−1.0	—	—
Coronary artery bypass	−1.0	−1.0	−1.6	−1.6
Morbid obesity surgery	−0.6	−0.5	—	—
Mastectomy	−0.4	−0.2	—	—

*Numbers shown are differences between two mortality rates expressed as percents. Dashes indicate that the volume at minimum mortality is estimated to occur before the end point of the interval. Estimated changes for hysterectomy are less than 0.1% for each interval shown.

Although there is generally a negative relation between volume and mortality, the regression analysis demonstrates that for any procedure, no more than 10% of the variance in mortality rates is explained by volume alone. For two procedures, delivery and nephrectomy, we found positive correlations between volume and mortality rates.

The observation that several hospitals performing high-mortality procedures (hip arthroplasty, coronary artery bypass, and nephrectomy) had no deaths while doing fewer procedures per year than did higher-mortality hospitals questions the validity of setting minimum levels for the procedure via a public regulatory process. In 1981, 42% of the hospitals from our sample performing coronary artery bypass were below the federal guidelines of 200 open-heart operations per year, and more than 80% were under the minimum mortality level of about 500. Our volume figures do not include valve operations; however, it is doubtful that their inclusion would bring many hospitals above 200. Similarly, virtually all hospitals were below the estimated minimum mortality volumes in 1981 (Table 13.3).

Regression analysis also allowed us to determine distinguishing factors of hospitals that experienced no deaths for a given procedure in 1 year. In general, hospitals experiencing 0% mortality had no teaching program and were located in nonmetropolitan counties with comparatively low proportions of board-certified specialists. These results are consistent with the view that hospitals with no surgical deaths took patients with a lower risk of dying. This pattern was much clearer for hip arthroplasty than for coronary bypass surgery or mastectomy.

The rise in hospital personnel per patient day and investments in sophisticated equipment may have contributed to the decline in mortality rates. The object of cost-containment approaches is to reduce the rate of growth in hospital expenditures by placing constraints on hospital employment and investment. To ascertain whether mandatory rate-setting programs, the most stringent cost-containment programs implemented during the 1970s, had an adverse effect on in-hospital mortality rates, we included variables representing such programs in our regressions (Appendix A). The rate-setting variables had statistically insignificant impacts on mortality in all regressions. Although these programs reduced the rise in hospital cost on the average,[7-9] they apparently did not constrain resources in such a way as to have an adverse effect on mortality.

Starting and Discontinuing Procedures

Table 13.5 shows how, under our scheme, a hospital's classification changed from 1972 to 1981 for the high-mortality procedures. For hip arthroplasty, the 39 hospitals with high mortality rates in 1972 had mainly moved into low (41%) or medium (44%) categories. Among the 67 hospitals that began the procedure after 1972, most had low or medium 1981 mortality rates, although this group of hospitals was more than twice as likely to have a high mortality rate in 1981 than were hospitals that had already performed this procedure by 1972. For coronary artery bypass, one out of 24 hospitals that did not perform the procedure in 1972 performed it in 1981 with no deaths. The vast majority had a medium rate in 1981. The high 1972 mortality hospitals appear to have achieved a better record in 1981 in that four of the five had moved into the medium category. One of the 10 low-mortality hospitals in 1972 had discontinued the procedure by 1981.

Nephrectomies appear to have had lower mortality rates in hospitals that began the procedure after 1972. Of the 47 not performing the surgery in 1972, only two were in the high-mortality group in 1981 and 44 had no deaths. Twenty-one of the hospitals classified as high in 1972 showed no deaths in 1981 and only five remained in the high category. Table 13.5 shows a trend for hospitals to move toward the medium category over time.

Table 13.6 examines hospital mortality rates and the length of time a procedure was performed at the hospital. The significance test in column 2 is for column 2 versus column 1. The test in column 3 is for column 3 versus column 1, and the test in column 4 is column 4 versus column 2.

Table 13.5:   Movement of Hospitals among Low-, Medium-, and
High-Mortality Categories between 1972 and 1981

		Low	Medium	High	Not Done	Total
Hip arthroplasty				1981		
	Low	67	67	24	9	167
	Medium	45	130	5	1	181
1972	High	16	17	5	1	39
	Not done	40	13	14	0	67
	Total	168	227	48	11	454
Coronary artery bypass						
	Low	0	7	2	1	10
	Medium	0	28	1	1	30
1972	High	0	4	1	0	5
	Not done	1	19	4	0	24
	Total	1	58	8	2	69
Nephrectomy						
	Low	163	61	32	37	293
	Medium	16	32	6	0	54
1972	High	21	15	5	0	41
	Not done	44	1	2	0	47
	Total	244	109	45	37	435

Hospitals that discontinued mastectomies or spinal fusions had a signifi-cantly higher mortality rate in 1972 than had those that retained the procedure. Significantly higher mortality rates are observed for hospitals that were relatively new at performing hip arthroplasties and spinal fusions. For most procedures, hospitals that continued to perform the procedure experienced a significant de-crease in mortality from 1972 to 1981. The only procedure to show an increase is nephrectomy. It would be expected that hospitals performing a procedure from 1972 to 1981 would have a lower mortality rate than those that started later. The difference in mortality rate was significantly lower only in hip arthroplasty and spinal fusion.

To determine whether deaths were procedure rather than hospital specific, we computed correlations for 1972 and 1981 between hospital mortality rates for coronary bypass surgery and the same hospitals' mortality rates for the other procedures. Because the sample of hospitals performing coronary bypass surgery was limited, we also correlated hip arthroplasty mortality rates with rates for the other procedures. If hospital-specific factors were important, we would have expected to find consistently positive correlations. However, the correlations varied in sign and almost none were statistically significant. This result suggests that hospital-specific factors (such as quality of nursing personnel and aseptic environment) are less important in explaining variations in mortality rates among hospitals than are those related to the procedure itself (such as physician profi-ciency and patient selection).

Table 13.6:   Relationship between Mortality Rate per Hospital and Length of
Time Procedure Has Been Performed at the Hospital

| | *Mean Mortality Rate (%)* | | | |
| | *Hospital Performed Procedure in 1972 and 1981* | | *Hospital Performed Procedure in 1972 but Not in 1981* | *Hospital Performed Procedure in 1981 but Not in 1972* |
Surgical Procedure	*1972*	*1981*		
Hip arthroplasty	6.1	4.0*	3.6	5.8‡
Coronary artery bypass	11.4	4.3*	5.9	5.2
Morbid obesity surgery	3.4	1.6	7.0	1.7
Hysterectomy	0.3	0.2*	0.0	0.0
Mastectomy	0.7	0.3†	2.8†	0.0
Nephrectomy	3.5	6.2	0.0	3.3
Spinal fusion	0.7	0.6	2.8†	1.6‡

*Significant at the 1% level (*t* test for differences between 1972 and 1981 mean values).
†Significant at the 5% level (*t* test for differences between 1972 and 1981 mean values).
‡Significant at the 10% level (*t* test for differences between 1972 and 1981 mean values).

DISCUSSION

The results presented here suggest that the relationship between surgical mortality and the frequency with which a procedure is performed is complex, likely reflecting a patient risk selection mechanism. By examining characteristics of hospitals at different points in the mortality rate distribution, we discovered a curvilinear relationship between mortality and volume-bed size, not reported heretofore. We found some relatively small hospitals with exemplary mortality records and other hospitals of comparable size with mortality rates at the top of the distribution. As some of our own regressions based on the full sample demonstrate, the existence of a cluster of small hospitals at the low end of the distribution could easily be obscured by fitting a straight volume-mortality line by means of regression analysis.[10-13] In none of the regressions based on the entire hospital sample does volume alone explain as much as 10% of the variation among hospitals in 1981 mortality rates, and in most cases, it explains far less than this. With a larger number of explanatory variables and the 0% mortality cases excluded, as much as three fifths of the variation in mortality is explained, and the explanatory power of our regression exceeds those reported in past work on this topic.[10-13]

Several factors could account for the favorable mortality records of certain small hospitals: favorable risk selection, clinical excellence, or luck. We found appreciable year-to-year variability in mortality rates. A hospital's rank in the 1972 mortality distribution was at best a weak predictor of its rank in 1981. In fact, we detected some convergence from both low and high groups to the medium mortality group. We also computed mean mortality rates for 1972 to

1974 for hospitals classified as low and high mortality for the procedure in 1972 and performed an identical calculation for 1979 to 1981 for hospitals that were low and high in 1981. Although there was some convergence toward the overall sample means, large and statistically significant differences in mortality remained.[*] Thus although there is an element of luck or misfortune in the data, some differences among hospitals in procedure-specific mortality are systematic.

The fact that many low-volume hospitals, which also tended to be small, had no teaching program of any sort, and were typically located outside metropolitan areas, often had a favorable mortality record suggests that an effective sorting mechanism for surgical patients may exist. The issue of patient selection merits much greater attention in understanding the volume-mortality relation.

The number of procedures performed by some hospitals is low by any conceivable standard and low by standards that have been set. In some cases, particularly coronary bypass surgery, it is difficult to accept the notion that a hospital that performs less than 10 procedures per year is delivering the same services as a 300-operation hospital. Certainly such heterogeneity should be considered in assessing how many "is enough." Also, there is reason to question the advisability of a certificate of need law that grandfathers in a 10-unit hospital at the same time it denies entry to one with many times this number of potential cases but that is below the numerical standard.

The statistical basis for minimum-volume standard setting appears weak at best. First, on the average, mortality rates decline with increases in volume. However, the decrease occurs along a continuum; there is no single level of cases above which there is a precipitous drop in mortality. Second, volume by itself is a poor predictor of differences in mortality rates among hospitals. With volume and a number of other independent variables, we were able to explain less than 10% of the variation in rates, using regression analysis on the full sample. With 0% mortality rate hospitals removed, the explanatory power of our regressions increased manyfold (Appendix A). However, the planner does not have the luxury of selecting subsamples but rather must deal with the entire set of hospitals under the agency's jurisdiction. Third, although direct evidence is lacking, many low-volume hospitals may take the better risks, and higher-risk patients may be accepted for treatment only after the institution has gained some experience with the procedure. Fourth, another rationale for minimum standards relates to cost. Unfortunately, with a few exceptions, there is very little evidence on the relationship between unit cost and volume.[14-16] Available cost studies are based on very small localized samples, and therefore generalization is difficult. In fact, there would appear to be few instances in which the procedure-specific fixed costs associated with specialized personnel and equipment are sufficiently large to generate meaningful economies of scale.[16]

The volume level at minimum mortality was well in excess of the volume

---

[*]Appendix B. *Mean In-Hospital Mortality Rates for Three-Year Periods*, filed with NAPS.

levels of most hospitals. The application of those levels of minimum mortality would have prevented most hospitals from performing high-mortality procedures in 1981.

Mandatory disclosure by hospitals of prices, mortality rates, and caseloads has appeal as a competition-enhancing strategy. However, our evidence suggests that there is some merit in the argument of those opposing such a policy. Not only may there be important case-mix differences, but also the year-to-year variability in hospital mortality rates is a reason for some caution. Furthermore, given the very low correlations among rates for specific procedures, one cannot properly generalize from data on a few procedures to the mortality experience for the hospital as a whole.

Finally, some additional caveats are in order. Discharge abstracts in general are subject to error.[17,18] The abstracts from CPHA did not record some patient–specific information that has been shown to affect mortality. However, even the most recent studies in this area that used advanced statistical techniques failed to include some potentially important hospital-specific variables or to measure changes in relationships over time.[10-13] We attempted to measure the effects of some characteristics of hospital medical staff on mortality but found no relationship, perhaps because our data on medical staff were inaccurate. Unfortunately, to date, data adequate for conducting such research have been available only for individual hospitals.[19] Generalization to larger groups of hospitals from such studies is risky. Analysis based on larger samples with emphasis on the physician merits high priority. In-hospital mortality rates are only one of several important measures of outcome. Others include deaths in the months after discharge as well as morbidity. Determinants of variation in these other measures of outcome should be studied as well.

We express our appreciation to Jeanine DeLay, Linda Knop, and John Lowe of the Commission on Professional and Hospital Activities for help in several phases of the study, to a physician panel convened for purposes of this study for advice in selecting the surgical procedures and risk factors and in interpreting the findings from the clinical standpoints of these physicians' individual specialties (Rudi Ansbacher, Paul Lichter, and Herbert Sloan, Ann Arbor, Mich.; Norman Neches, Chicago, Ill.; Sol Pichard, Detroit, Mich.; David Ransohoff, Cleveland, Ohio; Bernard Rineberg, New Brunswick, N.J., Carl VanAppledorn, Ypsilanti, Mich., and Richard YaDeau, St. Paul, Minn.), and to Jon Gabel and Lawrence Rose of the National Center for Health Services Research, for their advice based on reading an earlier version of this article.

REFERENCES

1. U.S. Department of Health, Education, and Welfare. Health planning: National guidelines. Fed Reg 43:1304–50, 1978
2. Committee on Professional Standards of the American College of Obstetricians and Gynecologists. Standards for obstetrical and gynecological services. Syracuse, 1974, American College for Obstetrics and Gynecology

3. Grosse RN: The need for health planning. *In* Havighurst C, editor: Regulatory health facilities construction. Washington DC, 1974, American Enterprise Institute, pp 27–31
4. Blumstein J, Sloan F: Redefining government's role in health care: Is a dose of competition what the doctor should order? Vanderbilt Law Rev 34:849–926, 1981
5. Havighurst C: Deregulating the health care industry. Cambridge, 1982, Ballinger
6. U.S. Department of Health and Human Services: International classification of diseases, rev. 9. DHHS Publication No. 80–1260. Washington, D.C., 1980
7. Coelen C, Sullivan D: An analysis of the effects of prospective reimbursement programs on hospital expenditures. Health Care Financ Rev 2:1–40, 1981
8. Morrisey MA, Sloan FA, Mitchell SA: State rate setting: An analysis of some unresolved issues. Health Affairs 2:36–47, 1983
9. Sloan FA: Rate regulation as a strategy for hospital cost control: Evidence from the last decade. Milbank Mem Fund Q 61:195–221, 1983
10. Flood AB, Scott WR, Ewy W: Does practice make perfect? Part I: The relation between hospital volume and outcomes for selected diagnostic categories. Med Care 22:98–114, 1984
11. Flood AB, Scott WR, Ewy W: Does practice make perfect? Part II: The relations between volume and outcomes and other hospital characteristics. Med Care 22:115–25, 1984
12. Luft HS: The relation between surgical volume and mortality: An exploration of causal factors and alternative models. Med Care 18:940–59, 1980
13. Luft HS, Bunker JP, Enthoven AR: Should operations be regionalized? The empirical relation between surgical volume and mortality. N Engl J Med 301:1364–9, 1979
14. Finkler SA: Cost finding for high-technology, high-cost services: Current practices and a possible alternative. Health Care Manage Rev 3:17–29, 1980
15. McGregor M, Pelletier G: Planning of specialized health facilities: Size vs. cost and effectiveness in heart surgery. N Engl J Med 299:178–81, 1978
16. Schwartz WB, Joskow PC: Duplicated hospital facilities: How much can we save by consolidating them? New Engl J Med 303:1449–57, 1980
17. Corn RF: Quality control of hospital discharge data. Med Care 18:416–26, 1980
18. Demlo LK, Campbell PM: Improving hospital discharge data: Lessons from the national hospital discharge survey. Med Care 19:1030–40, 1981
19. Garber AM, Fuchs VR, Silverman JF: Case mix, costs, and outcomes: Differences between faculty and community services in a university hospital. N Engl J Med 310:1231–7, 1984

Chapter 14

Patient or Hospital as the
Unit of Analysis?

$\mathbf{A}$n important issue in volume studies is whether to use the patient or the hospital as the unit of analysis. There arc two perspectives on this question, which are often reflected in two basic statistical methods. In a number of studies using each patient as one observation, individual risk factors available on the data set were used to control statistically for differences in the probability of death, and direct measures of hospital volume were included in the regressions.[1] Flood, Scott and Ewy's approach differs from those used in other studies. They used a sophisticated patient risk factor model to generate for each patient an expected probability of death based on his or her risk factors. To test for a volume effect, the patients were divided into two groups, those treated in hospitals with less than the mean volume of patients with that procedure or diagnosis, and those treated in hospitals with greater than the mean volume. The difference between expected and observed mortality (based on the total number of patients) was then evaluated with the chi-square statistic.

In many of the earlier studies, researchers used the hospital as the unit of analysis when individual patient data were unavailable or difficult to obtain.[2] Differences in case mix among hospitals were accounted for by creating a matrix of risk groups based on several demographic and clinical criteria, and by adjusting for each hospital's mix of patients. In some cases these matrices were used to compute the expected number of deaths (or the death rate) in the hospital, based upon its case mix. In the study by Sloan, Perrin, and Valvona (1986), however, the proportion of hospital patients in each risk category was included directly in the regression.[3] In most of the studies, regressions were weighted to adjust for the number of patients treated in each hospital, and the dependent variable was represented as various forms of the difference between actual and expected mortality rate. Luft used observed-minus-expected mortality, Williams used observed over expected, and Hughes, Hunt, and Luft used a Z-score, which is explained in some detail in Chapter 17.

As indicated in Chapter 4, the general findings with respect to the volume-outcome relationship are quite similar with the various approaches, although there are some subtle differences. The "degrees of freedom" problem can be dealt with by remembering that the appropriate figure for analysis of volume effects is based on the number of hospitals, not the number of patients. Risk-factor matrices are useful in that they can display interdependencies among the risk factors. For example, the effect of increased age may depend on the patient's gender. Using the risk-factor variables in a linear regression model will not take account of such interactions, but one can easily include them once they have been discovered. Perhaps the most flexible approach is recursive partitioning, which makes no assumptions about linearity (Blumberg 1986). Once homogeneous risk-factor categories have been identified, these can either be used to specify dummy variable categories for patient-level regressions or be aggregated to provide expected poor-outcome rates at the hospital level.

Assuming one has access to patient-level data, several factors influence the decision to use a single patient-level regression with hospital volumes as independent variables or a two-step approach in which regressions or risk-factor matrices are used to develop expected outcomes at the hospital level. In some cases, the hospital is the logical unit of observation because one is also trying to explain the volume level in the hospital.[4] Likewise, Sloan, Perrin, and Valvona (Study 18) asked whether observed hospital mortality rates justify certain types of regulations. In other instances, the results were intended for uses beyond just the estimation of a volume-outcome relationship. Williams has been publishing hospital-specific infant mortality rates for years, so the hospital is the natural unit of observation.

Sometimes the choice of the unit of observation depends on whether one wishes to discuss the risk-factor results. For example, neither Flood nor Sloan and their colleagues reported risk-factor results in their articles, although they are available in appendices. Kelly and Hellinger (1987) report their risk-factor findings, but not all the results are easily explainable.[5] Although this sometimes indicates a problem, it often merely suggests complex relationships that are not yet understood. Exploring the implications of such risk-factor variables may lead to a better understanding of medical care outcomes, but it is unlikely to affect the analysis of volume-outcome relationships.

NOTES

1. See, for example, Riley and Lubitz (1985), reprinted in Chapter 15; Kelly and Hellinger (1987), reprinted in Chapter 10; Roos et al. (1986), reprinted in Chapter 8; and Showstack et al. (1987), reprinted in Chapter 11.
2. See, for example, Luft (1980), reprinted in Chapter 16; Williams (1979), reprinted in Chapter 18; Hughes, Hunt, and Luft (1987), reprinted in Chapter 17; and Sloan, Perrin, and Valvona (1986), reprinted in Chapter 13.
3. See reprint of Sloan, Perrin, and Valvona (1986) study in Chapter 13 of this volume.
4. See, for example, Luft (1980), reprinted in Chapter 16.
5. See Kelly and Hellinger (1987), reprinted in Chapter 10 of this volume.

Does Practice Make Perfect?

Part I: The Relation between Hospital Volume and Outcomes for Selected Diagnostic Categories

Ann Barry Flood
W. Richard Scott
Wayne Ewy

It has long been suspected but only recently demonstrated that hospitals performing more treatments of a given type exhibit better patient outcomes than hospitals processing fewer patients.[1,2] This so-called "volume–outcome" relation, if supported by additional research, has important policy implications for the regionalization of hospital services, suggesting that important health advantages may be attained by promoting a more explicit division of labor among hospitals in the types of treatment they provide. Data are available that allow us to evaluate the volume–outcome hypothesis for a large sample of hospitals and for a different set of procedures than those previously investigated. The study by Luft and colleagues was restricted to surgical patients but investigated a broader set of surgical categories than those covered in the present study.[1] Breadth is an advantage for generalization; however, it makes less tenable the assumption that patients within a given category may be regarded as comparable to one another. That is, it interferes with attempts to adjust outcome measures for patient differences, a process described later.

Our approach is to combine data on hospitals and patients from several data systems; no new data were collected. Quality of care is assessed using a single outcome—death in the hospital—adjusted to account for differences in patient condition at the time of admission. A variety of diagnostic categories and patients undergoing both surgical and medical treatment are included. Volume is assessed

Reprinted from *Medical Care* 22, no. 2 (1984): 98–114, with permission from The J. B. Lippincott Company.

Supported by the National Academy of Sciences and the National Center for Health Services Research, DHHS.

An early version of this paper was presented at the Annual Meetings of the American Sociological Association, Toronto, Canada, August 1981.

Basic data for use in this study were supplied by the Commission on Professional and Hospital Activities, Ann Arbor, Michigan, and the identities of individual hospitals were not revealed. Any analysis, interpretation, or conclusion based on these data is solely that of the researchers, and CPHA specifically disclaims responsibility for any such analysis, interpretation, or conclusion.

in two ways, one based simply on hospital experience with patients in the same diagnostic category, and the other based on experience with patients at a similar risk level within the same diagnostic category. We first present the approach used to adjust quality of care accounting for patient mix differences and the evidence that there is significance variation in quality of care among United States hospitals. Then, using cross-tabulations and graphs for several diagnostic groups, we investigate the effects of volume or hospital experience on adjusted patient outcomes.

PROCEDURES

Selection of Hospitals

All hospitals included in this study participated in the hospital chart abstracting system of the Commission of Professional Hospital Activities (CPHA). We considered it desirable to demonstrate the ability to use data from a widely used and uniformly available existing system based on patient information obtained from records. Consistent with maintaining the anonymity of each of their reporting hospitals, CPHA performed some of the required analyses. Although 1,300 hospitals were participating in the CPHA system at the time of our data collection (1972), only those hospitals for which organizational data were also available from the Annual Survey conducted by the American Hospital Association (AHA), and for which participation in the full Professional Activities Study (PAS) had been ongoing for at least 1 year prior to the study were selected for examination. The study sample consisted of 1,224 hospitals, which represents approximately one fifth of all nonfederal acute care hospitals in the United States and accounts for approximately one third of all nonfederal patient discharges in the United States. The sample is not entirely representative of the United States population of nonfederal hospitals, being biased toward the larger, more expensive and more self-critical units, but is large and diverse enough for our purposes.

Selection of Patients

One of the major goals of the study was to compare mortality in hospitals across the country, after carefully controlling for differences in patient mix. For the analyses reported here, patients in 17 diagnostic categories were selected for detailed analysis, following the tracer method of assessing hospital effectiveness. The 17 categories were chosen on the basis of several criteria considered important for ensuring the most valid and reliable measures of standardized mortalities possible: 1) a high number of deaths because of either a high mortality or a large number of patients; 2) involvement of a variety of organ systems and surgical/ medical specialties; 3) representation of patients of both sexes and a broad range of age groups and physical conditions; and 4) both medical and surgical treatment of patients. For the 15 surgical categories, patients were selected on the basis of having undergone the requisite study surgery and having the corresponding study diagnostic category. In most cases, these categories coincided with the primary diagnosis explaining admission. When a patient had multiple diagnoses listed, the patient was placed in only one study category based upon the most important diagnosis-procedure listed. Patients who underwent more serious surgeries than the study procedure or whose diagnoses indicated secondary or unspecified malignancies were omitted from the study. For the two medical categories, the patients were selected on the basis of having the requisite study diagnoses and no surgical procedure except a diagnostic procedure. Patients with secondary or unspecified malignancies were similarly eliminated from medical study categories. In the present analysis, attention is focused on three classes of study patients: (1) selected surgical categories, containing patients who underwent one of nine relatively pure study procedures—pure in that (a) the majority of patients having the study surgery shared the same diagnosis and (b) the majority of patients in the diagnostic group who underwent any related, nondiagnostic procedure had the study procedure (nine study categories); (2) all surgical categories, containing patients in the nine selected surgical categories plus six other study surgeries; and (3) medical categories, including patients who were hospitalized for one of two study diagnostic groups (gallbladder disease and ulcer disease) but who were treated medically rather than surgically. The study patient categories are listed in Table 14.1 together with the number of patients and deaths and mortality for each. The order of presentation of the categories within selected surgery and additional surgery reflects the relative difficulty of each type of surgery as evaluated by a panel of surgeons.[3] In a related study, 550 surgeons were asked to rate the difficulty in terms of the complexity and uncertainty of 71 surgical procedures, using a scale of 1 (easy) to 9 (difficult). Using these ratings, the study categories would be ranked: abdominal aorta surgery (7.86 involving renal vessels and 7.16 without renal vessels), arthroplasty of the hip (6.81 for total hip), gallbladder surgery (5.71 involving common duct exploration and 4.11 without), gastric surgery (5.45), repair of fractured shaft of femur (5.02), large bowel operations (5.00), and amputation of lower limb (3.74).[3] In all, 331,749 surgical patients and 227,107 nonsurgical patients were studied. The two diagnoses for which both nonsurgical and surgical cases were studied are ulcer and gallbladder disease. Our data (Table 14.1) show that gallbladder disease was treated surgically more frequently than medically—60% of all patients with gallbladder diagnosis received surgery. In contrast, ulcer was more commonly treated medically—84% of patients were treated medically. The crude mortality was lower in each diagnostic category for the more common treatment; i.e., for gallbladder, the mortality was lower for surgical patients (1.1% vs. 2.8%); for ulcers, it was lower for medical patients (2.4% vs. 4.3%). This finding is consistent with the argument that greater experience with a given treatment leads to better outcome. However, it is also consistent with the argument that the "usual" form of treatment is preferred for routine cases, while more difficult cases receive

Table 14.1: Basic Patient and Hospital Statistics by Patient Category

	Patient Statistics			Hospital Statistics		
	Patients (n)	Deaths (n)	Mortality (%)	Hospitals (n)	Patients (Average n)	Significance Level: Test of Differences[a]
Selected surgical categories[b]	266,944	11,653	4.4	1,209	220.80	<0.0005
Intraabdominal artery operations	9,532	1,476	15.5	645	14.78	<0.0005
Arthroplasty of the hip	13,424	199	1.5	702	19.12	0.3410
Gallbladder operations	130,749	1,444	1.1	1,196	109.32	<0.0005
Stomach operations—ulcer diagnosis	26,688	1,138	4.3	1,100	24.26	0.0170
Large bowel operations—specified diagnosis[c]	16,110	517	3.2	984	16.37	0.0460
Hip fracture diagnosis—with other trauma diagnoses	6,925	554	8.0	886	7.82	0.3710
Hip fracture diagnosis—with no other trauma diagnoses	52,368	4,774	9.1	1,169	44.80	<0.0005
Amputation of lower limb—no current trauma or diagnosis	10,267	1,476	14.4	973	10.55	<0.0005
Amputations of lower limb—current trauma or diagnosis	881	75	8.5	217	4.06	0.5080
Additional surgical categories	331,749	15,618	4.7	1,216	272.82	<0.0005
Stomach operations—cancer diagnoses[d]	1,500	161	10.7	377	3.98	0.2910
Stomach operations—other diagnoses[d]	7,148	578	8.1	875	8.17	0.1190
Large bowel operations—cancer diagnoses	17,872	1,160	6.5	1,040	17.18	<0.0005
Large bowel operations—other diagnoses	6,575	817	12.4	858	7.66	0.1790
Fracture of the pelvis	18,033	687	3.8	1,113	16.20	0.1790
Fracture of the shaft of femur	13,677	562	4.1	976	14.01	0.2120
Medical categories	227,107	5,776	2.5	1,215	186.92	<0.0005
Gallbladder diagnosis—nonsurgical	88,839	2,477	2.8	1,210	73.42	<0.0005
Ulcer diagnosis—nonsurgical	138,268	3,299	2.4	1,214	113.89	<0.0005

[a]Based on χ^2 statistic using exact mean and variance for hospital level SMRs.
[b]Categories are arranged in order of relative difficulty from greatest to lowest.[3]
[c]Includes benign tumor, enteritis, colitis, and diverticulosis.
[d]Excludes secondary or unspecified malignancies.

"unusual" treatment. To distinguish whether experience is important in explaining variation in outcomes for both surgical and medical patients, it is necessary to account for patient condition.

Because comparison of hospital performance was a major goal of the study, we developed a method to predict the probability that each patient would die, given his or her health-related characteristics. This method is described below in more detail. For a given hospital, the ratio of actual deaths to the expected number of deaths (the Standardized Mortality Ratio—SMR) is a measure of performance that accounts for the number of deaths that could be expected on the basis of detailed information about patient mix. Before turning to the question of whether the volume of patients in a hospital has an effect, we determine whether there are significant differences in mortalities among hospitals that remain after accounting for patient condition. Much of the variation in hospital performance can be attributed to chance, particularly where the number of deaths observed in the total population of study hospitals is below 1,000. Using a chi-square statistic based on exact mean and variance, we examined the hospital level SMRs for each category to determine the level of significance; details are presented elsewhere.[4,5] The results of this test are reported in Table 14.1. It should be noted that the ability to detect differences in hospital performance using this test increases with the number of overall patient deaths in the category. For five of the six selected surgical categories with more than 1,000 deaths, the test for hospital differences was significant at the 0.0005 level or greater. The sixth category (stomach operations with ulcer diagnoses) was significant at the 0.017 level. Similarly, the one additional surgical category with more than 1,000 deaths revealed differences in hospital performances significant at the 0.0005 level. Both medical categories exhibited significant variation among hospitals. Summary measures for each of the three categories were likewise significant at the 0.0005 level.

In sum, there is considerable evidence that hospitals in our sample differ in their performance as measured by deaths in hospital, after rigorous adjustments to account for patient mix differences. For individual diagnostic-procedure categories, failure to demonstrate significant differences did not appear to be due to differences in the nature, i.e., difficulty, of the procedure but to differences in the number of observed deaths.

Next we describe the principal independent variables: measures of volume or hospital's experience in treating patients of a given type. Other hospital measures, used primarily as controls, are detailed below.

Volume Measures

Two measures of volume of cases treated were developed. Both are based on CPHA data and assess the extent to which the hospital treating a given patient is experienced in cases of that patient's type. Both measures are dichotomous, indicating whether or not the patient was treated in a hospital that has treated more than the average number of patients of each type—the average based on the combined year-long experience of all study hospitals with at least two patients in the study category.

The first volume measure, volume within category, is positive only if for each study patient the hospital treated more than the average number of patients in the same category. The categories used are those listed in Table 14.1. The second volume measure, volume within category and risk level, is more stringent in its definition of relevant experience: it is positive only if for each patient the hospital treated more than the average number of patients in the same category and at the same risk level as that patient. Risk level is a measure of severity of illness (estimated probability of death) and therefore represents a more refined measure of patient similarity. Because the calculation of risk level is an integral part of the process by which outcome measures are adjusted, this measure is discussed below in association with this topic.

Outcome Measure: Death in Hospital

The outcome measure employed is death in hospital. This indicator is not ideal: it does not account for many health status outcomes of interest (e.g., morbidity, return to function, quality of life); a sizable proportion of deaths following a hospitalization period occur not in the hospital but after discharge.[6] Further, because death is a relatively rare event, the power of statistical attempts to estimate its probability of occurrence is reduced.[6] Moreover, Luft[7] argues that mortality may exhibit spurious variation by region caused by differences in length of stay. Because average length of stay (ALOS) varies significantly by region (the shortest ALOS is in the West and the longest is in the Northeast), the number of deaths that occur outside the hospital and are thus unrecorded in the data base is likely to be higher in areas with the shortest ALOS. Luft also found that rehospitalization is higher in areas with the shortest ALOS. Because each hospitalization is treated as an independent episode in our analyses, areas with significantly higher rehospitalization could appear to have lower mortalities because of counting the same patient for multiple "survivals" of hospitalization. In separate analyses on a subset of study hospitals reported elsewhere, we examined the impact of the region of the country on our measures of outcome and found that region explained the differences in ALOS but did not account for the differences in mortalities among hospitals.[8] Finally, death within a specified number of days generally is regarded as a more appropriate indicator for surgery than for medical treatment. On the positive side, death can be reliably measured and is unarguably a valid indicator of an adverse health outcome.

It is well-known that patient mix varies greatly among hospitals.[9-12] If outcome measures, such as death, are to be regarded as valid indicators of quality of care, they must be adjusted (standardized) to take account for differences among patients in type of illness and general health status. A complex statistical model was developed to perform this adjustment; details are available elsewhere,[4] but the approach is summarized briefly below.

Predicting Death in Hospitals

To adjust observed outcomes for differences in patient mix we used indirect standardization, which involves the computation of estimated probability of death for each study patient. These estimates were derived empirically through the use of logistic equations relating patient-specific information to outcome measures. The first step was to separate the patients into the diagnosis-procedure categories detailed in Table 14.1. The empirical estimates for expected death were then derived separately for patients in each diagnostic category. In general, two types of information on patients were used: (1) up to 15 variables pertaining to the demographic characteristics or information obtained from the medical history or laboratory tests on admission were collected for each patient, specifically, age, sex, admission white blood cell count, admission systolic blood pressure, admission diastolic blood pressure, admission urine sugar, admission urine albumin, admission temperature, admission hemoglobin, surgical pathology report on most important operation, poverty indicator, height/weight index, oral anti-diabetics given, insulin given, and thyroid drugs given; and (2) three types of information pertaining to the patient's diagnoses and operations, including measures of the particular operative procedures performed, measures to identify the stage of disease at the time of hospitalization (these varied for each type of diagnosis), and measures of other diagnoses and operations (other than the primary diagnosis and related procedures). These variables were developed through extensive consultation with medical specialists and with the aid of sample data from CPHA used to determine those characteristics best able to gauge the risk of dying for an individual patient in each diagnosis-procedure category.[6] All of these data were drawn from the PAS abstract.

For each of the categories, the patient and diagnosis characteristics were used to develop a logistic prediction function that would estimate the probability of death in the hospital for any individual patient. The statistical fitting of the data was performed without regard to the particular hospital treating the patient. In the first step of the analysis, a stepwise linear regression was performed with death regressed on all available variables describing the initial patient condition and diagnosis. The actual number of potential variables differed for each category because of the staging variables, but between 40 and 65 variables were used in this first step. Second, the 15 best variables—best in terms of explained variance in outcome—were selected to be used as standardization variables for the logistic step. Third, these variables were combined into a multiple logistic model to permit the computation of probability of death for each patient, based on his or her observed characteristics. Finally, each patient was characterized by an adjusted mortality measure consisting of the difference of his or her observed outcome from that expected, i.e., predicted on the basis of the logistic model applied to his or her specific characteristics.

Risk Level of Patients

The expected outcome, the probability of dying in the hospital, also was used to rank each patient in each category to provide a measure of risk level. Patients were divided into three risk levels—low, medium, and high probability of dying—in such a way as to ensure that each level would contain approximately one third of the patients who died in the hospital within each category. The division of risk into levels was based upon the number of deaths to increase the statistical power of our tests for variation in rates per hospital. As already noted, for one of the two measures of volume, hospitals were differentiated by whether they treated more or fewer than the average number of patients at each risk level within a given category.

Levels of Analysis

For present purposes, the data analysis is performed at the level of the individual patient. (For other purposes, e.g., determining whether hospitals in the sample differed significantly in adjusted patient outcome as described above, patient data were aggregated at the hospital level.) The effect of this decision is to treat each patient as a separate case and to characterize him or her by the specific volume and other structural measures describing the hospital in which care was received. One important consequence of this approach is to weight these structural variables by the number of patients receiving care in each hospital. A second consequence of this decision is to place a limitation on the amount of explained variance possible in our analyses; we return to this point in Part II when we present our regression analyses.

The patient level seems most appropriate for the analyses reported here because not only are the outcomes and their adjusting variables measured at the patient level, but the measures of volume are assessed in terms of the experience of a given hospital with patient subgroups highly similar to the patient of interest in both diagnosis and risk level. Nevertheless, the patient level can be argued to overestimate the significance of differences observed, because it uses as the number of "independent" observations the number of patients rather than hospitals. To compensate for this aggregation bias, we employ fairly stringent tests of significance throughout these analyses.

FINDINGS

Volume and Outcomes

In the first set of analyses, we examine the impact of volume, or hospital experience with patients in the same diagnostic-procedure category, on patient outcomes as measured by SMRs (Table 14.2). We turn first to the results for each of the five individual diagnostic categories exhibiting more than 1,000 deaths in the set of study hospitals. As reported in Table 14.1, one of these categories— stomach operations, ulcer diagnosis—revealed significant differences among hospitals at only the 0.017 level. It is retained in this analysis to permit comparisons with ulcer patients treated medically. Within categories, rows indicate whether patients were treated in a high-volume (i.e., above-average number of patients treated in the same category) or low-volume hospital. The first three columns report number of patients involved, number of deaths observed, and number of deaths expected (i.e., the sum of the probability of dying for every patient in the low- and high-volume hospitals). As expected, there were more patients and, hence, more observed deaths in the high-volume hospitals. The next two columns report the average observed mortality and the average expected mortality for patients in low- and high-volume hospitals. For each of the surgical categories, the observed mortality was higher for low-volume hospitals. However, in all cases except gallbladder operations, the expected mortality was also higher in low-volume hospitals. This finding was unexpected in that it implies that the low-volume hospitals were more likely to treat more difficult patients. It also underscores the importance of accounting for patient mix when comparing mortalities. The same overall patterns were observed for the two groups of surgical categories—all selected and all surgical categories.

Turning to the two medical categories, ulcer diagnosis patients displayed a pattern similar to that of the individual surgical categories. Gallbladder patients, however, exhibited a lower mortality in low-volume hospitals that also tended to treat patients with more difficult cases.

In the last two columns of Table 14.2 are displayed the standardized mortality ratios (SMRs) and the results of a statistical test for differences between outcome performance in low- and high-volume hospitals. For chi-square analysis, we utilized the number of expected deaths from the logistic regression analyses. Because computation of the expected number of deaths was not based on cell margins, there is no loss of degrees of freedom over the number of cells.[4] Using the selected surgical categories as an example, we computed

$$\chi^2 = \sum_i \frac{(0 - E_i)^2}{E_i}$$

where $(0 - E_i)^2 = (\pm 300.2)^2$ and expected number of patients in each category is as follows: expected number of survivors—66,257.2 in low-volume hospitals, 189,033.8 in high-volume hospitals; expected number of deaths—3,357.8 in low-volume hospitals, 8,295.2 in high-volume hospitals. $\chi^2 = 39.54$ with four degrees of freedom. The SMR for patients treated in low- and high-volume hospitals can vary above 1, indicating more deaths than expected, or below 1, indicating fewer deaths than expected. Because of the model used to estimate deaths, the overall number of observed deaths equals the overall expected deaths in each category, and the SMR for all hospitals combined is 1.0.

Table 14.2: The Effects of Volume on Adjusted and Crude Outcome: Nonparametric Analyses

	Patients (N)	No. of Observed Deaths (D)	No. of Expected Deaths (E)	Observed Mortality (D/N)	Expected Mortality (E/N)	Standardized Mortality Ratio: SMR (D/E)	Ratio of SMRs, χ^2, P
Selected surgical categories							
Intraabdominal artery operations							
Low-volume	2,459	539	448.9	0.219	0.183	1.201	1.32
High-volume	7,073	937	1,027.1	0.132	0.145	0.913	$\chi^2 = 31.38$
Total	9,532	1,476	1,476.0	0.155	0.155	1.000	$P < 0.001$
Gallbladder operations							
Low-volume	33,818	456	384.4	0.013	0.011	1.190	1.27
High-volume	96,931	988	1,059.6	0.010	0.011	0.930	$\chi^2 = 18.38$
Total	130,749	1,444	1,444.0	0.011	0.011	1.000	$P < 0.005$
Stomach operations with ulcer diagnosis							
Low-volume	7,418	353	334.1	0.048	0.045	1.057	1.08
High-volume	19,270	785	803.0	0.041	0.042	0.977	$\chi^2 = 0.08$
Total	26,688	1,138	1,138.0	0.043	0.043	1.000	$P < 0.05$
Hip fracture diagnosis with no other trauma diagnosis							
Low-volume	13,627	1,411	1,357.0	0.104	0.100	1.040	1.06
High-volume	38,741	3,362	3,416.0	0.087	0.088	0.984	$\chi^2 = 3.32$
Total	52,368	4,773	4,773.0	0.091	0.091	1.000	$P > 0.05$
Amputation of lower limb with no current trauma diagnosis							
Low-volume	3,001	504	451.6	0.168	0.151	1.116	1.18
High-volume	7,266	972	1,024.4	0.134	0.141	0.949	$\chi^2 = 10.27$
Total	10,267	1,476	1,476.0	0.144	0.144	1.000	$P < 0.05$
All selected surgical categories (9)							
Low-volume	69,615	3,658	3,357.8	0.052	0.048	1.089	1.13
High-volume	197,329	7,995	8,295.2	0.041	0.042	0.964	$\chi^2 = 39.54$
Total	266,944	11,653	11,653.0	0.044	0.044	1.000	$P < 0.001$

Continued

Table 14.2: Continued

	Patients (N)	No. of Observed Deaths (D)	No. of Expected Deaths (E)	Observed Mortality (D/N)	Expected Mortality (E/N)	Standardized Mortality Ratio: SMR (D/E)	Radio of SMRs, χ^2, P
Additional surgical categories							
Large bowel operations with cancer diagnosis							
Low-volume	4,492	344	299.7	0.077	0.067	1.1484	1.21
High-volume	13,380	816	860.3	0.061	0.064	0.9487	$\chi^2 = 9.48$
Total	17,872	1,160	1,160.0	0.065	0.065	1.000	$P < 0.05$
All surgical categories (15)							
Low-volume	87,676	4,879	4,519.1	0.056	0.052	1.080	1.12
High-volume	244,076	10,739	11,098.9	0.044	0.046	0.968	$\chi^2 = 55.96$
Total	331,752	15,618	15,618.0	0.047	0.047	1.000	$P < 0.001$
Medical categories							
Nonsurgical gallbladder diagnosis							
Low-volume	28,036	759	834.9	0.027	0.030	0.909	1.21
High-volume	60,803	1,718	1,642.1	0.028	0.027	1.046	$\chi^2 = 10.7$
Total	88,839	2,477	2,477.0	0.028	0.028	1.000	$P < 0.05$
Nonsurgical ulcer diagnosis							
Low-volume	42,932	1,169	1,145.0	0.027	0.027	1.021	1.03
High-volume	95,336	2,130	2,154.0	0.022	0.023	0.989	$\chi^2 = 0.03$
Total	138,268	3,299	3,299.0	0.024	0.024	1.000	$P < 0.05$
All medical categories (2)							
Low-volume	70,968	1,928	1,979.9	0.027	0.028	0.974	0.96
High-volume	156,139	3,848	3,796.1	0.025	0.025	1.014	$\chi^2 = 2.10$
Total	227,107	5,776	5,776.0	0.025	0.025	1.000	$P > 0.05$

In each of the six surgical categories, the SMR indicates better outcomes (i.e., fewer deaths than expected) in more experienced hospitals. For four of the six comparisons, the differences are statistically significant at the 0.05 level or greater. One nonsignificant category, ulcer surgery, also was not significant in the test for hospital differences. For the two groups of surgical categories, the more experienced hospitals were more likely to have better outcomes, with a significance level of less than 0.001.

The last column of Table 14.2 reports the ratio of high- and low-volume SMRs, providing an indication of the percentage increase of deaths over what would be expected on the basis of patient condition. Among the significant categories, they range from a 32% increase in mortalities for less experienced hospitals for intra-abdominal aorta operations to an 18% increase for amputation of lower limb with no current trauma. The percentage increase in mortalities in the less experienced hospitals for all selected surgical categories combined was 13%.

For the medical categories, gallbladder patients unexpectedly had a better SMR (i.e., fewer deaths) in the low-volume hospitals, a finding significant at the 0.05 level. Neither ulcer diagnosis nor the combined medical categories was statistically different for the two types of hospitals.

In summary, for surgical categories we found strong evidence that treating a larger volume of patients in the same category was associated with better outcomes than would be expected on the basis of patient health characteristics. These results characterize both groups of surgical categories as well as all six individual surgical categories, although significant for only four. According to our data, the importance of experience of the hospital for improving surgical outcomes was not dependent upon the relative difficulty of the procedure. Medical outcomes were mixed: greater experience was not significant for explaining different outcomes in ulcer patients or in the combined medical categories, but was weakly related to poorer outcomes for gallbladder patients.

Volume, Risk Level, and Outcomes

Next we examine the effect of volume on outcomes when the patient's risk level is taken into account. First, we determine whether a hospital's overall experience in treating patients in a given category reveals differential benefits to patients at varying risk levels. That is, volume is assessed for the patient category as a whole, while outcomes are assessed accounting for the patient's risk level. Second, we qualify experience as well as outcome by the patient's risk level. Using the alternate measure of volume, experience has an effect only when a hospital treats patients in the same category and at the same risk level. We focus first on the surgical categories.

Our first question, then, is whether experience in treating patients in a given category is more or less beneficial for high-, medium-, or low-risk patient groups. Figures 14.1 through 14.6 and Table 14.3 present the results of our tests for the six surgical categories, exhibiting more than 1,000 deaths. Each figure graphs the SMR for each of the three risk groups in high- and low-volume hospitals, with volume defined as experience in treating patient in that surgical category. Also reported is the SMR for all risk groups combined. Recall that an SMR greater than 1 indicates that more deaths were observed than were expected; less than 1 indicates fewer deaths. Significance tests for each comparison indicate whether the differences observed between high- and low-volume hospitals are larger than would be expected by chance.

The pattern of findings for the six categories reveal both similarities and differences. It appears that high-volume hospitals exhibit fairly consistent effects on patient outcomes regardless of risk level (note the relative flatness of their graph line), with a possible exception of amputation of a lower limb (Fig. 14.6), while low-volume hospitals exhibit effects that interact with risk level. Focusing on the patterns in low-volume hospitals, we observe in general that low- or medium-risk groups seem to fare worse, while high-risk patients experience better outcomes (lower SMRs). It appears that, for patients in low-volume hospitals, those undergoing surgery for gallbladder, ulcer, and cancer of the large bowel (Figs. 14.2, 14.3, and 14.4), experience somewhat worse outcomes in the low-risk category compared with other risk levels. On the other hand, for patients

Figure 14.1:   Standardized Mortality Ratios for High- and Low-Volume Hospitals by Risk Level of Patients: Intraabdominal Aorta Surgery

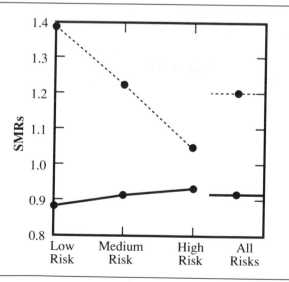

Broken line, treatment in low-volume hospital.
Solid line, treatment in high-volume hospital.
SMRs >1 indicate more deaths than expected.

Figure 14.2: Standardized Mortality Ratios for High- and Low-Volume Hospitals by Risk Level of Patients: Gallbladder Surgery

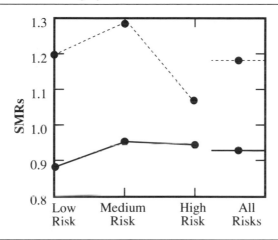

Broken line, treatment in low-volume hospital.
Solid line, treatment in high-volume hospital.
SMRs >1 indicate more deaths than expected.

Figure 14.3: Standardized Mortality Ratios for High- and Low-Volume Hospitals by Risk Level of Patients: Stomach Operations with Ulcer Diagnoses

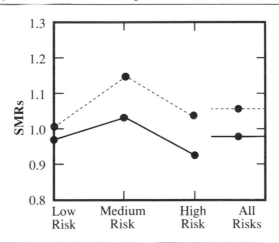

Broken line, treatment in low-volume hospital.
Solid line, treatment in high-volume hospital.
SMRs >1 indicate more deaths than expected.

Figure 14.4:   Standardized Mortality Ratios for High- and
Low-Volume Hospitals by Risk Level of Patients: Large
Bowel Operations with Cancer Diagnoses

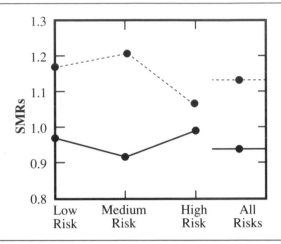

Broken line, treatment in low-volume hospital.
Solid line, treatment in high-volume hospital.
SMRs >1 indicate more deaths than expected.

Figure 14.5:   Standardized Mortality Ratios for High- and
Low-Volume Hospitals by Risk Level of Patients: Hip
Fracture Surgery with No Other Trauma

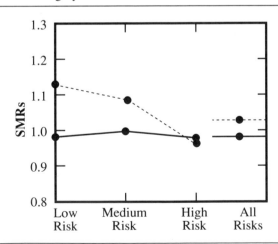

Broken line, treatment in low-volume hospital.
Solid line, treatment in high-volume hospital.
SMRs >1 indicate more deaths than expected.

Figure 14.6: Standardized Mortality Ratios for High- and Low-Volume Hospitals by Risk Level of Patients: Amputation of Lower Limb with No Current Trauma

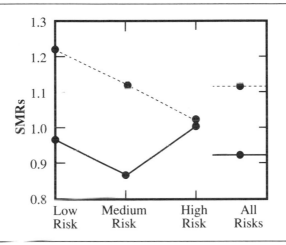

Broken line, treatment in low-volume hospital.
Solid line, treatment in high-volume hospital.
SMRs >1 indicate more deaths than expected.

in low-volume hospitals undergoing surgery for abdominal aorta, hip fracture, and amputation of a lower limb (Figs. 14.1, 14.5, and 14.6) in the medium-risk level have somewhat worse outcomes. Note, however, that many of the differences between high- and low-volume hospitals associated with risk groups are not significant, partly because of the smaller number of deaths in each subgroup. In no instance is the difference between high- and low-volume hospitals significant for high-risk patients. The greater fluctuation of SMRs by risk level for the individual categories (Figs. 14.1–14.6) for low-volume hospitals compared with high-volume could be due in part to the smaller number of cases being analyzed in the low-volume hospitals. We will examine the interaction between risk level and volume when we look at the combined study categories.

Before commenting further on these patterns, we determine if they persist when the second volume measure is employed. Is hospital performance improved by experience in treating *any* patient within a given category, or by treating only patients at the same risk level? If experience depends on risk level as well as category, we would expect to see stronger results in each of the risk levels for the second volume measure. And, in particular, we would expect experience to have an effect on high-risk patients. If risk level is an important qualifier of experience, then ignoring risk could be particularly misleading for high-risk patients, because they represent such a small percentage of all patients. For example, more than 90% of all gallbladder patients undergoing surgery were in the low-risk

Table 14.3: F and P Values Associated with Standardized Mortality Ratios by Risk Level of Patients and Diagnosis

	Low-Risk		Medium-Risk		High-Risk		All Patients	
	F	P	F	P	F	P	F	P
Intraabdominal aorta surgery (Fig. 14.1)	28.48	0.001	15.18	0.005	4.24	NS	31.37	0.001
Gallbladder surgery (Fig. 14.2)	9.14	NS	11.91	0.05	2.00	NS	18.38	0.005
Stomach operations with ulcer diagnoses (Fig. 14.3)	0.15	NS	2.92	NS	2.53	NS	1.58	NS
Large bowel operations with cancer diagnoses (Fig. 14.4)	3.36	NS	7.04	NS	0.99	NS	9.48	0.05
Hip fracture surgery with no other trauma (Fig. 14.5)	7.76	NS	6.30	NS	1.91	NS	3.32	NS
Amputation of lower limb with no current trauma (Fig. 14.6)	7.78	NS	9.73	0.05	0.03	NS	10.27	0.05
Nonsurgical gallbladder diagnoses (Fig. 14.9)	2.89	NS	2.23	NS	9.21	NS	10.72	0.05
Nonsurgical ulcer diagnoses (Fig. 14.10)	0.51	NS	1.78	NS	0.18	NS	0.79	NS

NS, not significant.

Table 14.4: F and P Values Associated with Standardized Mortality Ratios by Risk Level of Patients, Category, and Diagnosis

	Volume in Same Category								Volume in Same Category and Risk Level							
	Low-Risk		Medium-Risk		High-Risk		All		Low-Risk		Medium-Risk		High-Risk		All	
	F	P	F	P	F	P	F	P	F	P	F	P	F	P	F	P
Intraabdominal aorta surgery (Fig. 14.7)	28.48	0.001	15.18	0.05	4.24	NS	31.37	0.001	25.32	0.001	5.16	NS	0.83	NS	18.35	0.005
Selected surgeries combined (Fig. 14.8)	33.25	0.001	24.39	0.001	4.56	NS	39.54	0.001	28.34	0.001	32.98	0.001	3.75	NS	38.93	0.001

NS, not significant

category. Recall that patients were distributed among risk level groups to equalize numbers of observed deaths, not number of patients treated. Figure 14.7 and Table 14.4 demonstrate the relation between volume and outcome for patients undergoing abdominal aorta surgery by risk level for high- and low-volume hospitals, using two measures of volume: greater-than-average experience in treating any patient in the category (the same measure reported in Figs. 14.1–14.6) and greater-than-average experience in treating patients at the same risk level in the category. It appears that the effects of volume on outcome for each of the three risk groups are very similar for the two measures of volume. To the extent that there are any differences between the measures, use of the more refined volume measure tends to be associated with smaller, not greater, differences between the two types of hospitals. These results hold for the other surgical categories studied, with the exception of gallbladder surgery, for which differences between types of hospitals were slightly greater using the more refined volume measure.

To combat the problem of reduced numbers, we examine the relation be-

Figure 14.7: Standardized Mortality Ratios for High- and Low-Volume Hospitals by Risk Level of Patients: Intraabdominal Aorta Surgery

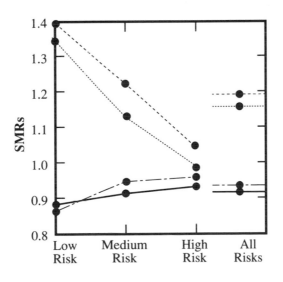

- - - - - - - - - - - , treatment in low-volume hospital.
——————————— , treatment in high-volume hospital.
·························· , treatment in low-volume hospital.
—— · —— · —— , treatment in high-volume hospital.
SMRs >1 indicate more deaths than expected.

tween volume, risk level, and outcomes for all selected surgical categories combined. The pattern of findings revealed by inspecting the individual categories is sufficiently similar to suggest that it is appropriate to examine them in combination. Results for all selected surgery are shown in Figure 14.8 and Table 14.4 for both volume measures. First we note that the general pattern for patients to have better outcomes in high-volume hospitals at each risk level is consistent with the results already noted, but that differences in SMRs between high- and low-volume hospitals are significant at the 0.001 level for both low- and medium-risk patients groups as well as overall. We conclude first that hospitals with more experience in conducting a given type of surgery produce better outcomes for their patients, particularly those at low or medium risk, than do hospitals with less experience. The results in Figure 14.8 also reveal an interactive relationship between risk level and volume. As before, SMRs for high-volume hospitals varied little by risk level. Low-volume hospitals, however, had the highest SMR and the greatest discrepancy from high-volume hospitals for low-risk patients, which was a significant difference. Medium-risk patients in low-volume hospitals had relatively better outcomes but still had significantly worse outcomes than their counterparts in high-volume hospitals. High-risk patients in low-volume hospitals had relatively better outcomes than either medium- or low-risk patients,

Figure 14.8: Standardized Mortality Ratios for High- and Low-Volume Hospitals by Risk Level of Patients: Selected Surgeries Combined

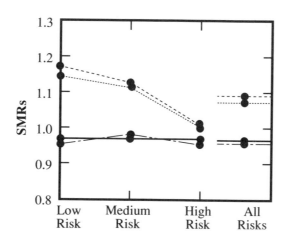

-----------, treatment in low-volume hospital.
———————, treatment in high-volume hospital.
......................., treatment in low-volume hospital.
—— - —— - ——, treatment in high-volume hospital.
SMRs >1 indicate more deaths than expected.

and they did not have significantly different outcomes than their counterparts in high-volume hospitals. We conclude, second, that there is support for the overall relationship between volume and surgical outcomes to be mitigated by the risk level of the patient (Fig. 14.8) and the type of diagnostic procedure involved (Figs. 14.1–14.6). Last, the results in Figure 14.8 demonstrate no difference between the two measures of volume. We conclude that there is no support for the effect of experience or volume in treating patients to depend upon treating surgical patients in the same category *and* and the same risk level.

Next we turn briefly to the two medical categories: gallbladder and ulcer patients treated medically rather than surgically. As reported in Figures 14.9 and 14.10 and Table 14.3, there are no significant differences in outcomes associated with differences in patient risk level. As already noted, high-volume hospitals performed no better than low-volume hospitals on ulcer, and, contrary to prediction, high-volume hospitals experienced poorer outcomes than low-volume hospitals for gallbladder patients, a difference significant at the 0.05 level for all risk levels combined.

For gallbladder medical patients, the relation between risk level and volume paralleled the pattern observed for surgical patients. That is, there is no evidence of an interaction between risk and outcome in the high-volume hospitals. For low-volume hospitals, on the other hand, high-risk patients appear to

Figure 14.9: Standardized Mortality Ratios for High- and Low-Volume Hospitals by Risk Level of Patients: Nonsurgical Gallbladder Diagnoses

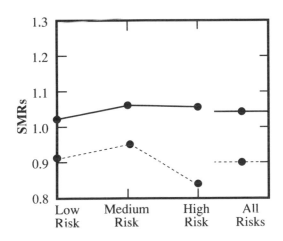

Broken line, treatment in low-volume hospital.
Solid line, treatment in high-volume hospital.
SMRs >1 indicate more deaths than expected.

Figure 14.10:   Standardized Mortality Ratios for High-
and Low-Volume Hospitals by Risk Level of Patients:
Nonsurgical Ulcer Diagnoses

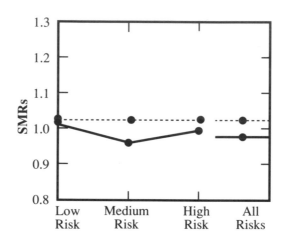

Broken line, treatment in low-volume hospital.
Solid line, treatment in high-volume hospital.
SMRs >1 indicate more deaths than expected.

fare better than either low- or medium-risk patients. As before, in no instance
were the differences between high- and low-volume hospitals significant for any
risk level. For ulcer patients, there was no evidence of an interactive effect
between risk level and outcomes. In analyses not reported here, we examined the
impact of using the second volume measure and found no differences from those
reported. We conclude that there is little consistent support for the effect of
experience or volume in treating patients for producing better outcomes for
medical patients.

DISCUSSION

We can only speculate on the bases of these patterns. The tendency for high-risk
surgical patients to fare somewhat better than low- or medium-risk surgical
patients in low-volume hospitals may indicate that these hospitals treat high-risk
surgical patients differently, perhaps by providing special facilities or arrangements, such as intensive care, that help to overcome the limitations of the hospital's general lack of experience. Alternatively, high-risk patients may not be
randomly distributed among hospitals performing these procedures but may be
concentrated in certain types of hospitals, e.g., teaching hospitals or larger
hospitals, that have arrangements that compensate for their low volume.

Many other factors may enter into these results to obscure any connection between volume, risk level, and outcomes for surgical patients. Surgical procedures vary greatly in complexity, and the benefits of experience may vary accordingly, although our data provide little support for this argument. Our measures of volume are crude, allowing us to assess only whether a hospital had more or less experience than the average among our study hospitals. For some procedures, this results in designating some hospitals as low-volume even though they treat, in absolute terms, a large number of patients. We are not able to redefine our measures of volume to test for this possibility because precautionary steps taken to protect the anonymity of the study hospitals, required by our contract with CPHA, preclude the redefinition of any measure. Finally, as already noted, death is not a sensitive measure of surgical outcome, and this is particularly the case for patients in low- and medium-risk groups.

The absence of strong outcome effects associated with volume and/or risk level for medical patients is consistent with several varying explanations. Experience in dealing with medical patients may not have the same positive impact on performance that it appears to have for surgical patients. Or it may be that in-hospital death is not a valid indicator of medical performance either in general or in the case of these two diagnostic categories. Alternatively, it is possible that the medical categories chosen are sufficiently frequent in occurrence that even those hospitals with below-average volume see sufficient numbers of patients to be experienced in their care. Finally, it is possible that volume is highly intercorrelated with other structural characteristics of hospitals affecting outcomes, so that the true effect of volume is masked in our results. This final explanation is one that we evaluate for both surgical and medical patients in Part II, using other data from the present study.[13]

ACKNOWLEDGMENT

The authors gratefully acknowledge the contributions of W. H. Forrest, Jr. and B. W. Brown, Jr., who were members of the original staff.

REFERENCES

1. Luft HS, Bunker JP, Enthoven AC. Should operations be regionalized? The empirical relation between surgical volume and mortality. New Engl J Med 1979;301:1364.
2. Shortell SM, LoGerfo J. Hospital medical staff organization and quality of care: results for myocardial infarction and appendectomy. Med Care 1981;19:1041.
3. Schoonhoven CB, Scott WR, Flood AB, Forrest WH Jr. Measuring the complexity and uncertainty of surgery and postsurgical care. Med Care 1980;18.893.
4. Forrest WH Jr, Brown BW Jr, Scott WR, Ewy W, Flood AB. Impact of hospital characteristics on surgical outcomes and length of stay. Final Report to National Center for Health Services Research, 1978. (DHHS, HRA 230–75– 0173).
5. Staff of the Stanford Center for Health Care Research. Comparison of hospitals with regard to outcomes of surgery. Health Serv Res 1976;11:112.

6. Staff of the Stanford Center for Health Care Research. Study of the institutional differences in postoperative mortality, Springfield, VA: NTIS PB 250–940, 1974.
7. Luft HS. Diverging trends in hospitalization: fact or artifact? Med Care 1981; 19:1979.
8. Flood AB, Ewy W, Scott WR, Forrest WH Jr, Brown BW Jr. The relationship between intensity and duration of medical services and outcomes for hospitalized patients. Med Care 1979;17:1088.
9. Lave JR, Lave LB. The extent of role differentiation among hospitals. Health Serv Res 1971;6:15.
10. Berry RE. Product heterogeneity and hospital cost analysis. Inquiry 1970;7:67.
11. Horn S, Schumacher D. Comparing classification methods: measurement of variations in charges, length of stay, and mortality. Med Care 1982;20:489.
12. Young WW, Swinkola RB, Zorn DM. The measurement of hospital case mix. Med Care 1981;20:501.
13. Flood AB, Scott WR, Ewy W. Does practice make perfect? Part II: The relation between volume and outcomes and other hospital characteristics. Med Care 1984;22:115.

Chapter 15

Sampling of Patient Data

The Medical Provider Analysis and Review (MED-PAR) data set that Riley and Lubitz used for their study was a 20 percent random sample of aged Medicare beneficiaries undergoing selected procedures. The study illustrates two problems that arise in assessing hospital volumes if one does not have data for all the patients undergoing the procedures. The first problem is generalizability and estimating volumes from a nonrandom sample. The second problem is the bias arising from unequal numbers of patients in hospitals.

First, Medicare beneficiaries over age 65 do not constitute a consistent proportion of any of the procedures studied. Although they account for a large number of prostatectomies and a majority of femur fracture reductions, hip replacements, and intestinal resections, they account for only a minority of coronary artery bypass graft, cholecystectomy, and hernia operations.

It is reasonable to consider the outcomes of certain patient subgroups, such as the elderly. Although aged patients present special surgical and management problems, surgical experience with non-aged patients is at least partly generalizable to aged patients. A hospital volume estimated from the number of Medicare patients however, may be a poor estimate of the total number of such patients, since hospitals may face dissimilar age distributions among their surgery patients. Clearly, the Medicare estimate is the lowest possible volume. Some hospitals, perhaps those in retirement communities, may have few non-Medicare patients, and other hospitals may have only a handful of elderly patients. Varying proportions of Medicare-eligible patients will make it more difficult to detect a true volume-outcome effect. It may even lend a substantial bias to the results.

Second, because the data are drawn from a 20 percent sample of patients, not all hospitals have an equal chance of being included in the sample. Hospitals with rather low patient volumes are quite likely to be excluded because none of their patients fell into the 20 percent sample. On the other hand, hospitals with higher volumes of Medicare patients are not likely to drop out.

The use of a 20 percent sample of Medicare beneficiaries may seem strange, but the authors recognize its limitations. Data for all Medicare beneficiaries are now available, so the 20 percent sampling problem can be avoided, but one must still contend with the fact that Medicare volumes may not be reliable estimates of total volumes for a procedure in a hospital. The Medicare data, however, are particularly valuable because they can be used to track posthospital outcomes. In some instances it may be possible to get total volume estimates from routinely collected discharge abstract data sets and link them to the Medicare data that would be used for the outcome analysis. However, if an insurer chose to use its own data for volume-outcome studies, either because discharge abstract data were unavailable or because follow-up claims data were used to measure outcomes, the sampling problem illustrated by Riley and Lubitz would reappear.

Sampling problems associated with various data sets raise issues of both generalizability and bias. For example, the average hospital volume of coronary artery bypass surgery patients in California is substantially below that of heavily regulated states, such as New York or New Jersey, where fewer institutions are granted state permission to operate open-heart surgery services. Therefore we do not know whether the volume-outcome relationship estimated by Showstack and his colleagues (1987) also holds for those other states, but the California data include many more low-volume hospitals.[1] Many studies have used data from the Commission on Professional and Hospital Activities.[2] Although this sample includes hospitals from across the nation, it overrepresents larger institutions and certain states. This imbalance alone threatens the generalizability of results, but the fact that subscribing to CPHA is usually voluntary also suggests that the hospitals may have been more concerned than most about quality.

If one can predict the implications and direction of a sampling bias, this information can be used to strengthen the analysis. The sampling in the Riley-Lubitz study could have led to a failure to detect a relationship between volume and outcome at very low volumes due to incomplete inclusion of low-volume hospitals. The fact that, even with this limitation, a relationship is often observable provides strong evidence for an effect.

NOTES

1. See reprint of Showstack et al. (1987) in chapter 11 of this volume.
2. See, for example, Flood, Scott, and Ewy (1984a), Part I reprinted in Chapter 14 of this volume; Luft (1980), reprinted in Chapter 16; and Sloan, Perrin, and Valvona (1986), reprinted in Chapter 13.

Outcomes of Surgery among the Medicare Aged

Surgical Volume and Mortality

Gerald Riley
James Lubitz

Surgical procedures performed on the aged account for a high percentage of all surgeries in the United States. A National Center for Health Statistics (NCHS) report (Pokras, 1983) estimates that in 1979 more than 20 percent of all procedures were for patients 65 years of age or over. The rate of all listed procedures per 10,000 population was estimated by NCHS to be 2,583 for the aged and only 1,371 for all ages in that year. Lubitz and Deacon (1982) have noted that the incidence of surgery among the Nation's aged increased at a faster rate between 1967 and 1977 than for younger people. Because mortality following surgery generally increases with age (Lubitz, Riley, and Newton, 1985; Jensen and Tondevold, 1979; and Gersh et al., 1983), postsurgical mortality among the aged is an important aspect of surgical outcomes.

Among hospitals, surgical outcomes can vary considerably in a manner not fully explained by measurable differences in individual patient characteristics. The National Halothane Study (National Academy of Sciences, 1966) examined the effects of halothane anesthesia on patients undergoing surgery. The study, adjusting for differences in procedures, age, and preoperative physical status, produced evidence of considerable variation in inhospital death rates among the 34 hospitals. The Stanford Center for Health Care Research (1974), using Professional Activities Study (PAS) data collected from 1,224 hospitals, studied differences in institutional mortality rates after indirectly standardizing for demographic and clinical differences in patient populations. The authors found significant differences in mortality rates among institutions. The study also addressed the relationship between various hospital characteristics (e.g., size, teaching programs, and staffing levels) and standardized mortality ratios (MR's) for various categories of procedures. The investigators found that standardized MR's differed according to hospital characteristics, but the nature and strength of the relationship varied strongly by procedure. In general, the amount of variation in

Reprinted from *Health Care Financing Review* 7, no. 1 (1985): 37–47, HCFA Pub. No. 03206. Office of Research and Demonstrations, Health Care Financing Administration. Washington. U.S. Government Printing Office, November 1985.

standardized MR's explained by hospital characteristics was rather small for each procedure.

Schumacher and Horn (1978) examined postoperative death rates among Maryland hospitals both for those located in standard metropolitan statistical areas (SMSA's) and those in non-SMSA's. Controlling for case mix, the investigators found an inverse relationship between cost per case and mortality rates in SMSA's, but did not find significant relationships between mortality rates and other hospital characteristics, such as number of residency training programs, hospital salary level, and presence of high technology facilities (e.g., coronary care units and intensive care units). The Commission on Professional and Hospital Activities (1970), using Professional Activity Study (PAS) data, found that after adjusting for differences in patient mix, cholecystectomy patients discharged from small hospitals experienced a much higher mortality rate than those discharged from large hospitals. Hospital size was defined in terms of total number of discharges.

Luft, Bunker, and Enthoven (1979) and Luft (1980) examined the issues of whether hospitals that perform large numbers of specific surgical procedures have different mortality outcomes than hospitals that perform relatively few of these procedures. From PAS data, hospital-specific mortality rates were compared with expected mortality rates, adjusting for age, sex, and presence of single or multiple diagnoses. Mortality rates decreased as volume of the specific operations increased for several procedures, including open heart surgery, coronary artery bypass graft, transurethral resection of the prostate (TURP), and hip arthroplasty (total replacement). This association was determined to exist independent of the effects of hospital size such as total admissions and total number of operations performed. No significant volume-mortality relationship was found for some procedures, e.g., vagotomy. Although the data suggest that greater surgical experience may lead to lower mortality rates for some procedures, Luft (1980) also provided evidence that suggests a referral effect may exist, i.e., that better outcomes may lead to more referrals and higher volume. Regardless of the exact nature of the relationship between volume and mortality, Luft, Bunker, and Enthoven (1979) have argued that the data support the concept of establishing regional referral centers for some procedures.

Additional evidence supporting the establishment of regional centers for performing certain procedures was reported recently by Flood, Scott, and Ewy (1984a and 1984b). They used 1972 data from the Commission on Professional and Hospital Activities, and found strong and consistent evidence that high volume is associated with lower inhospital mortality for surgical patients, after controlling for patient mix. In particular, low-volume hospitals were associated with poorest outcomes relative to expectations for low-risk surgical patients.

Our study examines the relationship between hospitals' postsurgical mortality rates and surgical volume for aged Medicare beneficiaries undergoing eight types of procedures in 1979 or 1980. The procedures are TURP, hip arthroplasty (total hip replacement and other arthroplasties are examined separately), femur fracture reduction,* resection of the intestine, cholecystectomy, inguinal hernia repair, and coronary artery bypass.

These procedures were chosen for several reasons. All, with the exception of coronary artery bypass surgery, are common among the aged. For five of the eight study procedures, more than half of all operations were performed on the aged. In 1979, 86 percent of all hip arthroplasties (not including total hip replacement), 74 percent of all TURP's, 69 percent of all femur fracture reductions, 57 percent of total hip replacements, and 52 percent of resections of the intestine were performed on the aged (National Center for Health Statistics, 1982). Between 23 percent and 28 percent of the coronary artery bypass surgeries, repairs of inguinal hernia, and cholecystectomies were performed on aged patients.

In addition, all these procedures, except for femur fracture reduction, are often of a nonemergency nature. This means that, aside from the decision to operate or not, there is often considerable discretion available as to which hospital the procedure will be performed in. Lastly, several of the procedures exhibit rather high mortality rates following surgery (Lubitz, Riley, and Newton, 1985). The association of volume and mortality rates is particularly important for the aged, because the relative frailty of this population and the frequent presence of co-morbidity may make the aged more sensitive to the effects of surgical experience.

DATA AND METHODS

Data for this study were obtained from two files of the Medicare Statistical System of the Health Care Financing Administration (HCFA): the Medicare provider analysis and review (MEDPAR) file and the enrollment file. The MEDPAR file contains information on discharges from short-stay hospitals for a 20 percent probability sample of Medicare beneficiaries (selected on the basis of their Medicare identification numbers). The information includes demographic data (e.g., age, sex), hospital data (e.g., size, location), and stay data (e.g., principal surgical procedure, principal diagnosis, and inhospital patient death). In 1979 and 1980, the principal surgical procedure and principal diagnosis were coded for each discharge using the *International Classification of Diseases, Ninth Revision, Clinical Modification* (ICD-9-CM). The records of hospital stays for the eight selected procedures were linked to the enrollment file to identify all deaths, regardless of where the death occurred, for 60 days following surgery.

---

*Although the *International Classification of Diseases, Ninth Revision, Clinical Modifications* (ICD-9-CM) surgical codes do not identify the specific part of the femur that is fractured, for elderly patients the majority of breaks occur at the neck of the femur. In this study, among patients for whom the principal diagnosis was a fractured femur, more than 90 percent of the cases had a diagnosis of fracture at the neck of the femur.

One hospital-specific variable was computed from the MEDPAR file. This variable, referred to in this article as VOLUME, is the annual number of surgeries of a given type performed on the Medicare aged in a specific hospital. VOLUME was derived by summing, for each hospital, the number of surgeries performed in the appropriate year and then multiplying by 5.

Several limitations are present in the data. First, the experience of many hospitals with a very low volume of specific surgeries is not represented in the analysis. This is true because, under the 20-percent sample selection criterion, no patients are selected from many hospitals that perform only a few operations of a specific type in a given year. Consequently, it should be more difficult to detect mortality-volume relationships that exist at a low range of surgical volumes. A related problem is that some error is present in the measurement of surgical volumes for individual hospitals because the MEDPAR file discharges are selected as a national sample and not on a hospital-by-hospital basis. This error can be substantial at very low sample volumes (Table 15.1). Second, the exact date of death is not always identified because, in the Medicare enrollment file, the date of death is sometimes coded as the last day of the month of death. This is most often true for railroad retirees, who constituted approximately 3 percent of our sample. Railroad retirees were therefore excluded from the analyses, and for the remainder of the sample it was estimated that 5 percent of all deaths were erroneously recorded as having occurred on the last day of the month. The effect of erroneously recorded death dates would be to slightly underestimate the number of deaths occurring within 60 days of surgery, but there is no reason to believe that this invalidates the results relating to mortality-volume relationships.

Third, there are known to be some problems with the reliability of diagnostic and surgical data in the Medicare statistical system (National Academy of Sciences, 1977). The problems uncovered in the National Academy of Sciences study are described in another article (Lubitz, Riley, and Newton, 1985). The study did not reveal any errors that would appear to systematically bias our study results.[*]

For six of the procedures, cases with a principal diagnosis of cancer for the stay in which the study procedure was performed were excluded from the sample; the six procedures are hip arthroplasty (total), hip arthroplasty (other), femur fracture reduction, inguinal hernia repair, cholecystectomy, and coronary artery bypass. Among beneficiaries undergoing these operations, there were few cancer patients (1.2 percent); their mortality experience was considerably different from that of the noncancer patients. Cancer patients were retained in the sample for TURP and resection of the intestine because there were significant numbers of such patients. The analyses control for the effect of a cancer diagnosis on mor-

---

[*]For this study, certain consistency edits were performed to identify other kinds of miscoding. For example, 2 percent of the TURP cases were identified as having been performed on women, and were excluded from the study.

Table 15.1:   Approximate Standard Errors Associated with Estimates of the Surgical Volume at an Individual Hospital, by Sample Sizes[1]

Sample Surgeries (Individual Hospital)	Population Estimate	Approximate Standard Error
3	15	7.75
6	30	10.95
10	50	14.14
15	75	17.31
25	125	22.35
40	200	28.26

[1]Taken from the 20-percent national Medicare provider analysis and review (MEDPAR) file.
   Source: Health Care Financing Administration, Bureau of Data Management and Strategy: Data from the Medicare Statistical System, 1979–80.

tality rates. The study also does not include Medicare beneficiaries entitled because of disability (all of whom are under 65), who constitute approximately 10 percent of the Medicare population.

The hospital discharge is the unit of analysis for this study. Discharges of aged beneficiaries with the appropriate ICD-9-CM surgical codes, occurring in 1979 and 1980, were selected and pooled across both years. If an individual underwent more than one hospitalization for the study procedures during 1979–80, each discharge was included as a separate observation. In addition to individual patient attributes for each discharge, such as age and sex, characteristics of the hospital in which the surgery was performed were appended to the unit record, including the annual number of procedure-specific surgeries from the MEDPAR file (VOLUME). Annual numbers of surgeries were computed for the year in which the discharge occurred. It should be noted that for patients undergoing either hip arthroplasty (total) or hip arthroplasty (other), VOLUME represents the sum of the operations of *either* type performed in a given hospital and year.

The surgical outcome focused on in the study was whether the patient died within 60 days of surgery. This time period was chosen because of evidence that high mortality persists for these procedures for at least 2 months after surgery (Lubitz, Riley, and Newton, 1985). The use of deaths within 60 days of surgery represents an important difference from earlier studies on the relation of surgical volume to mortality; those studies were limited to inhospital deaths (Luft, 1980; Flood et al. 1984a and 1984b). Following patients for 60 days removes any possible confounding effect of a relation between length of hospital stay and other variables. The associations between outcome and patient and hospital attributes were examined using multiple logistic regression, with the dependent variable defined as death within 60 days of surgery (1 = yes, 0 = no). Logistic regression is commonly used to ascertain the association between one or more independent variables and a binary response variable. The LOGIST procedure of statistical analysis system (SAS) was used to estimate the regression relationships (Harrell, 1983). Throughout the analyses, a significance level of .05 is used, although *p*-values are shown to indicate the strength of the relationships.

FINDINGS

The sample sizes of the eight study procedures are shown in Table 15.2, along with the number of deaths that occurred within 60 days of surgery. The most common procedure was TURP with 55,742 sample cases in 1979–80, and the least common procedures were coronary artery bypass, with 6,157, and hip arthroplasty (total), with 9,862. The remainder were in the range of 17,000 to 35,000. Mortality rates varied substantially by procedure. The highest mortality rates within 60 days of surgery were experienced by patients undergoing resection of the intestine (11.0 percent), and femur fracture reduction (10.2 percent). In the latter case, the high death rate is partly because of the advanced age of the patients (mean 80.4 years), as indicated in Table 15.3. The lowest death rate was for patients undergoing inguinal hernia repair (1.5 percent).

The independent variables examined in the study, with their mean values by procedure, are listed in Table 15.3. The number of hospitals represented is also given by procedure. Average annual surgical volume for aged Medicare patients for specific procedures (VOLUME) was highest for TURP, with an annual average of 84 such operations in hospitals performing one or more TURP's. The second highest surgical volume was attributed to coronary artery bypass, with 70 such procedures per hospital. This fact and the fact that only 990 hospitals are represented in our sample for coronary artery bypass suggest that this operation is concentrated in relatively few hospitals and that the volume of coronary artery bypass procedures tends to be large in these hospitals. The smallest procedure-specific surgical volumes were attributed to femur fracture reduction, with 34 mean annual operations, and resection of the intestine, with 36 mean annual operations. There is an unknown degree of upward bias in these average figures because some hospitals with a very low volume of specific procedures are not identified for the study, given the 20-percent sample size limitation of the MED-PAR file.

Coronary artery bypass differs from other procedures with respect to the hospital-specific variables. It tends to be performed in larger hospitals, as measured by bed size. More than 70 percent of coronary artery bypass operations were performed in hospitals with a medical school affiliation, compared with 52 percent for the next highest procedure, hip arthroplasty (total). The percentage of coronary artery bypass procedures performed in proprietary hospitals was somewhat lower (5 percent) than for any other procedure, and nearly all (98 percent) were performed in a hospital located in an SMSA area.

The percentage of patients dying within 60 days of surgery varied by surgical volume for several study procedures (Table 15.4). Mortality rates exhibited a rather consistent decrease as volume increased for resection of the intestine, coronary artery bypass, TURP, and hip arthroplasty (other). Mortality rates declined most sharply for resection of the intestine, from 12.4 percent for the lowest volume group to 9.7 percent for the highest. Hip arthroplasty (total) patients exhibited a substantial decrease in mortality among the highest volume hospitals. Repair of inguinal hernia patients exhibited a less consistent decline in mortality as volume increased, and femur fracture reduction and cholecystectomy patients did not show any consistent relation between death rate and surgical volume.

In Table 15.4, the percentage of procedures performed in low-volume and high-volume hospitals is shown. On the one hand, more than one-half of all operations on the Medicare aged for femur fracture reduction and resection of the intestine are done in low-volume hospitals (sample size of fewer than seven procedures). On the other hand, procedures for TURP, coronary artery bypass, and hip arthroplasty (total) are frequently performed in high-volume hospitals (sample size of more than 15 procedures). The relative concentration of these procedures in high-volume hospitals probably reflects the electiveness of these procedures. Even so, approximately 27 percent of coronary artery bypass and hip arthroplasty (total) operations were done in low-volume hospitals.

The number of surgeries performed does not represent any hospital's complete surgical experience for the study procedures, but rather that with aged Medicare beneficiaries. Consequently, the study focuses on the relationship between a hospital's institutional experience in the surgical treatment of aged patients and the mortality of those patients. Surgical care of aged patients often requires special attention to co-morbid conditions, and involves substantially greater risk of complications and death. Thus, surgical volume related specifically to aged patients is an important measure of experience.

The relationship between mortality rates and surgical volume is more clearly identified through the multiple logistic regression equations developed separately for each procedure (Table 15.5). Because the regression coefficients are not readily interpretable in a logistic regression equation, only the signs of the coefficients are given in Table 15.5 along with their approximate *p*-values. A negative sign indicates that mortality decreases with an increase in the value of the independent variable and vice versa. The natural logarithm of VOLUME was used to represent surgical volume. (The logarithm of VOLUME was used because previous research has shown that the curve describing the association between surgical volume and mortality "flattens" as surgical volume increases [Luft, 1980]). Dummy variables were used to indicate sex, geographic region, presence of specific principal diagnoses, medical school affiliation of the hospital in which the surgery was performed, proprietary status, and location in an SMSA area. For resection of the intestine, cholecystectomy, and inguinal hernia repair, an additional dummy variable was included to indicate whether or not the date of surgery and the date of admission were the same. Surgery on the day of admis-

Table 15.2:   Sample Size and Deaths Occurring within 60 Days of Surgery for Medicare Enrollees 65 Years of Age or Over, by Surgical Procedure: 1979–80

Surgical Procedure	ICD-9-CM[1] Codes	Sample Size	Number of Deaths within 60 Days of Surgery	Percent of Patients Dying within 60 Days of Surgery
Transurethral resection of the prostate	60.2	55,742	1,638	2.9
Femur fracture reduction	79.05, 79.15, 79.25, 79.35	20,161	2,057	10.2
Resection of the intestine	45.6, 45.7, 45.8	22,560	2,492	11.0
Cholecystectomy	51.2	34,693	1,468	4.2
Inguinal hernia repair	53.0, 53.1	32,721	482	1.5
Coronary artery bypass	36.1	6,157	398	6.5
Hip arthroplasty	81.5, 81.6	27,490	1,792	6.5
Total replacement	81.5	9,862	228	2.3
Other hip arthroplasty	81.6	17,628	1,564	8.9

[1]*International Classification of Diseases, Ninth Revision, Clinical Modification.*
Source: Health Care Financing Administration, Bureau of Data Management and Strategy: Data from the Medicare Statistical System, 1979–80.

Table 15.3:   Mean Values of Independent Variables, by Procedure for Medicare Enrollees 65 Years of Age or Over: 1979–80

Independent Variable	Transurethral Resection of Prostate	Femur Fracture Reduction	Resection of the Intestine	Cholecystectomy	Inguinal Hernia Repair	Coronary Artery Bypass	Hip Arthroplasty (Total)	Hip Arthroplasty (Other)
				Mean value				
Patient-specific								
Age	74.5	80.4	75.1	73.2	73.4	69.2	73.8	79.3
Sex[1]	1.00	.21	.42	.35	.88	.70	.34	.21
Emergency[2]	—	—	.06	.03	.06	—	—	—
Diagnosis[3]	.17[10]	—	.52[10]	—	.06[12]	—	.09[13]	.74[13]
	—	—	.13[11]	—	—	—	—	—

Geographic region:[4]								
Northeast	.22	.22	.27	.22	.23	.16	.22	.19
South	.32	.33	.29	.34	.32	.30	.22	.37
North-Central	.28	.29	.27	.28	.27	.28	.33	.28
Western	.18	.16	.17	.16	.18	.26	.23	.16
Hospital-specific								
MED[5]	.43	.43	.46	.38	.39	.72	.52	.43
SMSA[6]	.79	.77	.81	.73	.74	.98	.83	.79
PROP[7]	.09	.07	.08	.09	.09	.05	.06	.08
BEDS[8]	360	349	371	321	330	571	400	359
VOLUME[9]	84	34	36	41	42	70	59[14]	45[14]
Number of hospitals represented	7,081	5,960	6,403	8,280	8,168	990	6061[15]	

[1]Sex: 1 = Male; 0 = Female.

[2]Emergency admission is defined as one in which surgery was performed on the same day as admission to the hospital.

[3]Diagnosis: 1 = Presence of indicated diagnosis; 0 = Absence.

[4]Geographic region: 0 = Patient not residing in that region. Northeast: 1 = Patient residing in Northeast region. South: 1 = Patient residing in South region. North-Central: 1 = Patient residing in North-Central region. West: 1 = Patient residing in West region. This variable is not included in the regression.

[5]MED is medical school affiliation: 1 = Medical school affiliation; 0 = No affiliation.

[6]SMSA is standard metropolitan statistical area: 1 = Location in SMSA; 0 = Location other than SMSA.

[7]PROP is proprietary: 1 = Proprietary hospital; 0 = Nonproprietary hospital.

[8]BEDS refer to bed size.

[9]Number of surgeries of specific type performed on the Medicare aged. Inflated from 20-percent sample of discharges.

[10]1 = Principal diagnosis of cancer; 0 = Other principal diagnosis.

[11]1 = Principal diagnosis of diverticula of intestine; 0 = Other principal diagnosis.

[12]1 = Principal diagnosis of obstructed hernia; 0 = Other principal diagnosis.

[13]1 = Principal diagnosis of femur fracture; 0 = Other principal diagnosis.

[14]VOLUME represents number of arthroplasties performed of either type (total or other).

[15]All hip arthroplasties combined.

Table 15.4: Crude Mortality Rates for Medicare Enrollees 65 Years of Age or Over, by Procedure and Range of Volume: 1979–80

Procedure and Range of Volume[1]	Number of Sample Discharges	Percent Dying within 60 Days of Surgery
Transurethal resection of the prostate		
Total	55,742	2.9
Less than 9	15,687	3.2
9–14	13,951	3.0
15–22	12,213	2.8
More than 22	13,891	2.7
Femur fracture reduction		
Total	20,161	10.2
Less than 4	6,217	10.8
4–6	5,899	10.1
7–9	3,615	9.7
More than 9	4,430	10.0
Resection of Intestine		
Total	22,560	11.0
Less than 4	6,739	12.4
4–6	6,016	11.5
7–10	5,152	10.1
More than 10	4,653	9.7
Cholecystectomy		
Total	34,693	4.2
Less than 5	10,513	4.1
5–7	8,294	4.4
8–11	7,909	4.2
More than 11	7,977	4.2
Inguinal hernia repair		
Total	32,721	1.5
Less than 5	10,934	1.5
5–7	8,221	1.8
8–11	6,355	1.4
More than 11	7,211	1.2
Coronary artery bypass		
Total	6,157	6.5
Less than 7	1,697	7.3
7–11	1,524	6.6
12–19	1,437	6.1
More than 19	1,499	5.7
Hip arthroplasty (total)		
Total	9,862	2.3
Less than 6	2,643	2.6
6–9	2,391	2.2
10–15	2,407	3.0
More than 15	2,421	1.5
Hip arthroplasty (other)		
Total	17,628	8.9
Less than 4	4,233	10.0
4–7	5,248	8.5
8–12	4,054	9.1
More than 12	4,093	8.1

[1]Surgical volume figures are not inflated from the 20-percent national sample.

sion may indicate that the admission was for an emergency or urgent case. As further controls for patient mix, length of stay and total charges were considered for inclusion as independent variables; however, they were dropped because they could equally well be considered dependent variables, e.g., a poor surgical outcome often involves complications that increase length of stay as well as total charges. Dummy variables indicating proprietary status and SMSA location were excluded from the equation for coronary artery bypass because so few of these procedures were performed in proprietary hospitals or non-SMSA areas.

Under the model described above, surgical volume exhibits a significant association with mortality for several of the study procedures, with higher volumes being associated with a lower probability of mortality. Resection of the intestine patients ($p < .001$) and those undergoing TURP ($p = .017$) exhibit a highly significant relationship between volume and mortality. Patients undergoing coronary artery bypass or hip arthroplasty (other) also show a significant association between volume and mortality ($p = .031$ and $p = .043$ respectively). The regression coefficients for patients undergoing femur fracture reduction, cholecystectomy, repair of inguinal hernia, and hip arthroplasty (total) are not statistically significant with respect to LOG (VOLUME). It is interesting to observe that all eight of the regression coefficients with respect to LOG (VOLUME) are negative, which would not be expected in the absence of any volume-mortality relationships.

It cannot be determined with certainty whether the association between VOLUME and mortality reflects the effects of procedure-specific surgical volume or the volume of surgical cases in general. It is possible, for example, that general operating room experience acquired by hospital personnel may affect outcomes for certain procedures more so than experience with that particular type of procedure. If this is true, then our procedure-specific volume variable may only be a proxy for general surgical volume. We attempted to measure the effect of general surgical volume on mortality by introducing into the equations a general surgical volume variable measuring the number of all operations performed on the elderly; the high positive correlations among the general and procedure-specific volume variables and bed size (BEDS) (Table 15.6) produced substantial multicollinearity problems in the models, with the exception of coronary artery bypass. Thus, no firm conclusion could be drawn about the relationship between mortality and general surgical volume.

Several other variables exhibit consistently strong associations with postsurgical mortality in Table 15.5. Age exhibits a strong positive association with mortality for all eight procedures ($p < .001$). The regional dummy variables exhibit a consistent pattern for several procedures, with superior outcomes for patients residing in the West. (The West is the region excluded from the regression and therefore each regional dummy variable represents a comparison of that region with the West.) Patients undergoing TURP, hip arthroplasty (other), and femur fracture reduction in the West exhibit significantly better outcomes than patients undergoing the same procedures in most or all of the other three regions

Table 15.5:   Multiple Logistic Regression for Specific Procedures with Death within 60 Days as the Dependent Variable, by Log (VOLUME) and Other Independent Variables: 1979–80

	Procedure			
Independent Variable	*Transurethral Resection of the Prostate*	*Femur Fracture Reduction*	*Resection of the Intestine*	*Chole-cystectomy*
	Sign of the regression coefficient (p-value)			
Age	Pos. (<.001)	Pos. (<.001)	Pos. (<.001)	Pos. (<.001)
Sex[1]	([10])	Pos. (.350)	Pos. (.004)	Pos. (.001)
Age × sex	([10])	Pos. (.546)	Neg. (.022)	Neg. (.007)
Emergency[2]	([10])	([10])	Pos. (<.001)	Pos. (<.001)
Diagnosis[3]	Pos. (<.001)	([10])	Neg. (<.001)[11]	([10])
	—	—	Neg. (<.001)[12]	—
Geographic region:[4]				
Northeast	Pos. (.010)	Pos. (<.001)	Pos. (.362)	Pos. (.993)
Southern	Pos. (.014)	Pos. (.006)	Pos. (.039)	Neg. (.775)
North-Central	Pos. (.017)	Pos. (.003)	Pos. (.083)	Neg. (.698)
MED[5]	Pos. (.380)	Neg. (.926)	Pos. (.015)	Pos. (.601)
SMSA[6]	Neg. (.954)	Neg. (.102)	Pos. (.286)	Neg. (.247)
PROP[7]	Pos. (.379)	Pos. (.472)	Pos. (.536)	Pos. (.283)
BEDS[8]	Pos. (.984)	Neg. (.434)	Neg. (.315)	Pos. (.252)
Log (VOLUME)[9]	Neg. (.017)	Neg. (.723)	Neg. (<.001)	Neg. (.431)

[1]Sex: 1 = Male; 0 = Female.

[2]Emergency admission is defined as one in which surgery was performed on the same day as admission to the hospital.

[3]Diagnosis: 1 = Presence of indicated diagnosis; 0 = Absence.

[4]Geographic region: 0 = Patient not residing in that region. Northeast: 1 = Patient residing in Northeast region. South: 1 = Patient residing in South region. North-Central: 1 = Patient residing in North-Central region.

[5]MED is medical school affiliation: 1 = Medical school affiliation; 0 = No affiliation.

[6]SMSA is standard metropolitan statistical area: 1 = Location in SMSA; 0 = Location other than SMSA.

[7]PROP is proprietary: 1 = Proprietary hospital; 0 = Nonproprietary hospital.

[8]BEDS refer to bed size.

[9]VOLUME is inflated by a factor of 5.

[10]Not applicable.

[11]1 = Principal diagnosis of cancer; 0 = Other principal diagnosis.

[12]1 = Principal diagnosis of diverticula of intestine; 0 = Other principal diagnosis.

[13]1 = Principal diagnosis of obstructed hernia; 0 = Other principal diagnosis.

[14]1 = Principal diagnosis of femur fracture; 0 = Other principal diagnosis.

Source: Health Care Financing Administration, Bureau of Data Management and Strategy: Data from the Medicare Statistical System, 1979–80.

Table 15.5:   Continued

	Procedure		
Inguinal Hernia Repair	*Coronary Artery Bypass*	*Hip Arthroplasty (Total)*	*Hip Arthroplasty (Other)*
Sign of the regression coefficient (p-value)			
Pos. (<.001)	Pos. (<.001)	Pos. (<.001)	Pos. (<.001)
Neg. (.053)	Neg. (.190)	Pos. (.246)	Pos. (.554)
Pos. (.037)	Pos. (.299)	Neg. (.427)	Pos. (.465)
Pos. (.008)	([10])	([10])	([10])
Pos. (<.001)[13]	([10])	Pos. (<.001)[14]	Neg. (.165)[14]
—	—	—	—
Neg. (.420)	Pos. (.096)	Neg. (.364)	Pos. (.060)
Pos. (.905)	Pos. (.337)	Pos. (.658)	Pos. (.008)
Pos. (.221)	Pos. (.031)	Neg. (.789)	Pos. (.003)
Pos. (.002)	Pos. (.685)	Neg. (.037)	Neg. (.664)
Neg. (.762)	([10])	Pos. (.696)	Pos. (.233)
Neg. (.188)	([10])	Pos. (.360)	Pos. (.773)
Neg. (.455)	Pos. (.193)	Neg. (.807)	Pos. (.811)
Neg. (.184)	Neg. (.031)	Neg. (.759)	Neg. (.043)

($p < .05$ for the regional dummy variables). Similarly, for resection of the intestine and coronary artery bypass, patients in the West had the lowest mortality, although only one regional coefficient for each procedure is significant at the .05 level. These findings confirm those obtained from earlier univariate analyses on the same data set (Lubitz, Riley, and Newton, 1985). These findings are also similar to those reported by Luft, who found significantly better outcomes in the West for 7 out of 12 procedures studied. No evidence of a regional effect on mortality among cholecystectomy, hip arthroplasty (total) or inguinal hernia repair patients is shown in Table 15.5.

Medical school affiliation exhibits a positive association with mortality at the .05 level for resection of the intestine and inguinal hernia repair. For hip arthroplasty (total) patients, however, medical school affiliation is significantly associated with favorable outcomes. An often cited explanation for poorer outcomes in hospitals affiliated with a medical school is that the patients undergoing operations in these facilities tend to be in poorer health than those treated else-

Table 15.6:   Correlations between Procedure-Specific Volume
and Beds, and Procedure-Specific Volume and General Surgical
Volume, by Type of Procedure: 1979–80

Procedure	Procedure-Specific Volume and Beds	Procedure-Specific Volume and General Surgical Volume
Transurethral resection of the prostate	.62	.79
Femur fracture reduction	.63	.65
Resection of the intestine	.67	.80
Cholecystectomy	.66	.79
Inguinal hernia repair	.63	.76
Coronary artery bypass	.35	.29
Hip arthroplasty (total)	.42	.55
Hip arthroplasty (other)	.60	72

Note: Coefficients of correlation between beds and general surgical volume were between .78 and .86 for all procedures.

Source: Health Care Financing Administration, Bureau of Data Management and Strategy: Data from the Medicare Statistical System, 1979–80.

where. Our data do not permit a conclusion on this assertion. The dummy variable designating location of the hospital in an SMSA exhibits no consistent relationship for this set of procedures. Proprietary status yields positive regression coefficients for six of seven procedures, but none of the coefficients achieves statistical significance. Higher mortality is significantly associated ($p < .001$) with a principal diagnosis of cancer for TURP patients, with obstructed hernia for inguinal hernia repair patients, and with femur fracture for hip arthroplasty (total) patients. Patients undergoing resection of the intestine exhibit more favorable outcomes with a principal diagnosis of diverticula of the intestine, and, surprisingly, with a principal diagnosis of cancer. It is possible that the remaining patients, who exhibited a variety of principal diagnoses and who constituted only 35 percent of all resection patients, suffered from multiple conditions, and that cancer or some other serious illness was present, but not coded as the principal diagnosis associated with the hospitalization. It is also possible that many of the residual patients were nonelective cases, and constituted poorer risks for surgery than the cancer patients, who are commonly elective cases.

The predicted probability of death within 60 days of surgery is given for various levels of VOLUME for resection of the intestine, coronary artery bypass, TURP, and hip arthroplasty (other) (Table 15.7), which are the four procedures for which VOLUME was significant in Table 15.5. The probabilities are evaluated at the mean of the other independent variables. The predicted probability of death decreases substantially as VOLUME increases for resection of the intestine, coronary artery bypass, and hip arthroplasty (other). For resection of the intes-

Table 15.7:   Estimated Probability of Death within
60 Days of Surgery for Medicare Enrollees 65 Years
of Age or Over, by Type of Procedure and Volume,
Controlling for Other Independent Variables: 1979–80

Procedure and Volume	Estimated Probability of Death
Resection of the Intestine	
10	.109
25	.097
40	.091
Coronary artery bypass	
20	.067
40	.061
80	.056
Transurethral resection of the prostate	
20	.027
50	.025
100	.023
Hip arthroplasty (other)	
10	.081
25	.076
50	.072

Source: Health Care Financing Administration, Bureau of Data
Management and Strategy: Data from the Medicare Statistical System, 1979–80.

tine, a change in VOLUME from 10 to 25 operations decreases the predicted probability of death from .109 to .097 (a 11.0 percent decrease). An increase in VOLUME from 10 to 40 operations decreases the predicted probability of death from .109 to .091, or 16.5 percent. Similarly, an increase in VOLUME of coronary artery bypass surgeries from 20 to 40 results in a decrease in predicted mortality from .067 to .061 (a 9.0 percent decrease). An increase in VOLUME from 20 to 80 coronary artery bypass operations per year results in a decrease in the predicted probability of death from .067 to .056 (a 16.4 percent decrease). For hip arthroplasty (other), an increase in VOLUME from 10 to 25 reduces the predicted probability of death from .081 to .076 (or 6.2 percent); an increase from 10 to 50 operations reduces it from .081 to .072 (11.1 percent). For TURP, the impact of a change in VOLUME is considerably less. An increase in VOL-UME from 20 to 100 operations produces a decrease in predicted probability of death from .027 to .023. Although this represents a 14.8 percent decrease, the decline is not very substantial in absolute terms because of the relatively low mortality rate associated with TURP.

The models are not suitable for predicting individual probabilities of death. In these cases, outcome can be affected by many additional variables that cannot be controlled in a model of this type.

As mentioned earlier, previous studies of the volume-mortality relation looked at deaths during the initial stay for surgery; we developed an additional set of models using inhospital deaths as the dependent variable. As indicated in Table 15.8, the association between surgical volume and inhospital mortality is much stronger than it is between volume and mortality within 60 days of surgery. Five of the eight procedures show a statistically significant relation between volume and inhospital deaths and the relation approaches significance for a sixth. For TURP, hip arthroplasty (other), and hip arthroplasty (total), the magnitude of the regression coefficients is much greater for the model using inhospital deaths, and the *p*-values are considerably lower; both facts indicate a stronger volume-mortality relationship for inhospital mortality than mortality within 60 days of surgery. For coronary artery bypass and resection of the intestine, the two models exhibit a similar association between volume and mortality. This is not too surprising, given the fact that many deaths following these procedures occur in the hospital (Table 15.8) Luft (1980) found a significant inverse association between inhospital mortality and surgical volume for all four of the procedures common to both studies: TURP, cholecystectomy, coronary artery bypass, and hip arthroplasty (total).

The reasons for a stronger relationship between in-hospital mortality and surgical volume are not clear. Because most deaths that occur during the surgical stay happen earlier than 60 days following surgery, it is possible that the effects associated with greater volume are manifested shortly after surgery, and may not be as evident for longer postoperative periods. It is also possible that high-volume hospitals may tend to discharge ill patients sooner than low-volume hospitals, and that more of their postoperative deaths may occur following discharge from the surgical stay. This might happen if, for example, many low-volume hospitals were located in rural areas where there are relatively few opportunities to transfer patients to other hospitals or nursing homes.

CONCLUSIONS

Our findings indicate that for the aged, increased institutional volume of surgery is associated with lower postsurgical mortality for some procedures. A significant inverse association between volume and mortality was found for resection of the intestine, TURP, coronary artery bypass, and hip arthroplasty (other). No statistically significant relationship was found between volume and mortality within 60 days of surgery for cholecystectomy, inguinal hernia repair, hip arthroplasty (total), or femur fracture reduction. The inverse association between volume and mortality appears to be much stronger when inhospital deaths, rather than death within 60 days of surgery, are used as the mortality measure. Although procedure-specific volumes were used in the analysis, it is possible that some of the effects attributed to procedure-specific surgical volume may result from general surgical volume of any kind.

Table 15.8: Comparison of Log (VOLUME) Effects In Logistic Regression Models Using Death during Surgical Stay and Death within 60 Days of Surgery as the Dependent Variable, by Type of Procedure: 1979–80

| | Death during Surgical Stay | | Death within 60 Days of Surgery | | Percent of Cases Dying | |
| | | | | | During Surgical Stay | Within 60 Days of Surgery |
Procedure	Coefficient	p-value	Coefficient	p-value		
Transurethral resection of prostate	−.218	<.001	−.087	.017	1.0	2.9
Femur fracture reduction	−.064	.187	−.013	.723	5.0	10.2
Resection of intestine	−.176	<.001	−.147	<.001	7.2	11.0
Cholecystectomy	−.099	.072	−.034	.431	2.5	4.2
Inguinal hernia repair	−.191	.117	−.096	.184	0.5	1.5
Coronary artery bypass	−.149	.033	−.131	.031	4.7	6.5
Hip arthroplasty (total)	−.273	.038	−.030	.759	1.1	2.3
Hip arthroplasty (other)	−.163	.003	−.078	.043	4.2	8.9

Source: Health Care Financing Administration, Bureau of Data Management and Strategy: Data from the Medicare Statistical System, 1979–80.

Although every attempt was made to control for appropriate patient characteristics, the results could be attributable to differences in case mix not measured by this study. For example, Flood, Scott, and Ewy (1984a and 1984b) and Luft, Bunker, and Enthoven (1979) found expected mortality to be generally higher in low-volume hospitals. High mortality in low-volume hospitals could reflect the fact that their caseload may contain a higher proportion of emergency or urgent cases. This might happen if nonemergency cases are often referred to specialty hospitals. Lower mortality in high-volume hospitals could reflect less stringent indications for surgery and hence better results. On the other hand, it is also commonly alleged that "sicker" patients are often referred to larger specialty hospitals and that their case mix is worse than that for less experienced community hospitals. Although we have no way of determining whether this is the case, we can say that, if true, this phenomenon would tend to mask any underlying mortality-volume relationship rather than falsely suggest it.

There are outcomes other than mortality that may be affected by institutional surgical experience. Farber, Kaiser, and Wenzel (1981) found a significant inverse relationship between surgical volume and incidence of postoperative wound infection for six of seven procedures including cholecystectomy, colon resection, and herniorrhaphy. Some of our study procedures, particularly those with low mortality, may be sensitive to surgical volume in terms of morbidity outcomes or patient functioning, but not mortality.

Specific causation cannot be attributed to the volume-mortality relationship found in our study. One possible interpretation is that greater surgical experience leads to improved technique, which results in lower mortality rates over time. Another interpretation is that hospitals that exhibit the best outcomes will attract more referrals and thereby increase their surgical volume. Luft (1980) found evidence of this effect in his study. Determination of causal factors was beyond the scope of our study, however.

Further research is needed on the reasons for the mortality-volume relationship, particularly the importance of the operating surgeon's experience. For example, it is possible that hospitals with high surgical volume have more skilled or experienced surgeons on their medical staffs, which would account for their superior outcomes. They may also have more specialists, as opposed to general practitioners. The role of the anesthesiologist, the operating room team, and other hospital personnel needs to be investigated. High-volume hospitals may recruit more skilled staffs, or conversely, the personnel at such hospitals may develop superior skills with increased experience. It is also possible that high-volume hospitals may have more specialized facilities and equipment (e.g., ICU's, CCU's). It is also important to determine why some hospitals have low surgical volume. Some of these hospitals may be geographically isolated, and it may not be practical for them to either increase their volume or to refer certain kinds of cases to other hospitals.

The results of this study indicate that hospitals with low surgical volumes should be reluctant to undertake certain procedures on a nonemergency basis.

Although our study does not pinpoint the separate effects of specific surgical volume and general surgical volume, our findings support the concept of establishing guidelines that include minimum volume levels for hospitals that undertake certain kinds of surgeries. Whether minimum levels are developed for specific procedures or operations in general would depend on the nature of each procedure. Many other factors must also be taken into consideration in establishing recommended minimum levels, such as types of facilities and equipment and availability of services elsewhere.

Luft, Bunker, and Enthoven (1979) have called for regionalization of certain procedures, based on their volume-mortality data. Our results provide support for this idea. For example, our study found a significant volume-mortality relationship for coronary artery bypass, resection of the intestine, and hip arthroplasty (other), which are relatively complex procedures with substantial mortality rates among the elderly. It is these types of operations that would be the most likely candidates for regionalization. Before these or other specific procedures are recommended for regionalization, policymakers should do detailed analyses to insure that the volume-mortality relationship is not due to differences in patient risk factors that could not be taken into account in the present study.

The findings also suggest the desirability of making information available to patients and referring physicians on the number of operations by hospital and by surgeon as a guide to the choice of hospital and surgeon. Information on the outcomes of surgery, of course, would be even more valuable. But, at this stage, we are not sure if there is enough understanding of the factors that determine outcome, especially at the physician level, to assure the correct interpretation of outcome data. Without such understanding, publicizing outcome data may create an incentive for physicians to avoid risky cases. A goal of future research should be the development of sufficient understanding of the factors determining outcome to enable dissemination of outcome data and to guide action to correct instances of less than optimal outcome.

These findings also have possible applications under Medicare's new prospective payment system (PPS) for hospitals. There has been concern that under PPS the financial incentives for hospitals to economize might adversely affect quality of care. On the other hand, PPS could encourage hospitals to specialize in the procedures they do most efficiently and thereby increase the concentration of particular procedures in a smaller number of hospitals. Because of the volume-outcome relationship, this could improve surgical outcomes. Under PPS, HCFA is collecting information on up to three procedures and five diagnoses per hospital stay on 100 percent of in-patient stays in short-stay hospitals. Surgical outcomes could be monitored on a hospital-specific or area-specific basis, using HCFA's expanded data system. If poor outcomes following certain procedures are associated with a given hospital, a low surgical volume for these procedures may, in the context of other information, explain the reason for these unfavorable outcomes. Solutions might be found, in cooperation with other area hospitals, that would guarantee a minimum number of procedures in any hospital receiving

Medicare reimbursement for these procedures.

Lastly, more favorable outcomes were experienced by patients in the West for five out of the eight procedures studied. Because death within 60 days of surgery is the mortality measure used in this study, rather than inhospital deaths, this finding is not a function of the fact that length of stay tends to be shorter in the West. Further research is needed to determine why patients in the West fare so much better following surgery.

ACKNOWLEDGMENTS

The authors wish to thank Marian Gornick and Allen Dobson of the Health Care Financing Administration (HCFA), and Dr. Benjamin Barnes or Harvard University for their excellent comments on earlier drafts of the article. We also wish to thank Marilyn Newton of the Bureau of Data Management and Strategy, HCFA, who provided programming support. Lastly, we wish to express our appreciation to Lee Sadler for her administrative assistance.

REFERENCES

Commission on Professional and Hospital Activities: Cholecystectomy mortality. *PAS Reporter*, Vol. 8, No. 8. Apr. 20, 1970.

Farber, B., Kaiser, D., and Wenzel, R.: Relation between surgical volume and incidence of postoperative wound infection. *N Engl J Med* 305 (4):200–204, July 23, 1981.

Flood, A.B., Scott, W.R., and Ewy, W.: Does practice make perfect? Part I, The relation between hospital volume and outcomes for selected diagnostic categories. *Med Care* 22 (2):98–114, Feb. 1984a.

Flood, A.B., Scott, W.R., and Ewy, W.: Does practice make perfect? Part II, The relation between volume and outcomes and other hospital characteristics. *Med Care* 22 (2):115–125, Feb. 1984b.

Gersh, B., Kronmal, R., Frye, R., et al.: Coronary arteriography and coronary artery bypass surgery, Morbidity and mortality in patients ages 65 years or older—A report from the coronary artery surgery study. *Circulation* 67 (3):483–491, Mar. 1983.

Harrell, F.: *The LOGIST Procedure*. In *SUGI Supplemental Library User's Guide*, 1983 Edition. SAS Institute, Inc., Cary, North Carolina, 1983.

Jensen, J., and Tondevold, E.: Mortality after hip fractures. *Acta Orthop. Scand.* 50:151–167, 1979.

Lubitz, J., and Deacon, R.: The rise in the incidence of hospitalizations for the aged, 1967 to 1979. *Health Care Financing Review*. Vol. 3, No. 3. HCFA Pub. No. 03141. Office of Research, Demonstrations, and Statistics, Health Care Financing Administration. Washington, U.S. Government Printing Office, Mar. 1982.

Lubitz, J., Riley, G., and Newton, M.: Outcomes of surgery in the Medicare aged population. Mortality after surgery, *Health Care Financing Review*. Vol. 6, No. 4. HCFA Pub. No. 3205. Office of Research and Demonstrations, Health Care Financing Administration. Washington, U.S. Government Printing Office, Summer 1985.

Luft, H.: The relation between surgical volume and mortality, An exploration of causal factors and alternative models. *Med Care* 18 (9):940–959, Sept. 1980.

Luft, H., Bunker, J., and Enthoven, A.: Should operations be regionalized? The empirical relation between surgical volume and mortality. *N Engl J Med* 301 (25):1364–1394, Dec. 20, 1979.

National Academy of Sciences, National Research Council, Subcommittee on the National Halothane Study of the Committee on Anesthesia: Summary of the national halothane study. *JAMA*, 197 (10):121–134, Sept. 5, 1966.

National Academy of Sciences: *Reliability of Medicare Hospital Discharge Records.* Contract No. SSA 600-7-0159. Prepared for the Department of Health, Education, and Welfare. Washington, D.C. Institute of Medicine. Nov. 1979.

National Center for Health Statistics, Division of Health Care Statistics: *Detailed Diagnoses and Surgical Procedures for Patients Discharged from Short-Stay Hospitals, United States, 1979.* DHHS Pub. No. (PHS) 82-1274.1. Public Health Service. Washington. U.S. Government Printing Office, Jan. 1982.

Pokras, R.: Surgical and nonsurgical procedures in short-stay hospitals, United States, 1979. *Vital and Health Statistics.* Series 13, No. 70. DHHS Pub. No. (PHS) 83-1731. Public Health Service. Washington, U.S. Government Printing Office, Feb. 1983.

Schumacher, D., and Horn, S.: *Hospital Death Rates, Analyses from a Statewide Data System.* Contract No. 600–76–01–40 and Grant 18-P-97031. Technical Report No. 308. Prepared for DHEW by Johns Hopkins University School of Hygiene and Public Health, Baltimore, MD, Dec. 1978.

Stanford Center for Health Care Research: *Study of Institutional Differences in Postoperative Mortality.* Report No. NCHSR 76–318. Contract No. PH 43–63–65, National Academy of Sciences, Wash. Dec. 1974.

Chapter 16

Causal Direction

There are at least two possible explanations for the association between hospital volume and patient outcomes. Higher volumes may produce better outcomes, through a practice-makes-perfect effect or through a scale effect. Alternatively, hospitals with better outcomes may attract a higher volume of patients because of selective referrals by physicians or patients to specialists or hospitals with better outcomes or away from those with worse outcomes.

The cross-sectional methods in all the volume literature preclude a complete understanding of the determinants of hospital volume. Sloan, Perrin, and Valvona (1986) noted great variability in hospital outcomes from year to year.[1] In addition, changing indications for performance of procedures, changing technologies, increased numbers of providers, and changing distribution of disease in the population are all significant factors in determining hospital volume. Without a clear and readily observable model of how selective referrals are made, skeptics can readily argue that outcome differences, which are hard to detect even with the data available at the research level, would be even more difficult for the ordinary patient or physician observer to use for selective referrals. Luft, Hunt, and Maerki (1987) provided an extended discussion of the issues in identifying the causal linkages. The study by Luft in this chapter adds little to that discussion because its model is much less complete. However, it provides a key piece in the historical discussion of the relationship between volumes and outcomes.

Luft, Bunker, and Enthoven (1979) presented their results on the relation between volume and outcome in a very simple way—observed and expected mortality rates for patients operated on in hospitals of varying volume levels.[2] The graphs for each procedure were meant to be easily understood by readers with little statistical sophistication. It did not seem possible to control for other variables, such as hospital size and teaching status, and still present the results as clearly. Since they wanted to reach the broadest possible audience by publishing in the *New England Journal of Medicine,* they chose a dual strategy. Luft estimated the more complex regression models, testing both the effects of other variables in a "classic" volume-outcome formulation and also the possibility of selective referrals with a simultaneous-equation model. Fortunately, the addition of variables such as total surgical volume, hospital bed size, and teaching status did not alter the basic association between volume and outcome. Thus, the simple graphic presentations would not be misleading. Since the journal prohibited prior publication, this study was merely presented at a professional meeting and its results referred to in the Luft, Bunker, and Enthoven piece. After publication in *NEJM,* it was submitted to *Medical Care* so that the detailed results would be made available to the health services research audience.

The authors recognized the possibility that an article such as this in the *New England Journal of Medicine* could have significant influence on policymakers. They wanted to affect policy, but they were concerned that their results might be misinterpreted as indicating that higher volumes definitely lead to better outcomes. The alternative hypothesis, that the findings might be a reflection of referrals to institutions with better outcomes or to patient selection, was discussed at some length. In fact, the three explanations were combined in the same sentence in the abstract to reduce the chances of misinterpretation.

Luft estimated a set of simultaneous equations to test the joint importance of the volume-outcome relationship and selective referrals, but he presented the results as exploratory. Even though the equations were sufficiently well specified to be interpretable, they could hardly be seen as fully convincing. The sketchiness of the model was due to the fact that the basic data were obtained from the Commission on Professional and Hospital Activities as a correlation matrix to prevent the identification of individual hospital data. Therefore, it was impossible to add variables or change their formulation without substantial additional cost. A simultaneous-equation model had not been considered in the original design of the project, so additional variables to include in a referral model had not been captured. The study by Luft, Hunt, and Maerki (1987) was designed to provide a better and more convincing test of the referral hypothesis. Even though the authors were able to estimate a more complete model, they devoted a considerable portion of their paper to simple bivariate results, in order to demonstrate the plausibility of a referral effect to those uncomfortable with more complex models.

Conflicting conclusions sometimes arise when multiple approaches are applied to the same data. Although most of the findings in the two studies were in agreement or could be easily reconciled there were instances (such as for cho-lecystectomy) where Luft, Bunker, and Enthoven found no effect and Luft reported a significant effect. Since detailed hospital-specific data are not available, it is impossible to determine why such conflicts occurred, but it now appears likely that they were due to the effects of single "unexpected" deaths in each of a few very low volume hospitals.[3]

NOTES

1. See Sloan, Perrin, and Valvona (1986), reprinted in Chapter 13.
2. Luft, Bunker, and Enthoven (1979) is reprinted in Chapter 12 of this volume.
3. See Luft, and Hunt (1986), reprinted in Chapter 19.

The Relation between Surgical Volume and Mortality

An Exploration of Causal Factors and Alternative Models

Harold S. Luft

Ever since Codman's classic study of the quality of medical care, there has been substantial interest in the factors determining the wide variation in outcomes among hospitals.[1] More recently, the National Halothane Study and the Institutional Differences Study found large differences in procedure-specific outcomes even after controlling for a wide range of patient characteristics.[2-4] One variable that has not received much attention, in spite of the fact that one often learns by doing, is the potential influence of experience on outcomes. The "experience curve" describing a logarithmic decline in unit costs as a function of cumulative production experience is well documented in industrial economics.[5-7] Our earlier work indicates that there is, indeed, a strong negative relation between the volume of certain procedures in hospitals and the in-hospital postoperative mortality rate, and that a substantial number of deaths could be averted if all patients were treated in hospitals having results similar to those of high-volume hospitals.[8] The presence of such a relation lends strong support to arguments in favor of regionalizing certain surgical procedures. The approach to such regionalization, however, depends crucially on the nature of the observed relation; that is, whether volume leads to better outcomes, or better outcomes lead to more volume, whether large teaching hospitals produce better outcomes, and whether experience must be accumulated over many years. The focus of this article is on developing a better understanding of such factors that may lie behind the observed correlation.

There are two major tasks in taking the investigation beyond the identification of a strong correlation. The first task is to develop a better sense of the causal factors at play. For instance, do outcomes depend merely on the volume in the current time period or on experience accumulated over several years? Similarly, do outcomes for a specific procedure such as coronary artery bypass graft

Reprinted from *Medical Care* 18, no. 9 (1980): 940–59, with permission from The J. B. Lippincott Company.

This research was supported by a grant from the Henry J. Kaiser Family Foundation.

Presented at the 54th Annual Western Economic Association Meeting, Las Vegas, Nevada, June 1979.

(CABG) depend upon the experience with that procedure alone, or with the more general set of all open heart procedures? At a more fundamental level, one may ask whether a model focusing on volumes may be backward. That is, instead of better outcomes resulting from more operations, are more patients attracted to better quality hospitals through well-functioning referral patterns? This obviously raises the problem of simultaneity, and while some results from a simultaneous equation model will be presented, they must at this point be considered tentative. The second task is understanding the role of other variables that may influence outcomes or referral patterns. For instance, do house-staff training programs lead to better or worse outcomes? Similarly, one may ask whether hospitals in metropolitan areas receive a disproportionate share of riskier patients because they serve as referral centers? A third task, which remains beyond the scope of this article, is to determine causal factors *within* the hospital. For instance, to the extent that volume is important, is it the number of operations done by a particular surgeon, anesthesiologist or operating room team? By exploring the first two tasks, this article will lay the foundation for future studies addressing the third task.

DATA AND METHODS

Basic data for use in this study were supplied by the Commission on Professional and Hospital Activities (CPHA), Ann Arbor, Michigan.* All U.S. short-term general hospitals participating in the Professional Activity Study (PAS) during 1974 and 1975 were eligible for inclusion in the study. To test the hypothesis, surgical procedures and diagnoses of differing degrees of complexity and anticipated mortality were chosen (Table 16.1).

A total of 33,336 patients were excluded because they were transferred, discharged against medical advice or had missing data on age or sex. This resulted in 420,538 patients in 1974 and 437,147 in 1975. Patients were then classified by five age categories (0–19, 20–34, 35–49, 50–64, and 65 +), sex and whether there were single or multiple diagnoses coded on the abstract. People with multiple diagnoses are known to have substantially higher mortality rates.[9] For each of the resulting 20 cells for each operation or operation group, the mortality rate was computed as the number of in-hospital deaths divided by the number of patients in the cell. This set of mortality rates used the largest possible sample of patients and hospitals in order to increase the reliability of the figures. Subsequently, an additional 15,063 patients were excluded because they were in 35 hospitals that were missing certain data or were not on the Master Facility Index of the National Center for Health Statistics. Thus, the hospital-based

---

*In these data the identities of individual hospitals are not revealed in any way. Any analysis, interpretation or conclusion based on these data is solely that of the author, and CPHA specifically disclaims responsibility for any such analysis, interpretation or conclusion.

Table 16.1: Operations and Diagnosis Groups

Group	Number of Patients Included in the Estimation of Mortality Rates, 1974–75	CPHA List B Group Numbers	Operation Code Number(s)*
1	55,397	463	Operations on heart, pericardium, and heart vessels (35.0–37.6)
1a	34,505	463	Direct heart revascularization (36.1) (CABG)
2	91,343	468	Operations on blood vessels, except ligation and bypass (38.0–38.3, 38.5–38.7, 39.3–39.5, 39.7–39.9)
2a	9,613	468	Resection of vessel with graft (38.3) and abdominal aortic aneurysm (441.0, 441.3, 441.4, 441.9, 093.0)
3	17,932	479	Vagotomy (44.0)
3a	9,090	479	Vagotomy (44.0) and/or pyloroplasty (44.1) and/or bypass gastroenterostomy (44.2) AND ulcer of duodenum without hemorrhage or perforation (532.0)
4	73,427	483	Colectomy (45.5–45.6)†
5	330,473	497	Cholecystectomy (51.1)
5a	8,085	497	Cholecystectomy AND incision of bile ducts (51.1 and 51.3)
6	18,408	498	Operations on biliary tract and gall-bladder except cholecystectomy (51.0, 51.2 51.9)
7	176,337	522	Transurethral prostatectomy (60.2)
8	33,075	586	Total hip replacement (81.5)

*Numbers in parentheses are the surgical procedure codes XX.X or diagnosis codes YYY.Y from the Hospital Adaptation of the ICDA (Second Edition).

†A search for patients with complete colectomy and primary diagnosis of Malignant Neoplasm of Large Intestine Except Appendix and Rectum yielded only 505 cases for the 2-year sample and thus was not analyzed further.

mortality data presented here are drawn from 842,622 patients operated on during 1974 and 1975 in 1,498 hospitals.

To correct for differences in case severity, expected death rates for each hospital were calculated using the age-, sex- and single-or-multiple-diagnosis-specific death rates for the whole sample, weighted by the proportion of each hospital's patients who were classified in each of the 20 age-, sex-, single-or-multiple-diagnosis cells. The actual death rates for each hospital were also computed.

Data records containing the mortality experience for each hospital were augmented with data from the 1975 file of the National Center for Health Statistics Master Facility Index. These data included the following variables: the number of beds in the hospital (BEDS), total number of admissions (ADMS), total number of operations (OPS), the ratio of house staff (residents plus interns) per bed (RIB), a (0,1) dummy indicating whether the hospital was located in a Standard Metropolitan Statistical Area (SMSA), (0,1) dummies indicating the major geographic region in which the hospital was located, Northeast (NE), North Central (NC), South Central (SC) or West (W), and average total expenses per patient day (EXP/DAY). The distributions of these variables were examined and nine hospitals were excluded at this last step because of values that seemed clearly to be in error. For instance, one hospital had listed expenses per day of $479. (Three other hospitals which had expenses slightly over $400/day were retained because other characteristics suggested those figures were correct.) Likewise, six hospitals with expenses under $40/day that also were primarily long-term institutions were dropped.[*]

The wide range in surgical volumes and the relative infrequency of postoperative death suggests that substantial variation in mortality rates across hospitals will occur merely by chance. Moreover, this random component will be much greater for low-volume hospitals, merely because the denominators for the former are smaller. To reduce this effect, each hospital's observation was weighted by the following factor:

$$ \mathrm{WT}_{i,j} = \frac{(\mathrm{NPAT}_{i,j})^2}{\displaystyle\sum_{k=1}^{\mathrm{NPAT}_{i,j}} P_{i,j,k} \bullet (1 - P_{i,j,k})} $$

where $\mathrm{NPAT}_{i,j}$ = number of patients with procedure i in hospital j.

$P_{i,j,k}$ = expected probability of death for the kth patient with procedure i in hospital j based on the patient's age, sex, and single/multiple-diagnosis category.

This factor gives more weight to hospitals with higher volumes (thus larger numerators) and patient mixes with lower expected death rates (implying smaller expected denominators.)[3]

For each of the 12 operations investigated, a separate data set was devel-

---

[*]This editing was performed by CPHA personnel with consultation by the author, who did not have access to any other information about the hospitals.

oped based only on those hospitals with at least one instance in 1975 of the target operation. Thus, 1,473 hospitals are included in the data set for cholecystectomy and only 195 are included for coronary artery bypass graft (CABG). Table 16.2 presents the number of observations and mean values for dependent and independent variables for each procedure. For reasons of confidentiality, CPHA was unable to provide us with a copy of these data for each hospital, even though identifiers had been removed. CPHA was willing, however, to provide the correlation matrices, means and standard deviations of the variables for each data set. While this provides all the information necessary for doing regression analyses, all the variables and transformations had to be specified in advance. Thus, without substantial additional expense it is impossible to test some of the hypotheses or questions that arise after an analysis of the initial set of results. One of the purposes of this article, therefore, is to foster such second-round analyses.

Alternative Formulations of the Volume–Experience Relationships

Table 16.3 presents the regression results for a basic ordinary least squares model with the difference between actual and expected death rates, or "excess death rate," as the dependent variable. The log of 1975 patients volume is the crucial independent variable, controlling for total hospital admissions, operations, house staff, SMSA and geographic location, and expenses per patient day. The lower portion of the table shows the relationship between excess death rates and patient volume alone.

Several aspects of these results should be highlighted. The first is that the volume relationship is usually rather significant statistically and, in some cases, its *t*-ratio exceeds 10. The second is that this relationship between volume and outcomes is essentially the same whether or not other variables are included in the regression. That is, even though many of the other hospital characteristics have a significant impact in their own right, they do not diminish and are not proxies for the volume effect. In those instances when controlling for other variable shifts the coefficient for LPT75, the shift is towards a stronger negative relationship. The third finding is that there is little discernible volume relationship for some procedures, such as vagotomy for any reason, vagotomy and/or pyloroplasty for ulcer, cholecystectomy and incision of the common bile duct, and other biliary-tract surgery. All of these procedures had rather low overall mortality rates (Table 16.2), and this may partially explain the apparent lack of relationship. It should be noted, however, that some other low-mortality procedures do exhibit a clear volume relationship, e.g., total hip replacement.

Although the early work on the learning curve in the aircraft industry found a logarithmic relationship, it may well be the case that some other function provides a better fit in this instance. The simplest alternative is a linear relationship. When the log of patients in 1975 was replaced by a simple count of patients, the fit was substantially worse for the major procedures that had originally shown a clear relationship in the log specification. (For example, the $\bar{R}^2$ for

Table 16.2A: Mean Values of Variables

	Open Heart (1)	CABG (1a)	Vascular Surgery (2)	Resection and Graft for Abdominal Aortic Aneurysm (2a)	Vagotomy (3)
BEDS (total number of beds)	339	458	245	325	255
ADMS (total number admissions)	12,362	16,453	8,931	11,936	9,342
OPS (total number of surgical procedures)	6,823	9,311	4,733	6,601	4,995
RIB (ratio of house staff to bed)	.048	.091	.027	.040	.028
SMSA (1 = location in SMSA)	.846	.944	.667	.790	.679
NC (1 = location in North Central region)	.376	.374	.398	.376	.401
SC (1 = location in South Central region)	.206	.210	.220	.198	.228
W (1 = location in West region)	.196	.262	.188	.193	.189
EXP/DAY (expenses per patient day)	159	178	143	153	144
PT74 (number of patients with this procedure, 1974)	38	80	32	6	8
PT75 (number of patients with this procedure, 1975)	44	97	35	7	7
ZERO74 (1 = no patients with this procedure in 1974)	.259	.128	.054	.150	.099
AD7475 actual death rate, this procedure, 1974–75	.157	.077	.120	.234	.028
ADED74 Actual − expected death rate, 1974	.047	.026	.022	.027	.0019
ADED75 Actual − expected death rate, 1975	.056	.026	.011	.043	.0050
GRP74 Number patients in major procedure group, 1974	—	125	—	51	—
GRP75 Number patients in major procedure group, 1975	—	144	—	58	—
Number of hospitals with one or more procedures in 1975	675	195	1,344	748	1,164

CABG: coronary artery bypass graft.
TUR: transurethral resection.
These are unweighted means and include figures for 9 hospitals excluded at the final stage.

Table 16.2A: Continued

Vagotomy and/or Pyloro-plasty for Ulcer (3a)	Colectomy (4)	Cholecy-stectomy (5)	Cholecy-stectomy and Incision of Common Duct (5a)	Other Biliary Tract Surgery (6)	TUR (7)	Total Hip Replacement (8)
268	238	229	273	247	260	307
9,834	8,664	8,312	10,099	8,984	9,467	11,281
5,289	4,580	4,377	5,473	4,767	5,085	6,198
.028	.026	.025	.029	.027	.029	.037
.694	.653	.633	.710	.668	.714	.772
.420	.412	.407	.412	.405	.403	.372
.214	.223	.231	.194	.218	.197	.196
.187	.178	.182	.188	.184	.188	.210
144	141	140	145	142	146	152
4	25	109	4	7	69	18
4	26	111	4	7	72	20
.182	.025	.001	.160	.067	.024	.126
.013	.077	.010	.028	.090	.012	.032
.00029	.011	.00125	.00087	.0038	.0017	.0079
.00308	.006	.00003	.00225	.0022	.0011	.0136
8	—	—	136	—	—	—
8	—	—	139	—	—	—
1,032	1,407	1,482	981	1,322	1,231	858

Table 16.2B: Weighted Mean Values of Variables

	Open Heart (1)	CABG (1a)	Vascular Surgery (2)	Resection and Graft for Abdom- inal Aortic Aneurysm (2a)	Vago- tomy (3)
BEDS (total number of beds)	530	528	432	467	314
ADMS (total number admissions)	18,991	19,178	15,761	17,099	11,735
OPS (total number of surgical procedures)	10,907	11,092	8,872	9,838	6,412
RIB (ratio of house staff to bed)	.095	.086	.063	.058	.032
SMSA (1 = location in SMSA)	.977	.982	.883	.894	.757
NC (1 = location in North Central region)	.392	.409	.349	.366	.404
SC (1 = location in South Central region)	.229	.216	.263	.249	.273
W (1 = location in West region)	.275	.293	.202	.196	.182
EXP/DAY (expenses per patient day)	180	178	160	156	145
PT74 (number of patients with this procedure, 1974)	254	197	101	16	15
PT75 (number of patients with this procedure, 1975)	286	231	109	18	13
ZERO75 (1 = no patients with this procedure in 1974)	.005	.009	.003	.025	.032
AD7475 actual death rate, this procedure, 1974–75	.078	.046	.105	.184	.021
ADED74 Actual − expected death rate, 1974	.00120	.00349	.00514	−.00149	.00049
ADED75 Actual − expected death rate, 1975	−.00106	−.00046	−.00253	−.00432	−.00024
GRP74 Number of patients in major procedure group, 1974	—	276	—	113	—
GRP75 Number patients in major procedure group, 1975	—	312	—	121	—
Number of hospitals with one or more procedures in 1975	674	195	1,337	747	1,160

CABG: coronary artery bypass graft.
TUR: transurethral resection.
All observations are weighted by:

$$\frac{(\text{Total number of patients in hospital with Procedure i})^2}{\Sigma\, p\,(1-p) \text{ for all patients in hospital with Procedure i}}$$

Table 16.2B: Continued

Vagotomy and/or Pyloroplasty for Ulcer (3a)	Colectomy (4)	Cholecystectomy (5)	Cholecystectomy and Incision of Common Duct (5a)	Other Biliary Tract Surgery (6)	TUR (7)	Total Hip Replacement (8)
314	375	331	323	344	366	410
11,779	13,661	12,422	12,135	12,569	13,601	15,150
6,441	7,711	6,908	6,767	6,997	7,742	8,596
.030	.048	.038	.032	.045	.041	.050
.788	.827	.797	.770	.802	.804	.848
.433	.371	.433	.437	.396	.383	.419
.245	.212	.218	.154	.217	.238	.182
.193	.170	.142	.196	.162	.185	.240
146	153	147	147	150	150	154
9	48	173	7	12	129	45
7	49	177	7	11	133	45
.026	.003	.000	.088	.016	.001	.021
.0064	.067	.009	.021	.081	.010	.014
.00051	.00300	.00038	−.00076	.00038	.00045	.00016
.00015	−.00246	−.00018	.00160	−.00076	.00007	−.00037
15	—	—	170	—	—	—
13	—	—	172	—	—	—
1,029	1,398	1,473	978	1,319	1,227	858

Table 16.3:   1975 Actual-Expected Death Rates, Basic Model and Relationship with Volume Alone

	Open Heart (1)	CABG (1a)	Vascular Surgery (2)	Resection and Graft for Abdominal Aortic Aneurysm (2a)	Vagotomy (3)	Vagotomy and/or Pyloroplasty for Ulcer (3a)
Basic Model						
Intercept	.0705	.0642	.0745	.1035	.0065	−.0028
	(.0204)‡	(.0231)†	(.0103)‡	(.0377)‡	(.0092)	(.0078)
LPT-75	−.0247	−.0187	−.0231	−.0309	−.0018	.0002
	(.0023)‡	(.0028)‡	(.0025)‡	(.0080)‡	(.0020)	(.0017)
ADMS§ .10⁴	.0103	.0060	.0200	.0006	−.0009	.0163
	(.0065)	(.0064)	(.0059)‡	(.0192)	(.0068)	(.0059)‡
OPS§ .10⁴	−.0000	−.0032	−.0122	.0089	−.0016	−.0258
	(.0009)	(.0090)	(.0083)	(.0277)	(.0104)	(.0091)‡
RIB	(.0224)	−.0410	.0690	−.1002	.0719	.0031
	(.0268)	(.0312)	(.0218)†	(.0932)	(.0290)*	(.0285)
SMSA	.0247	.0080	.0080	−.0299	.0075	.0018
	(.0158)	(.0174)	(.0059)	(.0214)	(.0045)	(.0038)
NC	−.0129	.0019	−.0226	−.0527	−.0071	−.0008
	(.0088)	(.0094)	(.0051)‡	(.0180)†	(.0053)	(.0044)
SC	−.0119	.0020	−.0163	−.0446	.0005	−.0015
	(.0095)	(.0101)	(.0056)†	(.0204)*	(.0057)	(.0050)
W	−.0410	−.0206	−.0380	−.0892	−.0023	−.0039
	(.0095)‡	(.0103)*	(.0060)‡	(.0216)‡	(.0062)	(.0054)
EXP/DAY§ .10⁴	1.8143	1.3606	.4909	2.3076	−.3919	−.0025
	(.6824)‡	(.7253)	(.5031)	(2.0720)	(.5159)	(.4388)
DF	664	185	1327	737	1150	1019
R̄²	.222	.270	.128	.066	.014	.010
Relationship with volume alone						
Intercept	.1215	.0945	.0538	.0747	.0023	−.0004
	(.0118)‡	(.0136)‡	(.0072)‡	(.0153)‡	(.0041)	(.0030)
LPT-75	−.0232	−.0185	−.0134	−.0134	−.0012	−.0004
	(.0022)‡	(.0026)‡	(.0017)‡	(.0059)‡	(.0017)	(.0016)
R̄²	.155	.207	.046	.041	.000	.000

*p < 0.05.
‡p < 0.01.
‡p < 0.001.
§The coefficients for these variables are scaled by a factor of 10⁴; e.g., the actual value for ADMS in column 1 is 0.00000103.

open heart fell from 0.222 to 0.173.) The linear specification, however, did improve the fit for vagotomy, cholecystectomy and other biliary tract surgery. The greatest improvement in $\bar{R}^2$, however, was only 0.004, and the other coefficients in the model did not change substantially.* Given the exploratory nature of this research, it is not worth examining other minor variations on the curvilinear model.

---

*Copies of these and other regression results not presented here may be obtained from the author.

Table 16.3:   Continued

Colectomy (4)	Cholecystectomy (5)	Cholecystectomy and Incision of Common Duct (5a)	Other Biliary Tract Surgery (6)	TUR (7)	Total Hip Replacement (8)
.0425	.0050	− .0256	.0069	.0127	.0262
(.0101)‡	(.0028)	(.0152)	(.0155)	(.0031)‡	(.0078)‡
− .0153	− .0013	− .0045	− .0063	− .0025	− .0043
(.0028)†	(.0006)*	(.0034)	(.0046)	(.0006)‡	(.0015)‡
.0067	.0016	.0016	− .0005	− .0011	− .0046
(.0052)	(.0010)	(.0102)	(.0110)	(.0014)	(.0045)
− .0036	− .0019	− .0145	− .0065	.0025	.0058
(.0075)	(.0015)	(.0145)	(.0160)	(.0020)	(.0065)
.0691	.0133	.1246	.0744	.0018	.0047
(.0243)†	(.0041)†	(.0548)*	(.0477)	(.0067)	(.0170)
.0114	− .00019	.0024	.0147	.0022	.0080
(.0043)†	(.00076)	(.0078)	(.0085)	(.0010)*	(.0037)
− .0045	− .00005	.0165	− .0093	− .0016	− .0034
(.0039)	(.00071)	(.0076)*	(.0080)	(.0011)	(.0638)
− .0030	.0001	.0061	− .0030	− .0004	− .0007
(.0045)	(.0008)	(.0100)	(.0093)	(.0012)	(.0044)
− .0135	− .0013	− .0017	− .0214	− .0038	− .0021
(.0049)†	(.0009)	(.0091)	(.0101)*	(.0013)†	(.0043)
− .2710	.0356	1.9106	.2205	− .1442	− .5664
(.4571)	(.0824)	(.9536)*	(.8811)	(.1204)	(.3827)
1388	1463	968	1309	1217	848
.040	.020	.030	.013	.030	.023
.0238	.0033	.0104	.0068	.0088	.0163
(.0066)‡	(.0019)	(.0050)*	(.0080)	(.0023)‡	(.0045)‡
− .0073	− .0007	− .0059	− .0036	− .0019	− .0049
(.0018)‡	(.0004)	(.0028)*	(.0035)	(.0005)‡	(.0013)‡
.012	.002	.005	.001	.011	.017
.019	.017	.028	.011	.018	.014

Is It Volume or Experience that Matters?

More important than the precise shape of the curve is the question of whether the relationship depends on current volume or accumulated experience. If it is the latter, then policies to regionalize surgery would not achieve lower mortality rates until sufficient cumulative experience had developed. Unfortunately, surgical volumes are highly correlated from year to year.* Thus, a set of regressions including both the log of 1974 and the log of 1975 experience yielded approximately the same results as the basic model. In only one instance, open heart surgery, were both the coefficients for volume, LPT75 and LPT74, statistically

---

*This is particularly true in these regressions in which the observations are weighted, in part, by the number of procedures.

surgery, were both the coefficients for volume, LPT75 and LPT74, statistically significant. Whereas the coefficients for LPT75 were uniformly negative, in eight of twelve cases the coefficients for LPT74 were positive. This would suggest that, with volumes held constant in the current year, higher volumes in the preceding year (more experience) are associated with excess deaths. Such an explanation is implausible and these results probably reflect the collinearity of the two variables. In fact, in almost all cases, the simple algebraic sum of the coefficients for LPT75 and LPT74 equals the coefficients for LPT75 in the basic model.

These results do not necessarily mean that the crucial factor is volume rather than experience. Before such a conclusion can be reached, other regressions, not so susceptible to multicollinearity, must be examined. The equation might be respecified so that the *increase* in volume (either absolute or proportionate) were included instead of LPT74. Alternative formulations should also be considered before ruling out the role of experience. On the other hand, volumes of several hundred procedures in a year can provide a great deal of experience within a rather short period of time, so the practical difference between volume and experience may be small.

Volume of the Specific Procedures versus Related Procedures

Associated with the question of volume versus experience is whether outcomes are dependent on the volume of the specific procedure or of a broader set of related procedures. As indicated in Table 16.4, the volume of related procedures may be an important factor to examine, but statistical problems prevent a clear resolution of the question. When the total number of open heart procedures is included in the equation for CABG, its coefficient is positive and not quite significant ($p < 0.08$) and the coefficient for LPT75 doubles in absolute value. (Unfortunately, the correlation between these two variables—.963—is so high that it precludes accurately estimating their separate effects.[*] Problems of collinearity are not nearly as great for the other three procedures.) Resection and graft for abdominal aortic aneurysm exhibits quite the opposite pattern. Although the coefficient for the number of specific procedures remains negative, it is no longer significant, while the coefficient for the total number of vascular procedures is large, negative and highly significant. It may be the case that outcomes for this type of operation may depend more on some of the generalizable skills, such as the operating room team, life support and postoperative care, than the skills related to the specific surgery. Given the lack of significance for the other two procedures, it is probably best to ignore their particular results and instead

---

[*]The very high correlations can be explained by the weighting scheme and the fact that the sample is limited to those hospitals performing the "subset" procedure. For instance, 479 hospitals performing some open heart procedures but no CABGs are excluded.

suggest a more thorough examination of the importance of related procedures for other sets of operations.

The Role of Other Variables

Although initially included to "hold other things constant" so that a volume effect could be discerned, some of the hospital-specific variables are of substantial interest in themselves. Among these "background" factors are 1) measures of the pure size of the hospital, such as beds, operations of all types and admissions; 2) teaching status; 3) expense per day; and 4) geographic location.

Table 16.4: 1975 Actual Minus Expected Death Rates in Basic Model with Volume of Related Procedures

	CABG (1a)	Resection and Graft for Abdominal Aortic Aneurysm (2a)	Vagotomy (3a)	Cholecystectomy and Incision of Common Duct (5a)
Intercept	.0447	.2061	−.0002	−.0079
	(.0255)	(.0467)‡	(.0080)	(.0363)
GRP75	.0226	−.0539	−.0042	−.0044
	(.0128)	(.0147)‡	(.0022)	(.0083)
LPT75	−.0378	−.0042	.0034	−.0038
	(.0118)‡	(.0108)	(.0024)	(.0036)
ADMS 10^4	.0041	.0226	.0179	.0037
	(.0065)	(.0199)	(.0059)†	(.0109)
OPS 10^4	−.0017	−.0005	−.0269	−.0137
	(.0090)	(.0276)	(.0091)†	(.0146)
RIB	−.0573	−.0679	.0029	.1215
	(.0324)	(.0929)	(.0284)	(.0551)*
SMSA	.0096	−.0203	.0017	.0033
	(.0173)	(.0214)	(.0038)	(.0080)
NC	.0017	−.0435	−.0011	.0166
	(.0094)	(.0180)*	(.0045)	(.0076)*
SC	.0009	−.0264	−.0011	.0060
	(.0101)	(.0208)	(.0050)	(.0100)
W	−.0203	−.0759	−.0038	−.0022
	(.0103)*	(.0217)†	(.0053)	(.0092)
EXP/DAY 10^4	1.1128	3.6881	.0189	1.8942
	(0.7348)	(2.0891)	(.4384)	(.9545)*
DF	184	736	1018	967
$\bar{R}^2$	.282	.083	.013	.030
Simple correlation between GRP 75 and LPT75	.963	.829	.734	.592

CABG: coronary artery bypass graft.
*p < 0.05.
†p < 0.01.
‡p < 0.001.

Size of Hospitals

As indicated in Table 16.3, two overall measures of hospital size—total admissions and total operations per year—show little consistent relationship to the excess mortality rate, controlling for volume of the specific procedure in question. Admissions has a significant positive coefficient for vascular surgery and for vagotomy and/or pyloroplasty for ulcer. In the latter instance, there is also a significant negative coefficient for operations. Given the poor overall fit of this equation and the high correlation between ADMS and OPS, this may well be an artifact.

To provide a clearer test of the size factors, three additional sets of regressions were estimated, one using ADMS, one using OPS, and one using BEDS as the only measure of size. None of the three variables alone was significant in the vagotomy and/or pyloroplasty regressions, supporting the conjecture of the multicollinearity problem. Of the 36 regressions, the only statistically significant coefficients for the size variables occurred for open heart procedures and vascular surgery. For these two procedure groups, each of the size coefficients was statistically significant and positive, indicating that larger institutions have worse-than-expected outcomes, controlling for other factors. For open heart surgery, the coefficients for all the variables in the ADMS-only equation are essentially identical to those in Table 16.3. In fact, even the coefficients for ADMS are identical, but the standard error is larger in Table 16.3, making the estimated t-ratio too small to be significant. Similarly, the choice of size measure in the other equations does not have any substantial impact on the other coefficients. Overall, the size measures generally have a positive effect on excess deaths (8 of 12 instances for ADMS, 6 of 12 for OPS and 10 of 12 for BEDS), but given their lack of significance and the difficulty in identifying a reason for such results, it is more accurate to say the larger hospitals *do not have better* results, rather than to say that larger hospitals have worse results, controlling for the volume of the procedure in question.

Teaching Status

The influence of teaching programs on outcomes is difficult to analyze because it is impossible to be sure that severity of case mix is held constant. Thus, if the presence of house staff is associated with worse outcomes, then it may be claimed that teaching hospitals receive the riskier patients. This may be the case in these results but, as will be discussed below, other data provide only partial support for the case-mix explanation. Ten of the twelve procedures have positive coefficients for the ratio of interns and residents per bed, RIB (Table 16.3) and half of these are statistically significant.

It is sometimes difficult to place such results in perspective. Some of the equations explain only a very small fraction of the variance, in spite of having several statistically significant coefficients. This suggests that some variables may have been omitted or that most of the interhospital variation in excess mortality is attributable to random variation. However, when a variable has a consistent effect for a large fraction of the procedures, it warrants further examination. For instance, even ignoring the fact that five of the RIB coefficients were significant at conventional levels, if there were truly no effect, the probability of finding 10 of 12 coefficients of the same sign is less than 5 percent.

One way of testing the case-mix hypothesis is to examine regressions explaining the expected death rate in each hospital. Although this variable is implicitly included on the left-hand side of the basic model, it seems reasonable to expect that if some hospitals have a riskier mix of patients at some subtle, unmeasured level, they would also have a riskier mix based on age-sex-multiple diagnosis. Table 16.5 presents these regressions for the 1974–75 expected death rates.* Half the coefficients for RIB are negative and of the five statistically significant coefficients, three are negative. The patterns among the procedures, moreover, are not immediately obvious. For instance, a larger house-staff ratio is positively associated with a riskier mix of open heart and vagotomy patients and a less risky mix of vascular surgery, cholecystectomy, and total hip replacement patients. Since our perceptions are generally derived from simple observations rather than complex multiple regressions, it should be noted that the zero-order correlations between RIB and expected deaths follow essentially the same pattern as the regression coefficients. The only notable exception is a relatively large negative coefficient ($-.167$) for CABG. Thus, there is only limited support for the argument that teaching hospitals have riskier patients.

Expenses per Patient Day

Many of the same arguments that are used to explain positive relations between teaching and mortality are used to explain relations between expenses per patient day and outcomes. In this instance, too, the data in Tables 16.3 and 16.5 lend scant support to the argument that the more expensive hospitals have a riskier mix of patients which then explains their worse-than-expected outcomes. The expense data, however, are subject to a number of criticisms, and should not be overinterpreted. In particular, expenses per day are sensitive to practice patterns that influence length-of-stay and these, in turn, exhibit important geographic patterns.

Geographic Patterns

The substantial role of geographic factors was rather unexpected. Hospitals in the West have lower-than-expected death rates for all 12 procedures and this rela-

---

*The correlation matrices we requested did not include the 1975 expected death rate. They do include 1974–75 actual minus expected death rates, and these produced regressions very similar to the 1975 ones in Table 16.3. Thus, it is likely that the figures in Table 16.5 are close to what would be found using 1975 data alone.

Table 16.5:   1974–75 Expected Deaths

	Open Heart (1)	CABG (1a)	Vascular Surgery (2)	Resection and Graft for Abdominal Aortic Aneurysm (2a)	Vagotomy (3)	Vagotomy and/or Pyloroplasty for Ulcer (3a)
Intercept	.1148	.0640	.0984	.1850	.0116	.0072
	(.0051)‡	(.0066)‡	(.0028)‡	(.0056)‡	(.0017)‡	(.0008)‡
LPT-74-75	−.0040	−.0007	.0057	.0056	.0033	.00033
	(.0006)‡	(.0008)	(.0006)‡	(.0012)‡	(.0003)‡	(.00018)
ADMS 10^4	.0021	.0005	−.0035	−.0038	.0019	.0002
	(.0016)	(.0018)	(.0015)	(.0028)	(.0012)	(.0006)
OPS 10^4	.0028	−.0004	.0007	−.0004	−.0008	.0015
	(.0022)	(.0025)	(.0021)	(.0040)	(.0018)	(.0009)
RIB	.0217	.0012	−.0273	−.0208	.0103	.0020
	(.0065)†	(.0086)	(.0054)‡	(.0134)	(.0051)*	(.0027)
SMSA‡	−.0138	−.0118	−.0065	−.0079	−.0032	−.0014
	(.0038)†	(.0048)*	(.0015)‡	(.0031)*	(.0008)‡	(.0004)‡
NC‡	−.0023	9,0002	−.0047	−.0039	−.0015	−.0009
	(.0021)	(.0026)	(.0013)‡	(.0026)	(.0009)	(.0004)*
SC	.0019	.0020	−.0095	−.0061	−.0045	−.0022
	(.0023)	(.0028)	(.0014)‡	(.0029)*	(.0010)‡	(.0005)‡
W	.0115	.0111	−.0015	−.0001	.0007	−.0002
	(.0023)‡	(.0028)‡	(.0015)	(.0031)	(.0011)	(.0005)
EXP/DAY 10^4	−.2678	−.4360	−.3473	.1394	.1224	−.0648
	(.1662)	(.2010)*	(.1246)†	(.2994)	(.0910)	(.0418)
DF	664	185	1327	737	1150	1019
$\bar{R}^2$	.185	.220	.122	.052	.166	.061

CABG: coronary artery bypass graft.
TUR: transurethral resection.
*$p < 0.05$.
†$p < 0.01$.
‡$p < 0.001$.

tionship is significant in seven instances. For open heart procedures, with a weighted mean death rate of .078, Western hospitals have adjusted death rates of .056 in comparison to .097 in Northeastern hospitals (the dummy variable left out of the regression).* For resection and graft for abdominal aortic aneurysm, the West's effect is −.089 relative to an average death rate of .184. This implies an average death rate, adjusting for volume and other factors, of .143 in the West, in contrast to .232 in the Northeast. These differences are not only highly significant, but potentially important. Is it possible that medical practice varies so

*The calculation is as follows, using the coefficients from Table 16.3 and weighted means from Table 16.2B. The overall death rate is the weighted average of the rates in each region, but the regression coefficients are deviations from the Northeast value, X, rather than the mean. Therefore,

$$.392 \cdot (X - .0129) + .229 \cdot (X - .0119) + .25 \cdot (X - .0410) + .104 \cdot X = .078$$
$$(.392 + .229 + .275 + .104) \cdot X - (.392 \cdot .0129 + .229 \cdot .0119 + .275 \cdot .0410) = .078$$
$$X = .078 + .0191$$
$$X = .097 = \text{adjusted death rate in Northeast}$$
$$.097 - .041 = .056 = \text{adjusted death rate in West}$$

Table 16.5:   Continued

Colectomy (4)	Cholecystectomy (5)	Cholecystectomy and Incision of Common Duct (5a)	Other Biliary Tract Surgery (6)	TUR (7)	Total Hip Replacement (8)
.0571	.0073	.0096	.0743	.0105	.0104
(.0023)‡	(.0007)‡	(.0018)†	(.0037)‡	(.0005)‡	(.0012)‡
.0044	.0007	.0057	.0055	−.0000	.0010
(.0006)‡	(.0001)‡	(.0004)‡	(.0011)‡	(.0001)	(.0002)‡
−.0020	.0000	−.0010	.0050	.0002	−.0006
(.0010)*	(.0002)	(.0011)	(.0023)*	(.0002)	(.0007)
−.0015	.0002	−.0001	−.0038	−.0006	.0005
(.0015)	(.0003)	(.0016)	(.0033)	(.0003)	(.0010)
.0021	−.0019	.0099	−.0149	−.0006	−.0068
(.0048)	(.0009)*	(.0061)	(.0099)	(.0010)	(.0025)†
−.0001	−.0009	.0006	−.0038	−.00005	−.0008
(.0009)	(.0002)‡	(.0009)	(.0018)‡	(.00016)	(.0006)
−.0013	−.0009	.0013	−.0084	−.00003	−.0008
(.0008)	(.0002)‡	(.0008)	(.0017)	(.00017)	(.0006)
−.0052	−.0007	.0021	−.0141	−.0007	−.0010
(.0009)‡	(.0002)‡	(.0011)	(.0019)‡	(.0002)‡	(.0007)
−.0019	.0004	−.0012	−.0059	−.0003	.0001
(.0010)*	(.0002)	(.0010)	(.0021)†	(.0002)	(.0006)
−.2216	−.0586	−.0607	−.1836	−.0085	.0504
(.0907)*	(.0188)†	(.0183)	(.1827)	(.0182)	(.0559)
1388	1463	968	1309	1217	848
.079	.087	.239	.088	.032	.066

much across such large geographic areas? If so, then better dissemination of skill and technology could have a major impact on health status. Medical explanations for nearly twofold differences in adjusted death rates across regions seem unlikely, but worthy of further examination. One nonmedical explanation is suggested by another type of geographic variation—patterns in length-of-stay. Table 16.6 presents the average length-of-stay in PAS hospitals for the broad procedures examined here. Hospitals in the West consistently have the shortest stays, ranging from 12 to 29 per cent below the average, while hospitals in the Northeast have the longest stays, 9 to 23 per cent above the average. There also seems to be a relationship between the extent to which the length-of-stay is lower in the West and the negative effect of the West on mortality.[*]

While it is becoming fashionable to point out the adverse effects of longer

---

[*]There is a simple correlation of .55 between (a) the percentage differences in length-of-stay between the Northeast and West (from Table 16.6) and (b) the ratio of the coefficient for the West (Table 16.3) to the average rate (Table 16.2). For example, the value of (a) for open heart is $(15.2 - 21.7)/21.7 = -.299$, while that of (b) is $-.0410/.157 = -.261$.

Table 16.6: Length of Stay for Selected Procedures, All PAS Hospitals, 1975

Group	ICDA		U.S.	Northeast	North Central	South	West
1	463	Open heart	17.6	21.7 (21.9)	19.1 (19.2)	16.6 (16.7)	15.2 (14.9)
2	468	Blood vessels	15.4	17.8 (17.7)	16.3 (16.4)	14.9 (15.0)	12.6 (12.5)
3	479	Vagotomy	16.3	19.1	17.4	15.6	13.1
4	483	Colectomy	20.8	22.9	21.6	20.3	16.6
5	497	Cholecystectomy	11.7	12.7	11.9	11.9	9.6
6	498	Biliary tract excluding cholecystectomy	19.6	22.5	19.9	18.8	16.1
7	522	Transurethral resection	11.7	13.7	12.5	11.3	8.3
8	586	Total hip replacement	21.2	24.0	22.2	21.4	17.7

Numbers in parentheses show the regional length of stay adjusted to the age- and multiple-diagnosis-mix of the whole United States. In general, adjustment makes very little difference.
Source: reference 10.

hospitalization, a simpler explanation for this relationship may be found in the construction of the data. PAS mortality data are, by definition, limited to deaths within the hospital because there is no easy way to obtain information on postdischarge mortality. If the patterns of care are such that with the same health status, hospitals in the West discharge patients sooner than those in the East, then if complications subsequently manifest themselves, a larger fraction of the patients in the East will still be in the hospital to be included in the mortality data. The patients in the West who were initially discharged might then be readmitted and eventually have the same mortality rate as those in the East, but the second admission will not have a surgical procedure listed. Data from the National Health Interview Survey tend to support the hypothesis of shorter stays followed by more readmissions in the West. In 1972 people in the West who were admitted once to a hospital had a 16.5 percent chance of being readmitted within the year in contrast to only 14.8 percent in the Northeast.[11]

The Referral and Volume Effects: A Preliminary Simultaneous Equation Model

While the volume or experience effect may cause the observed relationship between outcomes and the number of procedures in each hospital, there may also be a causal link in the opposite direction: hospitals having better outcomes may attract more patients. That this second influence, the referral effect, may exist is suggested by several facts. Various professional societies have suggested regionalization of certain procedures and it is reasonable to expect that such efforts would attempt to concentrate the operations in the best hospitals in the area.[12,13] The data from this study indicate substantial concentration of operations. For instance, of the 1,498 hospitals in the study, 1,482 performed at least one cholecystectomy while only 195 performed coronary artery bypass grafts. (This differs from the 1,473 hospitals mentioned earlier because nine hospitals were excluded at the last stage of the data preparation.) More importantly, the 14 percent of the 1,482 hospitals having more than 200 annual procedures accounted for 35 percent of all the cholecystectomies, while the 8 percent of the 195 hospitals having more than 200 annual procedures accounted for 56 percent of the CABG operations.

To try to estimate the relative importance of the referral and volume effects, a simple simultaneous equation model can be specified. The volume equation (1) relates the log of patients with the procedure (LPT75) to the predicted outcomes in the hospital (ADED75) to test the hypothesis that hospitals with better outcomes attract more patients. In addition, the total number of operations (OPS) is included to give an indication of the importance of surgery in the hospital; teaching status (RIB) as an "obvious" indicator of quality that might attract referrals; SMSA location; and expenses per patient day (EXPDAY), again as an external indicator of quality. The outcome equation (2) relates the excess death rate (ADED75) to the predicted number of patients (logged) with that procedure (LPT̂75), holding constant teaching status and expenses per day as two influences on outcomes and the region dummies (NC, SC, W) to capture the geographic patterns of mortality. (While referrals may take place between nonmetropolitan and metropolitan areas, they are unlikely to be substantial between regions.[14])

$$LPT75 = a + b_1 \widehat{ADED}75 + b_2 OPS +$$
$$b_3 RIB + b_4 SMSA + b_5 EXPDAY \qquad (1)$$

$$ADED75 = a + b_1 \widehat{LPT}75 + b_2 RIB +$$
$$b_3 NC + b_4 SC + b_5 W + b_6 EXPDAY \qquad (2)$$

Table 16.7 presents the results for this simultaneous equation model using two-stage least squares techniques. From the outcome equation, it appears that much of the apparent relationship between volume and outcome seen in Table 16.3 has disappeared. The volume coefficients for open heart, CABG, transurethral resection (TUR), and total hip replacement are all insignificant, whereas they had been highly significant before. The coefficients for vascular surgery and resection and graft for abdominal aortic aneurysm are both substantially smaller, although still rather significant. (Not surprisingly, these six procedures all show highly significant effects of expected outcomes on volume in the referral equation.) With one exception, however, predicted volumes have a negative (beneficial) effect on the outcome variable and significantly so for vascular surgery, resection and graft for abdominal aortic aneurysm, colectomy, cholecystectomy and cholecystectomy with incision of the common duct.

What seems to be lost by the volume effect on outcomes is gained by the referral effect on volumes. As previously mentioned, it is rather striking and significant for six of the procedures. Moreover, these are precisely the procedures for which one would expect to observe interhospital referral patterns. Referrals for surgery are commonplace, but to produce the relationships observed here, referrals must result in a concentration of patients in a relatively small number of hospitals and hence a pattern quite different from that usually found in which internists refer to surgeons within the same hospital.

A simple measure of the extent to which operations are concentrated in a small proportion of hospitals is the Gini coefficient. The Gini coefficient is a measure of the extent to which one variable, surgical procedures in this case, is equally distributed with respect to another, such as hospitals. It is computed from a Lorenz curve, (Fig. 16.1) which shows the cumulative proportion of operations on the vertical axis and the cumulative proportion of hospitals on the horizontal axis, where hospitals are ranked by the number of procedures. The Gini coefficient is the proportion of the area under the diagonal that lies below the curve. Perfectly equal distribution is signified by a coefficient of 1, while total concentration is represented by 0.

As seen in Table 16.8, with the exception of TUR, the six procedures with significant referral effects in two-stage regressions also have substantially lower

Gini coefficients, an indication of greater concentration of operations in a few hospitals. The six procedures exhibiting evidence of referral patterns are more complex and require more specialized skills than others.* Thus, it may be the case that if an internist (or general surgeon) must find a thoracic surgeon, urologist or orthopedist anyway, then the usual intrahospital referral patterns may be broken. Furthermore, while the differences across hospitals in death rates may not be large enough for the practitioner to easily notice, increased mortality may be associated with increased nonfatal complications and less satisfactory outcomes in general.

Whereas the simultaneous equation model results in major shifts in the apparent volume effect, there are few important changes in the estimated effects of teaching status, expenses per day or geographic patterns on outcomes. In the volume equation, teaching has the expected positive sign in 8 of 12 equations and is significant in only two. Surprisingly, one of the equations with a negative coefficient is CABG. Location in an SMSA has the expected positive sign in every case and is highly significant in half of these.

SUMMARY AND CONCLUSIONS

This article is an exploratory exercise probing what lies behind the significant correlation between the volume of surgery and subsequent mortality rates. While it is an interesting academic exercise to undertake such explanations, in this case—where the correlation has substantial relevance for medical care policy—such probing takes on greater importance. For instance, should one regionalize operations into large medical centers or can smaller hospitals with high volumes of specific procedures do as well? Must one wait years to accumulate enough experience or does the learning take place quickly? Perhaps even more crucially, is the causal path from high volume to better outcomes, or do hospitals and surgeons with better outcomes attract more patients, so that we must be able to *identify* those more likely to succeed and channel more patients toward them? While this article can suggest initial answers to a few questions, clear answers to others remain to be found.

These preliminary findings suggest that the relationship between volume and mortality is curvilinear and can be represented by a logarithmic function. Although other curvilinear forms might provide a better fit, the improvement is likely to be small. In addition, for the procedures studied, there is little evidence that experience over several years is more important than the experience gained in a short period with a large number of operations. This point, however, should be

---

*Comprehensive data are not available, but a study of four medical market areas indicates that, omitting interns and residents, 97 percent of cholecystectomies were performed by general practitioners or general surgeons. In contrast, 93 percent of TURs were performed by urologists and 91 percent of total hip replacements were performed by orthopedists.[15]

Table 16.7:   Simultaneous Equation Model

	Open Heart (1)	CABG (1a)	Vascular Surgery (2)	Resection and Graft for Abdominal Aortic Aneurysm (2a)	Vagotomy (3)	Vagotomy and/or Pyloroplasty for Ulcer (3a)
LPT-75 (Equation 1)						
Intercept	3.2704	4.1191	2.4464	1.3107	1.4564	1.3936
	(.3268)‡	(.5050)‡	(.1113)‡	(.2066)‡	(.1080)‡	(.3381)‡
AD-ÊD-75	−14.3071	−16.2029	−9.9707	−4.7216	−6.2578	−45.7203
	(2.4707)*	(5.6597)†	(1.6525)‡	(1.2414)‡	(8.0714)	(59.1454)
OP-CT 10^4	.5282	.2336	1.0314	.8657	.9894	.6432
	(.0772)‡	(.1068)*	(.0476)‡	(.0712)‡	(.0831)‡	(.2391)†
RIB	1.0306	−.4893	1.7254	.5188	.1749	.2061
	(.4899)*	(.6915)	(.3329)‡	(.5352)	(.7674)	(2.1064)
SMSA	.7886	.4940	.5022	.0928	.0861	.1812
	(.2799)†	(.4280)	(.0798)‡	(.1385)	(.0937)	(.2539)
EXP/DAY	.0031	.0016	.0016	.0004	.00003	−.0021
	(.0010)†	(.0015)	(.0006)*	(.0011)	(.00082)	(.0026)
AD-ED-75 (Equation 2)						
Intercept	.0136	.0167	.0518	.0845	.0073	.0050
	(.0356)	(.0658)	(.0118)‡	(.0397)*	(.0111)	(.0100)
LPT̂-75	.0023	−.0025	−.0088	−.0270	−.0018	−.0018
	(.0083)	(.0158)	(.0025)	(.0140)†	(.0040)	(.0046)
RIB	.0193	−.0322	.0709	−.1018	.0672	.0164
	(.0293)	(.0323)	(.0222)†	(.0949)	(.0284)*	(.0265)
NC	−.0365	−.0127	−.0250	−.0521	−.0075	−.0003
	(.0121)†	(.0180)	(.0052)‡	(.0182)†	(.0054)	(.0046)
SC	−.0327	−.0107	−.0206	−.0463	−.0002	−.0007
	(.0128)*	(.0182)*	(.0058)‡	(.0209)*	(.0058)	(.0052)
W	−.0671	−.0355	−.0443	−.0899	−.0025	−.0034
	(.0130)‡	(.0191)	(.0061)‡	(.0220)‡	(.0063)	(.0055)
EXP/DAY 10^4	.6574	.9235	.0745	1.8309	−.1536	.0893
	(.7407)	(.7566)	(.4938)	(2.0395)	(.4932)	(.4256)

CABG: coronary artery bypass graft.
TUR: transurethral resection.
*p < 0.05.
†p < 0.010.
‡p < 0.001.

confirmed using functional forms that are less subject to multicollinearity. Whether the crucial factor is the volume of the specific procedure or more generalized experience with related procedures is still unclear. For CABG, specific experience seems to be of primary importance, while for resection and graft for abdominal aortic aneurysm, the volume of vascular surgery is the dominant variable. These differing results may reflect different medical situations, but further confirmation is necessary.

An exploratory study cannot be compared to a series of existing studies, so one must be particularly sensitive to the possibility that the chosen variables are serving as proxies for the true causal factors. One obvious concern is that the

Table 16.7: Continued

Colectomy (4)	Cholecystectomy (5)	Cholecystectomy and Incision of Common Duct (5a)	Other Biliary Tract Surgery (6)	TUR (7)	Total Hip Replacement (8)
2.3221	4.1906	.9275	1.1466	4.0756	3.8642
(.0729)‡	(.0755)‡	(.1328)‡	(.0784)‡	(.1028)‡	(.8608)‡
.2424	47.0580	−.7114	1.9198	−38.6891	−113.8430
(3.8001)	(43.3898)	(3.4926)	(2.9462)	(16.2209)*	(57.2209)*
1.0121	1.0930	.9800	.9323	.9039	.3882
(.0493)‡	(.0607)‡	(.0807)‡	(.0576)‡	(.0506)‡	(.3751)
.3994	−1.1578	−.8187	.2223	−.2540	.1146
(.4136)	(.7568)	(.6909)	(.4189)	(.3816)	(1.8271)
.3767	.3312	.3466	.2236	.0722	.0968
(.0490)‡	(.0536)‡	(.0744)‡	(.0677)‡	(.0696)	(.4243)
.0012	−.0013	−.0024	.00080	−.0012	−.0058
(.0005)*	(.0005)*	(.0010)*	(.00054)	(.0007)	(.0045)
.0251	.0046	−.0139	.0117	.0063	.0257
(.0111)*	(.0026)	(.0166)	(.0182)	(.0043)	(.0107)*
−.0066	−.0011	−.0140	−.0075	−.0007	−.0046
(.0026)*	(.0005)*	(.0053)†	(.0065)	(.0008)	(.0026)
.0667	.0146	.1146	.0669	.0007	.0016
(.0241)†	(.0040)‡	(.0517)*	(.0476)	(.0066)	(.0171)
−.0032	.0000	.0150	−.0103	−.0019	−.0035
(.0039)	(.0007)	(.0075)*	(.0080)	(.0011)	(.0041)
−.0014	.0003	.0020	−.0049	−.0010	−.0014
(.0044)	(.0008)	(.0097)	(.0092)	(.0013)	(.0044)
−.0126	−.0013	−.0036	−.0224	−.0043	−.0020
(.0049)*	(.0009)	(.0091)	(.0102)*	(.0013)†	(.0045)
−.2049	.0257	1.7954	.6036	−.0720	−.5205
(.4466)	(.0795)	(.9022)*	(.8576)	(.1173)	(.3767)

volume of procedures really represents the size of the hospital. However, various combinations of size measures (beds, admissions and operations) are generally insignificant and in the two procedures where they have a significant effect, open heart and vascular surgery, larger hospitals have worse outcomes, controlling for their procedure-specific volumes. A second potentially confounding variable is the role of teaching programs. Perhaps surprisingly, the larger the ratio of house staff per bed, the worse the outcomes. It may be the case that teaching hospitals have patients whose higher risk is not captured completely by the expected death rates included here. If true, we might expect teaching hospitals also to have a riskier mix of patients based on the age-, sex-, multiple-diagnosis measure, but the evidence on this question is mixed.

The attempt to control for other factors also led to the unanticipated finding of very substantial geographic differences in mortality rates. If these differences can be confirmed in future studies, then a careful investigation of the clinical

Figure 16.1:   The Lorenz Curve

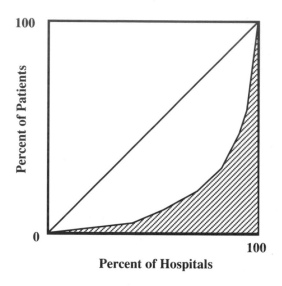

causes of such differences should be undertaken. Before such a major study is begun, however, we must first reject simpler explanations relating to differences in length of stay and its impact on data collection and interpretation.

Still unresolved is the major question of whether the observed relationship represents the effects of volume or experience on outcomes, or the attraction of more patients to centers having better-than-expected results. A simultaneous-equation model suggests that the second, or referral model, may be of crucial importance for some procedures. The results of any simultaneous equation estimation, however, depend upon the correct specification of the model, and in this particular case, there is little theory or experience to guide such specification. Furthermore, correlation matrices designed for simpler investigations do not include all the variables one would like to confidently estimate such a simultaneous model. While the two-stage regressions presented here may require modification, strong evidence of important referral patterns is provided by the high concentration of certain procedures in a small number of high-volume hospitals. If similar results are obtained with other data sets and alternative measures, then we can be more certain of the relative importance of the referral effect. Likewise, patient referral patterns in a geographic area should be examined to test the hypothesis.

Other important issues have not even been addressed in this research. Do the observed effects reflect the volume treated by a specific surgeon, anesthesiologist, operating room team, or the hospital staff in general? Are the very low-volume, poor-outcome hospitals in isolated rural areas or in the shadow of major medical centers? Are they for-profit or not-for-profit? Do they have certain life

Table 16.8: Gini Coefficients Measuring the Concentration of Procedures among All Hospitals in the Sample

1	Open heart	.0902
1a	CABG	.0611
2	Vascular surgery	.3630
2a	Resection and graft	.2594
3	Vagotomy	.4190
3a	Vagotomy and/or pyloroplasty for ulcer	.4174
4	Colectomy	.5128
5	Cholecystectomy	.6018
5a	Cholecystectomy and incision of common duct	.3972
6	Other biliary tract	.5168
7	TUR	.4535
8	Total hip replacement	.2720

support equipment? What happens over time in low-volume hospitals—do they attract more patients after several years and improve, or do they give up performing those procedures? To design informed policies concerning the appropriate sites for surgery, the answers to these and other questions must be had, but that will require further research.

ACKNOWLEDGMENT

We are grateful for the assistance of Wayne Ewy, Byron Wm. Brown and William Forrest in the early design of this study; to Walter Wood for his management of data processing studies at CPHA; and to Luke Froeb for his able research assistance. John Bunker, Alain Enthoven, Paul Newacheck and Nicole Urban provided valuable comments on earlier drafts.

REFERENCES

1. Codman EA. A study in hospital efficiency as demonstrated by the case report of the first five years of a private hospital. Boston: Thomas Todd, 1918.
2. Bunker JP, Forrest WH Jr, Mosteller F, Vandam LD, eds. The national halothane study. Bethesda: National Institute of General Medical Sciences, 1969.
3. The Staff of the Stanford Center for Health Care Research. Study of institutional differences in postoperative mortality, PB 250 940/LK. Springfield, Va.: National Technical Information Service, 1974.
4. Forrest WH Jr., Staff of the Stanford Center for Health Care Research. Comparison of hospitals with regard to outcomes of surgery. Health Serv Res 1976;11:112.
5. Wright TP. Factors affecting the cost of airplanes. Journal of the Aeronautical Sciences 1936;3:122.

6. Asher H. Cost-quantity relationships in the airframe industry. Santa Monica: Rand Corporation, 1956.
7. Boston Consulting Group. Perspectives on experience. Boston: Boston Consulting Group, 1972.
8. Luft HS, Bunker JP, Enthoven AC. Should operations be regionalized? An empirical study of the relation between surgical volume and mortality. N Engl J Med 1979;301:1364.
9. Commission on Professional and Hospital Activities. Hospital mortality: PAS hospitals United States, 1972–73. Ann Arbor: Commission on Professional and Hospital Activities, 1975.
10. Commission on Professional and Hospital Activities. Length of stay in PAS hospitals, by operation, United States, 1975. Ann Arbor: Commission on Professional and Hospital Activities, 1976.
11. U.S. National Center for Health Statistics. Persons hospitalized by number of episodes and days hospitalized in a year: United States—1972. Washington, D.C.: U.S. Government Printing office, 1977. (Vital and health statistics. Series 10, number 116.) [DHEW publication no. (HRA) 77–1544.]
12. Cardiovascular Committee of the American College of Surgeons. Guidelines for minimal standards in cardiovascular surgery. Ann Thorac Surg 1973;15:243.
13. Scannel JG, Brown GE, Buckley MJ. Report on the Inter-Society Commission for Heart Disease Resources: optimal resources for cardiac surgery: guideline for program planning and evaluation. Circulation 1975;52:A1.
14. Fuchs VR. The supply of surgeons and the demand for operations. J Hum Resour 1978;13(Supplement):35–56.
15. American College of Surgeons and the American Surgical Association. Surgery in the United States, 1976.

Chapter 17

Surgeon Volume

It is widely recognized that the volume of patients operated on by an individual surgeon may be an important factor in explaining the volume-outcome relationship at the hospital level. Yet results of physician volume studies remain largely inconclusive because of limitations in the availability of data on physician volumes. Researchers have been limited by ecologic measures of physician volume,[1] nonrepresentative data sets,[2] or small population size.[3]

The work by Hughes, Hunt, and Luft in this chapter demonstrates how interesting results can be obtained despite limited data. Two pieces of information were available to the authors from the data collected by the Commission on Professional Hospital Activities: (1) the number of surgeons in each hospital performing each procedure, and (2) the proportion of patients operated on by the surgeons doing the first, second, and third highest proportions. (CPHA was unwilling to provide physician- or patient-specific data.) Using this information, the authors determined surgeon volume as follows. When the number of surgeons performing a given procedure in a hospital was four or fewer, the exact volume per surgeon was determined from the CPHA data. They found that 74 percent to 98 percent of all patients were operated on in such hospitals. When the number of surgeons was five or more, an average volume was calculated for the fourth through last surgeon. Then the proportion of patients treated by surgeons doing less than the median volume per year was calculated for each hospital. The median number of procedures per surgeon ranged from 2 to 12. The authors then found that the higher the proportion of patients treated by low-volume surgeons, the poorer the outcomes at that hospital.

Shortell and LoGerfo (1981) also used CPHA data and were limited to an even more crude measure of surgeon volume than Hughes and his colleagues. For each hospital, they computed the average volume of acute myocardial infarction patients per internist and family practitioner on the active staff, and the average volume of appendectomies per surgeon and family practitioner. Pilcher and his associates (1980) had detailed data on each surgeon, but the study was limited to only eight hospitals and 26 surgeons.

Unlike Hughes and his colleagues, who used the hospital as the unit of analysis, Kelly and Hellinger (1987) used the patient as the unit of analysis with both hospital and physician volume measures.[4] Their results for coronary artery bypass graft surgery and cardiac catheterization were limited by their sample of 26 and 39 hospitals, respectively. In addition, physicians with fewer than 15 patient encounters per year were not included, to avoid attributing low volumes to physicians whose main practice sites were elsewhere. Kelly and Hellinger's mean physician volumes of 109 for CABG surgery and 97 for cardiac catheterization contrast with Hughes's mean volumes of 35 and 29. These striking differences in physician volumes may be contrasted with the figures for hospital volumes. Kelly and Hellinger reported volumes of 356 and 398, and Hughes reported volumes of 242 and 247. This discrepancy suggested that the 15-patient exclusionary rule may have dropped many very low volume physicians. Hughes and his colleagues focused their attention on the effects of those low-volume physicians. (Hughes offers a detailed discussion about other reasons for the difference in empirical results of these two studies.)

Hughes's measure of surgeon volume was plagued by numerous problems, only some of which can be solved by using more recently available data sets. Hospital discharge abstract data from over ten states included a physician license number, Medicare number, or unique statewide number. These data often are available for research after a review process and encryption of physician identifiers (Hughes and Lee 1990). Using such data, researchers can account for a surgeon's experience with related procedures, with the same operation during a previous period, and most important, with the same or related procedures at other hospitals. Even such improved data, however, will not allow researchers to identify house staff physicians or attending surgeons who have gained experience working as assistant surgeons but who were seldom coded as primary surgeons on the hospital discharge abstract form. Furthermore, in some teaching hospitals the attending physician is listed as the physician of record even if residents perform most of the work.

NOTES

1. See, for example, Shortell and LoGerfo (1981); and Hughes, Hunt, and Luft (1987), reprinted in Chapter 17.
2. See, for example, Pilcher et al. (1980) and Kelly and Hellinger (1986).
3. See, for example, Roos, Roos, and Sharp (1987).
4. The study by Kelly and Hellinger (1987) is reprinted in Chapter 10.

Effects of Surgeon Volume and Hospital Volume on Quality of Care in Hospitals

Robert G. Hughes
Sandra S. Hunt
Harold S. Luft

A growing body of evidence indicates that for certain surgical procedures, a relationship exists between the volume of surgical procedures performed at a hospital and the quality of care of those patients, as measured by their outcomes. This "volume-outcome" relationship, which takes patient mix into consideration, documents that having a higher volume of patients undergoing a particular procedure at a hospital is associated with better outcomes for those patients.

The volume of patients operated on by an individual surgeon may be an important component of the volume-outcome relationship, and the experience of surgeons may underlie the observed relationship between hospital volume and patient outcomes. That is, perhaps the proportion of patients operated on by high-volume or low-volume surgeons, and not the hospital volume, is important for outcomes; or both surgeon and hospital volume may be associated with patient outcomes. In this paper, we analyze the relative influence of hospital volume and the proportion of patients operated on by low-volume surgeons on patient outcomes for 10 procedures, controlling for other selected factors that may affect outcomes.

HOSPITAL VOLUME, PHYSICIAN CHARACTERISTICS, AND PATIENT OUTCOMES

Evidence documenting the relationship between the volume of patients treated at a hospital for a specific diagnosis or undergoing a specific procedure and their outcomes has been presented by Luft; Shortell and LoGerfo; Farber et al.; and Flood et al.[1-5] This volume-outcome relationship, observed at the hospital level of analysis, raises the question: how much of this relationship may actually be due to the experience of the individual surgeons?

Reprinted from *Medical Care* 25, no. 6 (1987). 489–503, with permission from The J. B. Lippincott Company.

Supported by Grant Number HS-04329 from the National Center for Health Services Research, Department of Health and Human Services, and a grant from the Pew Memorial Trust.

An earlier version of this paper was presented at the American Public Health Association's 114th Annual Meeting, Las Vegas, NV, October 1, 1986.

Attempts to investigate the importance of physician characteristics have been inconclusive.[6] Shortell and LoGerfo[2] found that the average volume of acute myocardial infarctions (AMI) per primary care physician in each hospital was related negatively with standardized mortality ratios, suggesting an experience effect, i.e., patients treated in hospitals in which physicians had more experience in treating AMI patients had better outcomes. However, an analogous measure for appendectomies, volume of operations per surgeon and family practitioner, was unrelated with the outcome (standardized percent of normal tissue removed). In a pilot study on total hip replacements, Fowles et al. found surgeon volume more strongly related to patient mortality than hospital volume, and both were equally related to major complications; however, none of these associations was statistically significant.[7]

Other researchers have failed to find significant relationships between surgeon characteristics and outcomes, especially in a group of studies based on the Study on Institutional Differences in Postoperative Mortality conducted at Stanford.[8] Flood et al.[9] investigated how surgical outcomes that were based on mortality and morbidity for patients in 17 hospitals were related to five physician characteristics. Four of them—extent of specialization, board certification, number of residencies, and years of experience—were not significantly related to outcomes. Only the percent of each surgeon's practice carried on at the study hospital was significantly related to outcomes; the higher the percentage, the better the patient outcomes. This relationship was controlled for case mix, but other variables, such as hospital expenditures per patient day, were not included. The relationship became insignificant when these variables were introduced into the regression. In this 1978 paper, Flood et al. used physician characteristics as control variables; their focus was on the relative power of groups within the hospital. In a 1982 paper using the same data source, Flood et al. directly examined the relative importance of hospital and surgeon characteristics on patient outcomes.[10] In this analysis, the number of residencies and the percent of practice carried on in the study hospital were related to outcomes. However, these associations did not significantly add to the explained variance of patient outcomes once hospital size, expenditures, and teaching status were taken into account. They concluded that "differences in the quality of surgical care seem to be more closely associated with features of the hospital setting in which care is delivered and features of the surgical staff as a corporate body than with the characteristics of individual surgeons"[10] (p. 361).

Still additional evidence from the Stanford study, using mortality data from 1,224 hospitals, on the relationship between surgeon characteristics and patient outcomes was presented by Flood et al.[11] in a reply to a comment[12] on their volume-outcome papers.[4,5] They described four different measures of physician experience, each based on the number of patients per surgeon per year, i.e., the total number of operations performed by each surgeon regardless of the diagnosis or procedure. None of the four experience measures was related to patient outcomes based on mortality.

Most recently, Kelly and Hellinger[13] directly examined the effect of surgeon volume and board certification on mortality for four patient groups classified by principal diagnosis and primary surgical procedure. They found some evidence that board certification is related to outcomes, but found no support for the hypothesis that individual surgeon volume of patients is significantly related to patient mortality.

Despite these findings, which are consistent in failing to detect a surgeon volume effect, it seems plausible that physician volume may have some effect on patient outcomes, particularly for low volumes of a given operation. Maintaining proficiency of skills through an adequate volume of cases is a recognized concern of surgeons, despite the virtual absence of procedure-specific guidelines for minimum numbers necessary to maintain competency. Such reasoning underlies the volume requirements for certification of surgery residencies. Requirements for the accreditation of general surgery programs, for example, state "While the number of operations to be performed by each resident is not specified, experience has shown that an acceptable range, in most instances, is from 500–800 total cases and from 150–300 cases as the 'Surgeon, Senior Year.'"[14] For specific operations, a consensus has emerged only for heart surgery, with the American College of Surgery guidelines stating that "the performance of at least 150 open-heart operations per year by an independent team is desirable to maintain an adequate standard."[15] The recommendation did not provide numeric guidelines for individual surgeons.

Residency program requirements aim at establishing minimum competence levels among the surgical residents for subsequent practice. Yet these requirements are usually not procedure specific; they refer to total operations. When a surgeon operates, however, experience with particular types of operations may be more important than operative experience generally. For example, a surgeon who performs 300 operations a year, yet only one or two cholecystectomies, may be less proficient at cholecystectomies than another surgeon who performs 150 operations per year, half of which are cholecystectomies. Thus it may be important to examine *procedure-specific* surgeon volume when analyzing the relationship between surgeon volume and patient outcome.

It is also important to consider the volume levels that can reasonably be expected to be associated with different outcomes. The volume-outcome relationship for many procedures at the hospital level is not linear; instead, there is a pronounced effect at low volumes, and a flattening of the curve at higher volumes.[1] This makes intuitive sense for individual surgeons as well. We expect that there may be a substantial difference in the performance of surgeons undertaking two total hip replacements a year in contrast to those doing 12 a year, but there may be little difference between those undertaking 50 versus 60 per year. Thus differences in volume are likely to have more of an effect on outcomes at the very low volumes. This argument applies to the volume of yearly operations needed to maintain skills as well as to the initial acquisition of those skills. Thus we will focus our empirical analysis of surgeon volume on low numbers of procedures, expecting that, in general, the fewer operations of a specific type performed by a surgeon in a given year, the more likely patients will experience bad outcomes. At the hospital level, the greater its proportion of patients operated on by low-volume surgeons, the more likely its patients will have poorer outcomes.

METHODS AND DATA

We use multiple regression with ordinary least squares for each of 10 procedures to analyze the relationship between the proportion of patients operated on by low-volume surgeons, hospital volume, and patient outcomes. Our patient outcome measure (described below) is the dependent variable; measures for low physician volume, hospital volume, and a set of control variables (some of which are procedure specific) are independent variables. In other papers, we have explored the notion that causality may lead both from higher hospital volumes to better outcomes and from better outcomes to higher hospital volumes through referrals.[16,17] There is evidence to support both causal linkages. Unfortunately, our data do not allow us to identify separate equations for hospital and low surgeon volume simultaneously. Thus, we are using the more conventional model in which outcome is the dependent variable, but one should recognize that better outcomes may also lead to more referrals.

This study uses the hospital as the unit of analysis. Thus, our measure of low surgeon volume, described below, is a hospital level variable. This approach was selected for conceptual and pragmatic reasons. Assessments of quality require a sufficient volume of patients before any especially good or bad performers can be identified. Luft and Hunt[18] have described the statistical limits, determined by patient volume and diagnosis-specific death rates, that preclude making meaningful evaluations of a hospital's performance. Since individual surgeon volumes are much lower than hospital volumes, the ability to assess quality using individual surgeons as the unit of analysis is even more difficult. Even using hospital level data, assessments of quality are controversial, as exemplified by the recent release of data from the Health Care Financing Administration.[19] A pragmatic reason for using the hospital as the unit of analysis is that our data do not link surgeons and patients, and we do not have exact patient volumes for all surgeons.

Data for this study come from four sources. Data on patient outcomes, hospital volume, surgeon volume, and other patient characteristics were derived from the discharge abstracts of the Professional Activity Study of the Commission on Professional and Hospital Activities (CPHA). Data on relevant specialized hospital services, personnel, and facilities were derived from the 1983 Survey of Specialized Clinical Services (SSCS).[20] Additional hospital variables were taken from the 1983 American Hospital Association Annual Survey,[21] and variables describing each hospital's county characteristics were taken from the Area Resource File (ARF).[22]

Hospitals were included in the analysis if they subscribed to the CPHA Professional Activity Study in 1982, admitted at least one patient for any of the 10 procedures selected for analysis, and responded to the 1983 SSCS. The final overall study sample included 757 short-term general hospitals representing 503,662 patient records. These hospitals are described in Table 17.1. The 757 hospitals are slightly larger than average, are somewhat more likely to be not-for-profit, and are more often affiliated with a medical school than the population of short-term general hospitals.

The 10 procedures selected for this study are listed in Table 17.2, along with the ICD-9CM codes used to define them. These procedures were selected to represent a spectrum of procedures with varying outcomes; bad outcomes (deaths and patients staying longer than the 90th percentile) for each procedure are also listed in Table 17.2. Patient records for any of the 10 procedures were excluded if data were missing on age, sex, discharge status, or length of stay. To maintain confidentiality, all data were aggregated to the hospital level and hospital identifiers were removed by CPHA before we received the data.

Differences in case mix across hospitals were measured by developing a risk factor matrix, as has been done in previous research,[2,17] based on characteristics known to be associated with mortality rates, including age, sex, type of procedure or diagnosis, and secondary diagnoses. These matrices are then used to develop the dependent variables. The number of classification cells in the matrices ranged from 9 for stomach operations, which was subset by age and admission diagnosis (a 3×3 matrix), to 48 for cholecystectomy, which was subset by age, sex, type of procedure, and single/multiple diagnosis (a $3 \times 2 \times 2 \times 4$ matrix). Admission blood pressure was originally used to develop

Table 17.1: Selected Characteristics of 757 Study Hospitals and All U.S. Community Hospitals

	Study Hospitals	All U.S. Community Hospitals
Average number of beds	210	166
Affiliated with a medical school	18%	15%
Region		
East	12%	15%
Northcentral	42%	29%
South	26%	37%
West	20%	19%
Ownership		
Voluntary	76%	58%
Public	20%	29%
Proprietary	4%	13%

Source: Hospital Statistics, 1983 Edition. Chicago: American Hospital Association, 1983.

Table 17.2:   Hospital and Patient Statistics for 10 Selected Procedures

	Hospitals	*Patients*	*Bad Outcomes[a]*	*ICD9-CM Code*
Cardiac catherteization	150	76,584	8,364 (896)	37.2–37.23
				88.50–88.58
Appendectomy	646	39,545	3,367 (38)	47.0
Coronary artery bypass graft	120	29,503	3,495 (1000)	36.10–36.19
Cholecystectomy	742	80,587	7,994 (903)	51.21–51.22
Hernia repair	742	78,377	7,638 (93)	53.00–53.05
				53.10–53.17
Hysterectomy	736	105,550	9,140 (94)	68.3–68.7
Intestinal operations	708	28,486	4,614 (1887)	45.71–45.79
				45.8
				45.92–45.94
				46.10–46.14
				46.20–46.24
Stomach operations	656	9,442	1,800 (892)	43.6, 43.7
				43.9
				44.0–44.03
				44.2
				44.44–44.42
Total hip replacement	501	13,767	1,271 (158)	81.5
Transurethral prostatectomy	631	41,821	4,106 (193)	60.2
Totals	757	503,662	51,789 (6154)	

[a]Bad outcomes include deaths and patients staying longer than the 90th percentile for the diagnosis or procedure based on all CPHA patients with this procedure. Deaths are shown in parentheses.

the risk-factor matrix for some procedures, but was later dropped because of poor reporting. Additional case-mix differences, such as the proportion of patients with a secondary diagnosis of hypertension, are measured as independent variables.

DEPENDENT VARIABLES

The first step in developing the dependent variables (one for each procedure) is counting the actual number of deaths in each hospital. This is compared with the expected number of deaths in each hospital given its distribution of patients among the cells in the case-mix matrix. To compute this indirectly standardized mortality rate, data from all the hospitals are combined to obtain cell-specific death rates. Each of these cell-specific death rates is then multiplied by the number of patients in the corresponding cell for each hospital; the sum over all cells is that hospital's expected number of deaths. This represents the number of deaths the hospital would have if its performance were equal to the national average, adjusted for case-mix differences.

A second component of the outcome measure is the number of patients with very long length of stay, as an indicator of complications. A very long length of stay is defined as greater than the 90th percentile length of stay for patients undergoing that procedure who were discharged alive. These percentiles were based on all CPHA hospitals; the 90th percentile cutoff for each procedure is listed in Table 17.3. Actual and expected values for long-stay patients are computed in a fashion analogous to that used for deaths.

Note that we are not using average length of stay as a component of the outcome variable. Well-documented regional variations in average length of stay make this an inappropriate outcome measure and dictate that average length of stay be used as a control variable (see below) so that the very long length-of-stay measure we are using reflects excessive morbidity due to complications. Alternative measures of morbidity due to complications based on discharge abstract data are difficult to interpret because it it not possible to determine if patient conditions existed at the time of admission or were acquired during a hospital stay; therefore, we chose very long length of stay as an approximation to bad outcomes for patients discharged alive. Other researchers have developed outcome measures combining mortality and morbidity,[10] but the morbidity component depended on (nurse) assessments and could thus be obtained for only a small number of hospitals. Our measure has the advantage of being based on routinely collected discharge abstract data.

These four steps result in four measures for each hospital: actual deaths, expected deaths, actual long-stay patients, and expected long-stay patients. We add actual deaths to actual long-stay patients to obtain total bad outcomes for each hospital. We also add expected deaths to expected long-stay patients to obtain total expected bad outcomes. Combining deaths and long length of stay patients, a proxy for morbidity, allows us to investigate volume-outcome relationships that are not detectable using deaths alone because of the low overall death rates for some procedures. When outcome rates and/or volumes are very low, it is impossible to identify statistically good performers, and even poor

Table 17.3:   90th Percentile Cutoffs for Very Long
Length of Stay for 10 Procedures

Procedure	*90th Percentile Number of Days*
Cardiac catheterization	12
Appendectomy	7
Coronary artery bypass graft	24
Cholecystectomy	18
Hernia repair	8
Hysterectomy	11
Intestinal operations	32
Stomach operations	32
Total hip replacement	25
Transurethral prostatectomy	18

performance is difficult to assess reliably.[18] Another reason to combine bad outcomes to assess quality is that mortality rates have declined in the decade. For example, the death rates for coronary artery bypass graft (CABG), total hip replacement (THR), and transurethral prostatectomy (TURP), all fell by more than 40% between 1972 and 1982, with the death rate for CABG falling from 6.71% to 3.56%, the death rate for THR falling from 5.06% to 1.17%, and the death rate for TURP falling from 1.19% to 0.45%.[23] Thus, outcome evaluations should focus increasingly on measures of morbidity.

For each hospital and each procedure, we then take the three numbers— bad outcomes, expected bad outcomes, and number of patients—and, using the binomial distribution, calculate the probability that the observed bad outcomes are different from expected bad outcomes. In the final step, this probability is converted into a Z-score for each hospital. This conversion standardizes the measure across procedures and assigns a negative value if results for the hospital are better than expected and a positive value if results are worse than expected.

PHYSICIAN VOLUME

To assess the relationship between low physician volume and hospital outcomes, we calculated the proportion of patients treated by low-volume physicians at each hospital. We expected that the higher the proportion of patients operated on by low-volume physicians, the poorer the outcomes at that hospital. The median number of procedures per surgeon per year, which we used as the cutoff to differentiate less experienced surgeons from others, is listed for each of the 10 procedures in Table 17.4. The distributions tend to be highly skewed, so the mean number of procedures per surgeon is far greater than the median.

Ideally, data on the exact number of patients operated on by each surgeon in a hospital would be used to calculate the proportion of patients treated by low-volume surgeons. However, our data were organized at the hospital level of analysis and did not link surgeons with individual patients, neither did we have exact patient volumes for all surgeons. Instead, CPHA provided us with a count of the number of different surgeons in each hospital performing each procedure and the proportion of patients for each procedure operated on by the surgeons doing the first, second, and third highest proportions. When the number of surgeons in a hospital performing the procedure was one to four, we were able to determine the exact number of surgeries performed by each surgeon. When the number of surgeons was five or more, the number of patients remaining after subtracting those operated on by the top three surgeons was divided by the remaining number of surgeons, giving an average number of operations for these surgeons. The proportion of patients for which we know the exact number of operations by each surgeon is listed for each procedure in Table 17.4.

Once each surgeon's volume was determined, the proportion treated by

Table 17.4: Total Number of Surgeons and Median Number of Procedures Used as Cutoffs to Define Less Experienced Surgeons, Mean Number of Procedures per Surgeon, and Proportion of Patients in Which the Exact Number of Operations for All Surgeons Is Known

Procedure	Total No. of Surgeons Performing Procedure	Median No. Procedures per Surgeon per Year	Number of Patients Treated per Surgeon per Year		Proportion of Patients in which Exact No. of Operations for All Surgeons Is Known
			Mean	SD	
Cardiac catheterization	2,987	11	28.64	46.87	0.938
Appendectomy	6,434	4	6.00	6.17	0.751
Coronary artery bypass graft	800	12	35.08	53.73	0.982
Cholecystectomy	7,062	7	11.12	12.72	0.762
Hernia repair	7,476	6	10.28	11.59	0.752
Hysterectomy	8,027	8	12.86	15.69	0.741
Intestinal operations	5,436	3	5.00	5.22	0.799
Stomach operations	3,735	2	2.32	2.17	0.838
Total hip replacement	2,301	3	5.34	9.71	0.929
Transurethral prostatectomy	2,892	7	12.78	15.94	0.915

surgeons doing less than the median volume for our sample per year was calculated for each hospital by putting all patients operated on by low-volume surgeons in the numerator and total patients in the denominator. This variable is designed to focus on the hypothesized relationship between low physician volume and poor patient outcomes by measuring the proportion of a hospital's patients that are operated on by surgeons with relatively little experience with that procedure.

HOSPITAL VOLUME

Hospital volume was measured by taking the log of procedure volume to account for a nonlinear effect. The proportion of patients treated by low-volume surgeons and hospital volume are the two independent variables of primary interest in this analysis. The mean and standard deviation of both variables for each procedure are listed in Table 17.5.

The relationship between the two volume variables is important methodologically and theoretically. Hospitals with very low volume will, of necessity, have a high percentage of their patients operated on by low-volume surgeons. As hospital volume increases, so does the opportunity for surgeons to have high volume in that hospital; thus, the proportion of patients operated on by low-volume surgeons decreases. In fact, across all 10 procedures, the higher the hospital volume, the lower the proportion of patients operated on by low-volume surgeons.

Table 17.5:   Mean and Standard Deviation of Hospital Volume and Low Surgeon Volume (Proportion of Patients Treated by Low Volume Surgeons) for 10 Procedures

	Hospital Volume		Low Surgeon Volume: Proportion Patients Treated by Surgeons Below Cutoff	
Procedure	*Mean*	*S. D.*	*Mean*	*S.D.*
Cardiac catheterization	246.25	348.3	0.122	0.206
Appendectomy	53.01	41.5	0.262	0.299
Coronary artery bypass graft	241.83	243.3	0.260	0.388
Cholecystectomy	107.88	87.8	0.246	0.300
Hernia repair	104.92	86.9	0.221	0.270
Hysterectomy	142.44	157.4	0.310	0.336
Intestinal operations	39.78	38.5	0.288	0.338
Stomach operations	14.11	12.7	0.454	0.350
Total hip replacement	27.15	34.6	0.345	0.377
Transurethral prostatectomy	65.76	57.7	0.230	0.332

HYPOTHESIZED RELATIONSHIPS

Following past research, we expected that higher hospital volume would be related to better patient outcomes. Since our outcome measure is constructed such that poor outcomes have positive values and good outcomes have negative values, the hospital volume coefficients will be negative and significant if our expectations regarding hospital volume are confirmed.

The surgeon volume variable is constructed such that we expect the higher its value (the higher the proportion of patients treated by less experienced surgeons), the more likely the hospital will have poorer outcomes. Since poor outcomes have positive values in the dependent variable, this variable's coefficients will be positive and significant if our expectations regarding surgeon volume are confirmed.

CONTROL VARIABLES

Surgeon volume and hospital volume are not the only factors likely to influence patient outcomes. We have included in the regressions a set of control variables that may influence outcomes for all procedures, as well as procedure-specific control variables.

Three types of control variables were selected. One type of variable is aimed at detecting differences in the types of patients that are admitted to a hospital to control for the possibility that observed differences in hospital outcomes are due to differences in patient mix not already captured in the risk-factor matrix, rather than to characteristics of the hospital itself. These variables measure patient characteristics, such as secondary diagnoses, and hospital characteristics, such as proportion of patients transferred from another hospital, that may be associated with more severely ill patients. A second type of control variable is directed at measuring differences in hospital organization, other than volume or low surgeon volume, that may be related to outcomes independent of patient differences. A third type of variable attempts to account for differences in the hospital's environment, such as population density, that may influence outcomes. The control variables are sometimes of interest in themselves, but our primary focus in this paper is low surgeon volume and hospital volume.

While it is conceptually helpful to consider the three types of reasons for the control variables, in practice specific variables may capture multiple effects. For example, region of the country may pick up differences in epidemiologic patterns and patient differences in disease severity, but it may also measure differences in practice patterns. For the purpose of investigating low surgeon volume, it is preferable to include variables, especially those that previous research has shown are empirically related to outcomes, to increase confidence that the estimated coefficients for the relationship between low surgeon volume and outcomes are not biased by omitted variables, even if each of those variables does not have a simple theoretical justification. Finally, many of the control variables are relevant only for specific procedures. These were determined on the basis of clinical relevance. To the extent we have selected control variables that accurately measure the concepts of interest, they give us more confidence that any relationships we find between hospital volume or low surgeon volume and the dependent variable are not caused by other, unmeasured, factors.

Hospital length of stay is included as a variable to control for the potential effects of overall length of stay on procedure specific length of stay. In particular, the proportion of patients staying beyond the 90th percentile length of stay will be influenced by geographic and other factors generally increasing the average length of stay. By including the average length of stay of all patients in each hospital, the general effects are removed statistically and the focus is on the extreme, procedure specific cases. Population per square mile, percent of population that is black, and region of the country (measured by dummy variables) were included because in past research they have been shown to be associated with outcomes,[16,24] although the underlying causes for these associations remain largely unexplained. Hospital ownership (measured by dummy variables) and medical school affiliation are included to control for hospital characteristics that may be related to outcomes. Some policy makers are concerned that proprietary hospitals may skimp on quality and public hospitals may be the recipients of high-risk patients. Teaching hospitals are expected to have better-quality attending physicians, but their residents may be inexperienced, and they may attract the higher-risk patients. (We also used residents per bed as an alternative measure of involvement in medical education, and found no significant difference in results.) The proportion of generalist physicians on the total medical staff addresses overall specialization of hospital services and personnel.

We included two types of procedure specific control variables. One type focuses on additional patient risk factors such as proportions of patients with specific secondary diagnoses and proportions of patients transferred to and from other hospitals. These variables were selected to control for differences in patients not controlled for in the risk-factor matrices because dividing the matrices into too many cells reduces the stability of the cell-specific rates. The proportion of patients with the procedure transferred into a hospital controls for those hospitals that attract a disproportionate share of complicated cases referred from other hospitals. Hospitals with a very high proportion of patients referred to other acute care institutions may have artifactually low rates of poor outcomes because patients with complications are transferred elsewhere. Specific secondary diagnoses were selected for each procedure in conjunction with our physician consultant to reflect higher risk of bad outcomes, e.g., the proportion of hernia repair patients with hypertension. The second type of procedure-specific control variable focuses on hospital characteristics, such as the grouping of all urology patients in a specific area; these variables were selected to control for other organizational characteristics that may be related to outcome.

In the regressions, the hospital observations were weighted by a factor that gives more weight to hospitals with higher volumes and with patient mixes having lower expected bad outcome rates, thus addressing the problem of having a large number of small-volume hospitals dominate the regression analysis even though they account for a small percentage of total patients.[*]

RESULTS

The regression results for one procedure, transurethral prostatectomy, are presented in Table 17.6 as an example of a complete model. In order to examine succinctly the relationships of primary concern, Table 17.7 presents the coefficients and standard errors only for the proportion of patients operated on by low-volume surgeons and hospital volume variables, along with the adjusted R^2 and N for each regression. (Full regression results are available from the authors.)

In Table 17.6 we see that both low surgeon volume and hospital volume are significant and in the expected directions; i.e., hospitals with larger volumes of patients undergoing a transurethral prostatectomy (TURP) are likely to have better outcomes, and hospitals with a higher percentage of their TURP patients operated on by low-volume surgeons are likely to have worse outcomes.

Among the control variables, higher county density and a greater percentage of the county population being black are related to worse outcomes, as is the average hospital length of stay. In addition, two of the region dummy variables are significant. Regional factors are associated with differential mortality rates both during hospitalization and postdischarge[24] in addition to well known geographic differences in length of stay. Note, however, that average length of stay for all patients in the hospital is already included in the equation. Controlling for volume, hospitals in which urology patients are grouped in a special unit are likely to have better outcomes, possibly because nursing staff is thus able to develop more expertise with such patients. Hospitals with a higher proportion of TURP patients transferred in from other hospitals are likely to have worse outcomes, probably reflecting a more severe case mix.

As shown in Table 17.7, the coefficients for the log of hospital volume are highly significant ($P < 0.01$) and in the expected direction for 8 of the 10 procedures, controlling for other selected factors, including the proportion of pa-

---

[*]The weighting factor is defined as follows:

$$WT_{i,j} = \frac{(Vol_{i,j})^2}{Vol_{i,j}}$$

$$\sum_{k=1} P_{i,j,k} \cdot (1 - P_{i,j,k})$$

where $Vol_{i,j}$ = number of patients with procedure i in hospital j, and $P_{i,j,k}$ = expected probability of bad outcomes for the kth patient with procedure i in hospital j based on the national estimate for that patient's case-mix cell category.

Table 17.6:   Regression Coefficients for Patient Outcomes Transurethral
Prostatectomy

Variable	*Coefficients (Standard Error)*	
Log of hospital volume	−0.587	(0.134)[a]
Proportion of patients operated on by low-volume surgeons	0.983	(0.456)[a]
Average length of stay	0.135	(0.040)[a]
East	−0.245	(0.264)
South	−0.959	(0.201)[a]
West	−2.178	(0.214)[a]
Public hospital	−0.400	(0.258)
Proprietary hospital	0.466	(0.384)
Medical school affiliation	0.050	(0.179)
Ratio of generalist MDs to total medical staff	0.095	(0.724)
Population per square mile in county	0.037	(0.009)[a]
Percent population black in county	0.034	(0.007)[a]
Emergency cardiologist always in house	−0.031	(0.296)
Emergency anesthesiologist always in house	−0.299	(0.212)
Urology department or division	0.291	(0.169)
Urology patients grouped on special unit	−0.553	(0.182)[a]
Proportion patients transferred from other hospital	5.729	(1.967)[a]
Proportion patients transferred to other hospital	−11.752	(11.287)
Proportion patients with second diagnosis:		
Hypertension	5.504	(15.080)
Diabetes	−11.541	(12.799)
Hypertension and diabetes	14.996	(65.518)
Proportion patients given blood	−1.718	(1.457)
Proportion patients with surgery within 6 hours	−2.053	(1.857)

R^2, adjusted R^2 = 0.407, 0.385
N = 631
[a]$P < 0.05$

tients operated on by low-volume surgeons. The coefficients for low surgeon volume are significant ($P < 0.10$) and in the expected direction for 6 of the 10 procedures. For three of the procedures, low surgeon volume was not significant, although the coefficients were positive. For one procedure, coronary artery by-pass graft, low surgeon volume was significant ($P < 0.10$) and negative, a finding opposite to our hypothesis. (In another study, we have determined that analyses of unselected CABG patients, such as is the case here, are skewed by a small proportion of patients also undergoing mitral valve surgery. The latter patients have substantially higher mortality rates and are concentrated in high-volume hospitals, thus creating a bias that may explain these unexpected results.[25]) Overall, the results for low surgeon volume are not as definitive as those for hospital volume, but they are generally consistent with our hypothesis.

DISCUSSION

The results indicate that both hospital volume and the proportion of patients operated on by low-volume surgeons are related to quality of care as measured by

Table 17.7: Physician Volume and Hospital Volume Coefficients and Standard
Error, R^2 and N for Overall Regression for 10 Procedures

Procedure	(Log) Hospital Volume	Surgeon Volume	R^2
Cardiac catheterization	-2.3021^c (0.3552)	4.8976^c (1.3926)	0.655
Appendectomy	-0.32180^c (0.989)	0.4515^b (0.2302)	0.357
Coronary artery bypass graft	-1.7543^c (0.3588)	-4.2107^a (2.2757)	0.651
Cholecystectomy	-0.1466 (0.1083)	0.5236^a (0.2877)	0.352
Hernia repair	-0.4750^e (0.1407)	0.9427^c (0.3484)	0.362
Hysterectomy	-0.7998^c (0.1239)	0.4663 (0.3692)	0.497
Intestinal operations	-0.5625^c (0.965)	0.3358 (0.2387)	0.348
Stomach operations	-0.0773 (0.0798)	0.1708 (0.1850)	0.184
Total hip replacement	-0.4782^c (0.0862)	0.5457^a (0.2996)	0.518
Transurethral prostatectomy	-0.5867^c (0.1336)	0.9829^b (0.4555)	0.407

[a] $P < 0.10$.
[b] $P < 0.05$.
[c] $P < 0.01$.

patient outcomes. The findings regarding hospital volume are consistent with
earlier research and add an additional set of procedures using more recent data to
the evidence for a general "volume-outcome" relationship at the hospital level of
analysis. These relationships were found even with the proportion of patients
operated on by low-volume surgeons variable in the model, indicating that however important this variable may be in and of itself, it does not explain the
hospital volume-outcome relationship. Indeed, hospital volume was, overall,
more significantly associated with outcomes than the proportion of patients operated on by low-volume surgeons.

The physician volume results are noteworthy because of the crudity of the
measure used. It fails to account for a surgeon's total experience with other
operations, with similar (but not identical) operations, with the same operation
before the year-long study period, or, perhaps most important, with the same
procedure performed at other hospitals during the study period. Each of these
shortcomings makes it more difficult to detect an association, for some surgeons
with more experience were probably included in the less experienced group.

Our measure of surgeon volume also may be imprecise because it accepts
that the surgeon of record on the discharge abstract actually performed the
operation. This assumption neglects experience a surgeon may acquire as an

assistant operating team member, and it may misrepresent operations that are actually performed by residents or in which residents assist. However, both possibilities would make it harder to detect a significant difference. The surgeon who may be classified as low-volume despite greater experience as a team member would presumably dilute the low-volume association. Likewise, if residents, who may be at the beginning of their learning curve and thus more likely to have patients with bad outcomes, have their patients attributed to a high-volume surgeon, this would suggest results opposite to those observed.

The proportion of patients operated on by low-volume surgeons may reflect a variety of organizational processes. For example, after controlling for hospital volume, a high proportion of patients operated on by low-volume surgeons indicates a hospital in which many physicians compete for patients, which, in turn, may lead to bad outcomes because of a lack of medical staff cooperation. Our data do not allow analysis of intrahospital variation, but it appears a reasonable area for further investigation.

With the exception of the Shortell and LoGerfo[2] findings for AMI patients, our results differ from previous research, notably the recent work of Kelly and Hellinger,[13] and possible explanations for these differences are worthy of detailed consideration. First, the levels of analysis differed: Kelly and Hellinger used the patient; we used the hospital. Using the patient as the unit of analysis puts more weight on hospital characteristics, because hospital effects are counted separately for each patient. Thus, the characteristics of high-volume hospitals have more weight in the regressions. Second, our measure of physician volume differed. Kelly and Hellinger used the exact number of procedures per physician in their regression, while we used the proportion of patients operated on by low-volume surgeons. Their measure investigates the potential of a linear relationship; our measure focused on the role of low-volume surgeons, implicitly assuming a curvilinear relationship. In fact, they excluded physicians with extremely low volumes, which is reasonable when focusing on physician effects but less necessary when the hospital is the unit of observation. Third, the two studies used different data sources, different methods of control for case mix, and different measures of patient outcome.

The two studies actually ask slightly different questions. The Kelly and Hellinger paper purposefully excluded patients of physicians with very small numbers of patients in the study hospitals. They, in essence, are asking whether physician volume has a separate effect from hospital volume; and to do so, they would like to approximate the surgeon's total volume in multiple hospitals; therefore, they exclude surgeons who occasionally practice in the study hospital. In contrast, our focus is on the average results for patients treated in hospitals, including the impact of the occasional surgeon in those hospitals. For example, the Kelly and Hellinger analysis is very helpful in answering questions about selected individual surgeons; our results are more oriented toward the selection of individual hospitals.

Even with all of these differences, it is noteworthy that, when investigating the same operations, the two studies' results are consistent. Three of the four groups of patients analyzed by Kelly and Hellinger overlap patients classified as undergoing intestinal operations or stomach operations in our analysis. These were two of three procedures for which the proportion of patients operated on by low-volume surgeons was not significantly related to patient outcomes. Overall, the two studies may be viewed as being not inconsistent, especially given the differences in methods.

The surgeon results in Table 17.7 are consistent, if not statistically significant, for all procedures except coronary artery bypass graft (CABG). The CABG result invites special scrutiny by its exception. Several factors may contribute to what seems a counterintuitive result. CABG physician volume has the highest median of all procedures; thus the differences between low-volume surgeons and others may be either diluted or inconsequential because there are few truly low-volume surgeons. In addition, CABG is ordinarily performed by a team with at least two surgeons and an organized staff, at a distinct facility, and with specialized equipment. Thus the success or failure of an operation is not as likely to be related to the experience of a single surgeon as when one surgeon operates with relative autonomy, less constrained by the complex social and technical organization surrounding heart surgery. Also, operating with other surgeons submits a surgeon to direct peer observation of skills, a stimulus to increase quality and a constraint on repeated poor performances. The team approach also means that our measure of low surgeon volume probably greatly underestimates true surgical experience. In addition, CABG is also the only surgical procedure for which the ACS has provided guidelines with regard to minimum number necessary to maintain standards. These recommendations may have had the effect of precluding surgeon volumes that might be sufficiently low to adversely affect outcomes, i.e., one purpose of the guidelines—to ensure quality through an adequate volume of procedures—may have been achieved. Finally, the results may be a statistical artifact due to multicollinearity between hospital volume and the proportion of CABG patients operated on by low-volume surgeons. The correlation for these variables is -0.915. This value is well above 0.7, a rough standard that was not exceeded by the R-values for the volume variables for any of the other procedures.

The results for the other operations raise questions concerning physician characteristics other than volume. For example, some operations are performed almost exclusively by specialists (total hip replacement—orthopedic surgeons, transurethral prostatectomy—urologists), some are performed primarily by general surgeons (cholecystectomy, hernia repair, appendectomy), and some are performed by different types of physicians (abdominal hysterectomies by obstetric gynecologists, general surgeons, and general practitioners). The extent to which operating surgeons are physician specialists and the relationship (if any) with patient outcomes are fruitful areas for further investigation.

Overall, these findings suggest it is premature to argue that surgeon volume is unimportant for patients outcomes; rather, these results suggest that the effects of surgeon volume on patient outcomes remain an area worthy of additional research. Such research and clinical assessment might be directed usefully at refining our understanding of the relationship between low surgeon volume and poor patient outcomes. It should be noted that our measure of low surgeon volume, the proportion of patients operated on by less experienced surgeons, does not address directly the quality of individual low-volume surgeons; rather, it indicates that the relationship of individual surgeon volume, especially low volume, with patient outcomes is worthy of investigation. Ideally, future research should use data on the procedure-specific exact patient volumes by physician across hospitals and over time to identify thresholds or volume ranges that are related to patient outcomes. Although current evidence is inconclusive, if further research confirms that low volumes of procedures by surgeons are related to poor outcomes, then professional associations, governmental bodies, and payers of health care costs that are concerned with quality will need to begin the difficult process of transforming this general finding into guidelines and recommendations for minimum volumes of procedures per year for the maintenance and improvement of overall clinical performance. Note that such recommendations should not be used as an excuse to undertake unnecessary procedures in order to meet a quota. Instead, systems may have to be designed to channel patients toward those surgeons with good outcomes and high volumes, and away from those without the necessary experience or with poor results.

Previous analyses have documented that many surgeons have modest work loads, performing far fewer operations than is their capacity and performing many specific operations less than once a month.[26] Such findings in the past have been examined for their surgical manpower planning implications.[27] With the observed relationship between the proportion of patients operated on by low-volume surgeons and patient outcomes, the extent of surgery performed by low-volume surgeons may become important not only for those concerned with a rational manpower policy and cost containment, but also for those concerned with the quality of the care provided. A variety of institutions are currently interested in controlling utilization, including surgical operations. The association between the proportion of patients operated on by low-volume surgeons and poor patient outcomes suggests that careful attention be given to the methods by which utilization is controlled in order to ensure that quality of care if preserved or enhanced.

ACKNOWLEDGMENTS

We thank several anonymous reviewers for their careful comments and helpful suggestions for improving this paper.

REFERENCES

1. Luft HS, Bunker, J, Enthoven A. Should operations be regionalized? An empirical study of the relation between surgical volume and mortality. N Engl J Med 1979;301:1364.
2. Shortell S, LoGerfo J. Hospital medical staff organization and quality of care: results for myocardial infarction and appendectomy. Med Care 1981;19:1041.
3. Farber B, Kaiser D, Wenzel R. Relation between surgical volume and incidence of postoperative wound infection. N Engl J Med 1981;305:200.
4. Flood AB, Scott WR, Ewy W. Does practice make perfect? I. The relation between hospital volume and outcomes for selected diagnostic categories. Med Care 1984;22:98.
5. Flood AB, Scott WR, Ewy W. Does practice make perfect? II. The relation between hospital volume and outcomes and other hospital characteristics. Med Care 1984;22:115.
6. Palmer HB, Reilly ML. Individual and institutional variables which may serve as indicators of quality of medical care. Med Care 1979;17:693.
7. Fowles J, Bunker J, Oda M, et al. Outcomes of total hip replacement using Northern California Medicare claims data: a pilot study. Final Report, National Center for Health Services Research Grant Number HS-04853, August 6, 1985.
8. Stanford Center for Health Care Research. Study of institutional differences in postoperative mortality. Springfield, VA: National Technical Information Service. U.S. Department of Commerce, December 15, 1974.
9. Flood AB, Scott WR. Professional power and professional effectiveness: the power of the surgical staff and the quality of surgical care in hospitals. J Health Soc Behav. 1978;19:240.
10. Flood AB, Scott WR, Ewy W, Forrest WH, Jr. Effectiveness in professional organizations: the impact of surgeons and surgical staff organizations on the quality of care in hospitals. Health Services Research 1982;17:341.
11. Flood AB, Scott WR, Ewy W. Letter in reply to Dranove, D. A comment on "Does practice make perfect?" Med Care 1984;22:969.
12. Dranove D. A comment on "Does practice make perfect?" Med Care 1984;22:967.
13. Kelly JV, Hellinger F. Physician and hospital factors associated with mortality of surgical patients. Med Care 1986;24;785.
14. Accreditation Council for Graduate Medical Education. 1985–86 Directory of Residency Training Programs. Chicago: American Medical Association, 1985.
15. Guidelines for Minimal Standards in Cardiac Surgery. ACS Bulletin 1984;67.
16. Luft HS. The relation between surgical volume and mortality: an exploration of causal factors and alternative models. Med Care 1980;18:940.
17. Luft HS, Maerki SC, Hunt SS. The volume-outcome relationship: practice makes perfect or selective referral patterns. Institute for Health Policy Studies. Health Services Research, 1987;22:157.
18. Luft HS, Hunt SS. Evaluating hospital quality through outcome statistics. JAMA 1986;255:1780–2784.
19. U.S. distributing lists of hospitals with unusual death rates. New York Times, March 2, 1986.
20. Survey of Specialized Clinical Services, 1983. Chicago, IL: Hospitals Data Center, American Hospital Association, 1983.
21. American Hospital Association Annual Survey of Hospitals, 1982. Chicago, IL: Hospital Data Center, American Hospital Association, 1982.

22. Area Resource File. Sponsored by the Bureau of Health Professions. Available through Natural Technical Information Service, Springfield, Virginia.
23. Commission on Professional and Hospital Activities. Profession activities study, 1972 and 1982. Ann Arbor, MI: Commission on Professional and Hospital Activities, 1972, 1982.
24. Riley G, Lubitz J. Outcomes of surgery in the Medicare population: mortality after surgery. Health Care Financing Review 1985;6:103.
25. Showstack JA, Rosenfeld KE, Garnick DW, et al. The association of volume with outcome of coronary artery bypass graft surgery: scheduled versus nonscheduled operation. JAMA 1987;257:785.
26. The American College of Surgeons and The American Surgical Association. Surgery in the United States. A Summary Report of the Study on Surgical Services for the United States. Vol. I. Chicago: The American College of Surgeons and The American Surgical Association, 1976.
27. Nickerson RJ, Colton T, Peterson O, et al. Doctors who perform operations. N Engl J Med 1976; 298:982.

Chapter 18

Use of Data for Quality of Care

In the following study, Williams made innovative use of linked birth and death data to derive hospital characteristics associated with better outcomes. After adjustment for differences in patient risk and chance variation, the author found several important hospital factors associated with improved perinatal outcomes.

The existence of data linking infant births and deaths is critical to this research because interhospital transfers to neonatal intensive care units are common for acutely ill infants. Currently, most statewide hospital discharge data bases lack unique patient identifiers—if patients are transferred to other hospitals, their ultimate outcome is lost. The receiving hospitals would be penalized by accepting many high-risk infants. With linked data, a death can be attributed to the hospital of birth in an analysis of possible problems in delivery. Furthermore, not all transfers indicate worsening status; many tertiary referral centers transfer babies back to their "home" hospitals when they are well enough to be discharged from a neonatal intensive care unit but not well enough to go home.

Although deaths were counted up to 28 days after birth, and could take place at a hospital other than the hospital of birth, Williams actually assessed care in the immediate period around the delivery, plus effects that might have been due to the transfer. Transfer of infants in itself may be an independent predictor of poor outcomes, but it is potentially preventable if there is proper recognition of high-risk pregnancy. Hospitals with inordinately high transfer rates of newborns (inborn babies transferring out rather than in) may provide poorer care if they fail to recognize in a pregnant woman the potential for a complicated birth. Williams did not include the transfer variable in his analysis, as either a risk factor or a dependent variable, but it would be easy to do so.

The high predictive capability (R^2 in excess of .4) of the case-mix measures distinguishes this study from other types of outcome studies. This research was successful because a single factor, birth weight, accounts for much of the variation in death rates. Birth weight is an easily measured and recorded statistic and is consistently the most important predictor of poor outcome in newborns. Infants weighing less than 2,500 grams are only 7 percent of births but account for almost 70 percent of deaths. Williams went to great lengths to use small birth-weight intervals (250 grams) with cross-classification by race and gender to get as sensitive a measure as possible. The 190 cells in this case-mix system were able to account for much more of the variation between hospitals than is the case for the other studies in this volume. Partially because the system provides a valid and convincing measure of case-mix differences between hospitals, birthweight-adjusted indexes of outcome are regularly generated in some states, including California and Michigan.

Williams also focused on the fact that neonatal death is a rare event, and the number of deaths in a hospital is a Bernoulli variable; that is, it can take on only the value 0, 1, 2, 3, . . . He used this property to calculate the variance associated with the observed probabilities of death in each hospital. This method allowed him to estimate that about 40 percent of the observed variability in indirectly standardized mortality rates is attributable to ordinary sampling variability. This finding highlights the often forgotten fact that, even when patient risk factors are well controlled, much of the variability in outcomes among hospitals is due to chance. Luft and Hunt (1986) also addressed the problem of identifying hospitals with particularly good or poor results.[1]

NOTE

1. The Luft and Hunt (1986) study is reprinted in Chapter 19 of this volume.

Measuring the Effectiveness of Perinatal Medical Care

Ronald L. Williams

Following an extended period during which attention was devoted primarily to measures of medical care quality based on structure and process, researchers have begun to focus their efforts on outcomes. The reasons for this change in emphasis as well as a conceptual framework for developing outcome measures have been reported by Brook et al.[6] In short, structural and process variables may often be invalid, yet because outcome measures are relatively less developed, little is known about their comparative validity and reliability.

Within the framework proposed by Brook, this study falls into the Retrospective Group Policy category in that it utilizes perinatal mortality statistics based on linked birth-death record cohorts, takes hospitals as the basic unit of observation, and aims at addressing quality assessment in the realm of policy recommendations. The study cannot formally be termed "disease" specific since it focuses on what is now viewed as a normal physiologic process rather than a pathologic condition.[11] Nevertheless, in spite of the fact that most women experience a medically-uneventful pregnancy, the newborn remains exposed to a relatively high risk of death and disease during and shortly following birth; i.e., during the "perinatal" period.

The growing interest in perinatal mortality rates reflects a departure from the traditional emphasis on mortality among live-born infants. It has been recognized that the factors responsible for the bulk of deaths in early infancy are often present before delivery or are brought about by unfavorable conditions during the birth process. Moreover, there is evidence of systematic differences concerning the manner in which physicians and hospital personnel classify a "live" birth.[22] For these and other reasons, the perinatal death rate has become more widely used as an outcome indicator. In California, perinatal deaths are defined as fetal deaths of 20 or more weeks gestation combined with neonatal deaths, with the latter including deaths to live-born infants under 28 days of age.

Reprinted from *Medical Care* 17, no. 2 (1979): 95–109, with permission from The J. B. Lippincott Company.

Supported in part by Maternal and Child Health (Social Security Act, Title V) Grant No. MC–R–060390–01/02 from the Bureau of Community Health Services The research reported herein was conducted in cooperation with the staff of the Maternal Child Health Branch of the California Department of Health.

This definition has the advantage of minimizing artifacts resulting from the classification of a live birth, as well as tending to measure the effects of both intra- and postpartum care, yet it also has several important limitations. While California's birth registration is considered to be virtually complete, and its death registration nearly complete, underreporting may occur for deaths under one year of age, particularly those occurring during the first day of life; fetal deaths are more subject to underreporting than are neonatal deaths. Also, there is significantly more missing data describing newborn characteristics for fetal deaths than for live births.

Despite these limitations, the use of perinatal mortality as an outcome measure retains several important advantages. By combining fetal and neonatal deaths, the probability of observing an adverse event in small hospitals is increased. And, by using large numbers of routinely-recorded birth and death certificates, it is possible to overcome the small probability of death (about 2 percent) by aggregating large numbers of births. The routine collection, matching, and coding of birth and death statistics by an increasing number of state health departments have now made that procedure economically feasible on a widespread basis. More importantly, however, a review of the epidemiology of perinatal mortality reveals a unique situation regarding the measurement of the impact of intervening variables.

Briefly, the multiple effects of a large number of behavioral, genetic, and environmental factors can be captured by a single universally-measured variable: the weight of the newborn at birth. Birth weight thereby serves as a primary risk-adjusting factor. Additional attributes such as sex, race and plurality, which too are available from vital records, may also be considered in order to further adjust each hospital's observed perinatal mortality rate for its patient risk characteristics.

PERINATAL MORTALITY, BIRTH WEIGHT, AND SOCIOECONOMIC-ENVIRONMENTAL CONDITIONS

One of the most important threads running through the fabric of infant and perinatal mortality is the critical role of maturity at birth. Although "premature" or low birth weight (less than 2501 g) infants comprise about 7 percent of all births, they account for almost 70 percent of all perinatal deaths. In the first large-scale study of the dependence of newborn mortality on birth weight and other factors, Shapiro[18] found that the variation of neonatal mortality with birth weight was considerably greater than for any other single variable. While a combination of birth weight and gestational age presently appears to be a more accurate predictor of fetal maturity, and therefore perinatal mortality, birth weight has been found to play the dominant role.[21,23] Indeed, in every study of the determinants of neonatal or perinatal mortality, birth weight was consistently the most important predictor. For example, Abernathy et al.[1] found that birth weight was by far the most important of the 28 variables tested in the North Carolina

Perinatal Study. In an analysis of 108,852 infants, Shah and Abbey[17] concluded that birth weight was the most important factor in neonatal mortality, and that adjustments for other variables had little or no effect. Kessner et al.[10] performed a multiple regression analysis of 140,000 births in New York City and found that 26.4 percent of the variance in infant mortality rates could be explained. Of that, almost all (26.3 percent) could be attributed to birth weight alone since the remaining 6 independent variables contributed only 0.1 percent.

In turn, the accumulated evidence has revealed a strong relationship between birth weight and socioeconomic-environmental variables. Some of the most important correlates of birth weight are: the mother's age, parity, and race; maternal socioeconomic and marital status; the timing and frequency of prenatal medical care; maternal health-related habits, such as smoking; and maternal nutrition. Indeed, Gruenwald[9] has suggested that fetal growth may serve as a sensitive indicator of socioeconomic change. He hypothesizes that many low-weight births are caused by chronic fetal distress resulting from the mother's continued inability to provide nutrients through the placental supply line at the rate necessary for optimal fetal growth. Poverty, nutritional deficiency, disease, adolescent pregnancies, drug abuse, and other adverse conditions tend to lower the maternally-imposed fetal growth constraint, and ultimately the birth weight. Evidence supportive of this hypothesis includes the association of lower socioeconomic conditions with retarded intrauterine development.[9,25]

In summary, birth weight can be considered to be the crucial intervening variable in a causal sequence that leads from the condition of the fetus to perinatal mortality. This feature allows the use of a quantitative, routinely-measured, descriptive variable to measure the many diverse factors known to influence perinatal mortality.

RESEARCH METHODS

The methodology presented here conceptually partitions the variation in unadjusted perinatal mortality rates between hospitals into three components:

1. That resulting from risk differentials in patient populations;
2. That caused by binomial variations;
3. That attributable to differences in medical care.

The concept of using "expected" mortality rates for purposes of adjusting observed rates has long been used in biometry, as for example the common instance of age-adjusted mortality rates. However, the concept has been recently generalized by basing the expected rates on multiple factors.[16,19,23,24] While a multiple logistic regression model may be used to compute the expected rate based on individual patient characteristics, it is not the central feature of the technique. Rather, the essential concept is to identify all those factors which might produce differences in the observed rate independent of the medical care system. Outcomes are then evaluated by comparing observed outcomes with those that would be expected on the basis of the identifiable exogenous patient factors.

Rate Standardization

The outcome measure studied here adjusts for patient risk using a method closely related to the technique of rate standardization. Let $f(1), f(2), \ldots f(m)$ be the fractions of all newborns in a particular hospital falling into m different birth weight groups, and let $r(k)$ be the mortality rate for the k-th birth weight group in a particular hospital. Assume that $F(1), \ldots F(m)$ correspond to the fractions of all newborns in a standard population to be used as a basis for comparison. Similarly let $R(1), R(2), \ldots R(m)$ be the birth weight- specific mortality rates for the standard population. Then the crude rate for the hospital population is

$$r(*) = \sum_k f(k)\, r(k)$$

For the standard population the crude mortality rate is

$$R(*) = \sum_k F(k)\, R(k)$$

The hospital mortality rates can then be weighted by the standard population birth weight characteristics (direct standardization):

$$D = \sum_k F(k)\, r(k)$$

Alternatively, the standard population rates can be weighted by the hospital population birth weight distribution (indirect standardization):

$$I = \sum_k f(k)\, R(k)$$

Using either method, it is possible to standardize the study population rate to obtain either the directly adjusted rate

$$DA = R(*)\, r(*)/D$$

or the indirectly adjusted rate,

$$IA = R(*)\, r(*)/I$$

In each case, ratios $r(*)/D$ and $r(*)/I$ may be considered to be adjustment indexes since the numerator is the actual study rate, and the denominator is an expected rate. For this study the indirectly adjusted rate is preferred to the directly standardized since the $r(k)$'s in the directly standardized rate are subject to considerable sampling error because they are based on relatively small samples for a rare event. On the other hand, the R(k)'s used in the computation of the indirectly standardized rate (I) are usually derived from a much larger standard population. For example, in this study the R(k)'s are based on a total of 1,730,702 births. The r(k)'s, on the other hand, would be based on a ten-year aggregate for individual hospitals, which record totals ranging from a few hundred to approximately 30,000 births, but averaging only about 7,000 births. When individual hospitals are evaluated for single years, the sampling error for the r(k)'s becomes even larger and in fact there are likely to be no perinatal deaths for some birth weight groups.

Observed-Expected Indexes

The measure of effectiveness adopted here is r(*)/I, i.e., the observed rate divided by the indirectly adjusted rate. However, rather than adjusting for a single risk factor such as birth weight (k), multiple risk factors (k, l, . . . , m) are accounted for by:

$$I = \Sigma \ldots \ldots \Sigma \quad f(k, \ldots, l) \quad R(k, \ldots, l)$$
$$k \ldots l$$

The R(k, l, . . . , m)'s, referred to as the Statewide reference rates, are based on a previous study of 1,730,702 births in California from 1966 through 1970. Perinatal mortality rates were tabulated in 250 g birth weight intervals for single births by sex for the total population and for three major ethnic groups. Separate reference rates were also computed by birth weight and sex (but, owing to the smaller sample size, not by ethnic group) for multiple births. The 190 distinct reference perinatal mortality rates which resulted are tabulated in Table 18.1.

Using perinatal mortality rates as measures of hospital performance, the index of medical care effectiveness may be defined as

$$ISPMR = r(*)/I = OBPMR/EXPMR$$

where OBPMR is the observed perinatal mortality rate, EXPMR is the perinatal mortality rate that would be expected given the characteristics of the hospital's population and the standard population mortality rates, and, following terminology previously suggested,[19] ISPMR is the Indirectly Standardized Perinatal Mortality Ratio. Note, however, that the ISPMR index has a reverse meaning in the context of medical care effectiveness or quality: the smaller the index the greater the effectiveness.

The observed perinatal mortality rate is then computed as

$$OBPMR(i) = PDTH(i)/BRTH(i)$$

where BRTH(i) is the total number of births over the sample period and PDTH(i) is the observed number of perinatal deaths, i.e.,

Table 18.1: Reference Perinatal Mortality Rates (per 1,000 Births) Based on 1,730,702 California Births During 1965–1970

Birth Weight (Grams)	Single White Male	Single White Female	Single Spanish Male	Single Spanish Female	Single Black Male	Single Black Female	Single Total Male	Single Total Female	Multiple Total Male	Multiple Total Female
<501	1000.	1000.	1000.	1000.	1000.	1000.	1000.	1000.	1000.	1000.
501–750	984.0	974.1	967.1	963.2	938.0	951.6	970.7	967.4	984.7	974.6
751–1000	923.1	845.3	907.7	836.8	844.2	773.8	903.6	830.6	888.6	805.0
1001–1250	747.7	620.7	759.5	625.9	611.9	503.3	725.2	592.6	650.4	485.3
1251–1500	547.9	441.5	558.7	509.9	420.4	355.7	526.7	432.0	410.3	286.7
1501–1750	376.8	289.0	377.9	293.9	276.6	207.8	358.9	273.8	193.9	126.9
1751–2000	249.9	166.2	236.7	194.3	156.7	109.3	228.2	159.5	92.51	57.29
2001–2250	129.7	85.04	133.2	97.53	89.98	60.09	121.6	81.56	51.19	29.11
2251–2500	65.84	38.10	65.60	38.74	43.25	28.12	60.71	36.00	27.80	19.10
2501–2750	27.33	15.47	27.07	17.15	19.54	13.42	25.33	15.20	14.42	11.04
2751–3000	13.08	8.222	12.92	10.06	10.13	6.414	12.37	8.293	11.82	9.187
3001–3250	8.044	5.487	8.110	6.929	7.949	6.978	7.887	5.294	11.47	10.78
3251–3500	5.629	4.512	6.187	5.570	8.317	5.155	5.886	4.764	7.692	9.709
3501–3750	5.033	4.031	7.123	5.335	7.114	5.678	5.546	4.403	11.56	9.434
3751–4000	4.460	4.159	5.890	7.371	8.668	7.513	5.069	5.108	16.61	16.61
4001–4250	5.400	4.574	9.905	8.978	14.09	12.07	6.852	5.893	67.96	67.96
4251–4500	5.842	5.376	12.29	16.66	15.47	13.72	7.727	8.145	66.66	66.66
>4500	10.97	13.80	27.41	35.49	51.05	46.58	16.34	19.95	263.2	263.2
Unknown	695.2	670.4	603.8	610.6	738.2	698.0	682.3	665.6	785.1	785.1

$$PDTH(i) = X(i, *) = \sum_j X(i, j)$$

where $X(i, j) = 0$ if the j-th newborn survives the perinatal period, and $X(i, j) = 1$ if the j-th newborn dies (in the i-th hospital). Then, given the Statewide reference rates and specific characteristics $(k, \ldots, l)$ for the j-th infant in the i-th hospital, it is possible to find $R(i, j)$. Each $R(i, j)$ is then assigned to the hospital of birth and the expected number of deaths in the i-th hospital computed as

$$EDTH(i) = R(i, *) = \sum_j R(i, j)$$

The medical care effectiveness index is then defined as

$$ISPMR(i) = OBPMR(i)/EXPMR(i) = PDTH(i)/EDTH(i)$$

Because the $X(i, j)$'s are Bernoulli variables with probabilities $R(i, j)$, $PDTH(i)$ will have the associated binomial variance

$$var[PDTH(i)] = \sum_j R(i, j) [1 - R(i, j)]$$

assuming the $X(i, j)$'s are independent events, as indeed they are likely to be. Because $EDTH(i)$'s are based on the standard population rates, it is reasonable to assume either that they are fixed numbers or that their variance is very small compared to $var[PDTH(i)]$. The sample variance for $ISPMR(i)$ then follows directly as

$$var[ISPMR(i)] = var[PDTH(i)]/[EDTH(i)]^2$$

An interesting approximation to the variance of $ISPMR(i)$ is possible when the $R(i, j)$ are all taken to be equally small. Under those conditions it can be shown that

$$var[ISPMR(i)] = 1/EDTH(i)$$

That is, the variance of the effectiveness index is determined largely by the inverse number of expected deaths.

Statistical analyses of the measured quality indexes for the 504 California hospitals took place on two levels. First, the variation of the indexes was tested independently of any hospital characteristics; the primary objective was to determine if the observed differences in the measured indexes could be attributed to an actual underlying variation in the quality of perinatal medical care and not merely to chance. On the second level, the measured indexes were evaluated relative to hospital structural and process features. The purpose of this mode of analysis was to identify those hospital characteristics that were associated with high quality care for purposes of medical care policy and planning.

The chi-square test statistic for the null hypothesis that all hospitals perform equally well is

$$\text{CHISQ} = \sum_i [[\text{PDTH(i)} - \text{EDTH(i)}]]^2/\text{var[PDTH(i)]}$$

Under the null hypothesis PDTH(i) = EDTH(i), the test statistic CHISQ has a chi-square distribution as EDTH(i) becomes large.

For the second level of analysis the Aitken[2] Generalized Least Squares (GLS) estimator was applied. As stated above, 1/EDTH(i) is a reasonable approximation for var[ISPMR(i)] when the OBPMR(i) are uniformly small. Under these conditions the Aitken GLS technique is equivalent to weighted least squares, using the square root of EDTH(i) as weights. This procedure has intuitive appeal since it gives those hospitals having more expected perinatal deaths a greater weight than the smaller hospitals with fewer expected deaths.

DATA SOURCES

The primary data source for the study was the linked vital record file compiled by the California Department of Health. Some selected characteristics of the California file through 1973 are presented in Table 18.2. It is noteworthy that the number of neonatal deaths has declined more rapidly than have fetal deaths. The basic study file consisted of birth certificate information for 3,441,996 live births and 39,407 fetal deaths recorded in California in 1960 and in 1965 through 1973. Added to this is the death certificate information for the 46,437 infants who died during the first year of life. Linkage of the birth and infant death records is believed to be substantially complete with fewer than one percent of infant deaths remaining unmatched. The natality characteristics of this small fraction, many of whom were abandoned newborns, have been estimated. By mutual agreement with other states, copies of death certificates for infants who died out of California were obtained and linked to the birth records.

Table 18.2:   Selected Characteristics of Total Population of California Births

Year	Total Births	Number of Hospitals	Total Fetal Deaths	Total Neonatal Deaths	Total Perinatal Deaths
1960	377,778	459	4,758	6,317	11,075
1965	360,910	527	4,520	5,638	10,158
1966	343,092	545	4,086	5,160	9,246
1967	342,077	535	4,028	4,827	8,855
1968	344,716	448	4,066	4,769	8,835
1969	358,208	443	4,113	4,772	8,885
1970	367,960	438	4,093	4,569	8,622
1971	334,356	434	3,538	3,885	7,423
1972	310,601	427	3,157	3,480	6,637
1973	301,790	433	3,048	3,020	6,068
Total	3,441,448	634	39,407	46,437	85,844

Of the 3,441,996 births studied, 548 were stillbirths weighing less than 500 g with gestations of less than 20 weeks, reducing the total to 3,441,448. Additionally, 21,028 were nonhospital births, and 11,245 were births which occurred in other U.S. states or in foreign countries, further reducing the total file to 3,409,215 records. Finally, 20,543 births occurred in hospitals which could not be identified, leaving a total of 3,388,672 records in 634 hospitals. However, a significant number of the 634 were hospitals without normal maternity services where emergency births occurred or were hospitals with small maternity services that have closed in recent years. Clearly, many of these hospitals having very few deliveries were not representative of hospitals with maternity services. It was decided, therefore, to delete such unrepresentative hospitals by using the arbitrary minimum standard of the presence of at least one bassinet. Because of their extreme characteristics, two additional hospitals were also deleted, leaving 504 hospitals in the basic study sample containing 3,370,338 births.

Selected parental and newborn characteristics were abstracted from each birth-death record and coded onto computer tape. These included birth weight, sex, race, and plurality. Perinatal outcomes, i.e., fetal deaths and neonatal deaths, were also extracted. Additionally, information related to type of delivery (e.g., by cesarean section) and type of hospital ownership was retained. Information concerning hospitals meeting standards for Infant Intensive Care Units was obtained from the Crippled Children Services Section of the California Department of Health. Size of delivery service was measured by the average annual number of deliveries obtained by dividing the total number of deliveries over the sample period by the number of years that a hospital had a viable maternity service. Hospital geographical location, i.e., either urban or nonurban, was determined using the U.S. Bureau of Census definition of what constitutes an "urbanized area."

The secondary source of information describing maternity hospital characteristics was the 1968 National Study of Maternity Care performed by the American College of Obstetricians and Gynecologists (ACOG). A comprehensive questionnaire[3] was mailed to all hospitals in the United States providing maternity services in 1967; a total of 316 California hospitals responded. Although the questionnaire was quite extensive, only a few questions produced high completion rates in areas relevant to the present study. Four hospitals had low rates of completion in several important areas and were therefore dropped from the study, leaving a total of 312 sample hospitals. Abstracted were questions as to whether or not Apgar scores were routinely recorded and whether or not the hospital had a perinatal mortality and morbidity study committee. To obtain an index of specialization, the number of board-certified and other obstetrician-gynecologists was divided by the number of general practitioners and general surgeons. And, as an indicator of the quality of nursing services, the presence of a registered nurse 24 hours a day, 7 days a week was used.

There were generally two classes of independent variables used to analyze the effectiveness index: either continuous or categorical variables. For example, the size of a delivery service as measured by the average annual number of births is clearly a continuous variable. On the other hand, the presence of an infant intensive care unit is a qualitative one; such a dichotomous variable can assume only two arbitrary values and can therefore be represented in a regression as a single binary variable. Other categorical variables, e.g., type of hospital ownership, may have more than one category; i.e., they are polychotomous. If a polychotomous variable has N categories, then it can be represented by N-1 binary variables in a regression equation.

RESULTS

Table 18.3 lists the sample means of the study variables according to their mnemonic names used to facilitate the discussion. The anticipated algebraic sign of the correlation of each study variable with the ISPMR index is indicated in parentheses. The observed first-order correlation coefficients are also reported along with their levels of significance. The validity of the ISPMR index is indicated by the remarkable agreement between the anticipated and observed correlations. As will be discussed later, this result differs markedly from previous studies.

It is clear from Table 18.3 that the characteristics of the ACOG sample and the main study sample are similar in most respects, and hence it is reasonable to assume that the ACOG sample is representative of the larger population of maternity hospitals. Note that the binary variable results are reported in proportions, rather than percentages; e.g., the fraction of hospitals recording Apgar scores in 1968 was 0.7019, or about 70 percent.

As discussed earlier, the statistical analyses were performed on two levels: (1) the variation in the effectiveness indexes was tested independently of any hospital characteristics, and (2) the indexes were evaluated relative to the hospital characteristics listed in Table 18.3. On level 1, the primary objective was to ascertain whether or not the observed variation in the measured indexes could be attributed to actual variation in the "true" efficacy of perinatal medical care between hospitals and not simply to sampling error. If it could be established that there were actual variations in the impact of perinatal medical care between hospitals, then the extent of variation was also of interest. On level 2, the measured effectiveness indexes were evaluated relative to hospital structural and process features using multiple regression analysis. In that phase the purpose of the analysis was to identify those hospital characteristics that were associated with increased efficacy in preventing perinatal deaths.

Testing for Differences in the Effectiveness of Perinatal Medical Care

Whereas the unadjusted perinatal mortality rates spanned a 16-fold range (from 5.4 to 88.6 per 1000) the measured ISPMR index varied over an 8-fold range

Table 18.3: Definition of Study Variables and Descriptive Statistics for Main and ACOG Samples

Variable Mnemonic Name	Description	ACOG Mean (N=312)	Main Mean (N=504)	Anticipated Correlation with ISPMR	Observed Correlation with ISPMR (N=312)	PROB>|R| Under HO: RHO=0 (N=312)
APGAR	Routine APGAR score: 1—Yes, 0—No	0.7019	...	(—)	−0.3132	0.0001
BIRTHS	Births (in 1000s) per annum	0.8261	0.7210	(—)	−0.3628	0.0001
BLACK	Per cent Black deliveries	6.3555	6.7403	(+)	−0.0960	0.0906
CSECTION	Per cent Cesarean sections	6.000	5.9935	(—)	−0.2004	0.0004
EXPMR	Expected perinatal mortality rate	23.8274	24.3216	...	−0.0610	0.2828
FEDERAL	Federal government ownership: 1—Yes, 0—No	0.0609	0.0476	...	−0.0796	0.1606
KAISER	Kaiser Foundation ownership: 1—Yes, 0—No	0.0352	0.0278	...	−0.0892	0.1158
LOCAL	Local government ownership: 1—Yes, 0—No	0.2500	0.2282	(+)	+0.1136	0.0450
MDSCHOOL	Medical school affiliation: 1—Yes, 0—No	0.0801	0.0615	(—)	−0.1610	0.0044
NICU	Neonatal intensive care unit: 1—Yes, 0—No	0.0449	0.0317	(—)	−0.1227	0.0302
NPROFIT	Nonprofit ownership: 1—Yes, 0—No	0.4200	0.4028	(—)	−0.1950	0.0005
OBPMR	Observed perinatal mortality rate	24.8978	26.0922	...	+0.6233	0.0001
PROFIT	For-profit ownership: 1—Yes, 0—No	0.2211	0.2817	(+)	+0.2126	0.0002
RNHRS	RN on duty 24 hrs., 7 days: 1—Yes, 0—No	0.7244	...	(—)	−0.1898	0.0008
SPANISH	Per cent Spanish surname deliveries	20.5114	19.2916	(+)	+0.2399	0.0001
SPECIAL	Specialist-to-generalist ratio	0.9542	...	(—)	−0.1677	0.0030
STUDYCOM	Perinatal study committee: 1—Yes, 0—No	0.4360	...	(—)	−0.2588	0.0001
TEENAGE	Per cent teenage (<20) deliveries	19.0367	18.8566	(+)	+0.1776	0.0016
URBAN	Urban hospital location: 1—Yes, 0—No	0.6827	0.6786	(—)	−0.2949	0.0001
WHITE	Per cent White non-Spanish deliveries	69.2837	70.2127	(—)	−0.1339	0.0180

(from .46 to 3.74) for the main study sample of 504 hospitals. For comparison, the expected perinatal mortality rates spanned a 6-fold range from 11.8 to 67.3 per 1000. It appears, therefore, that there are considerable differences in the quality of obstetric and newborn care in California hospitals even after adjusting for hospital variations in patient risk. However, a portion of the variation may be attributed to binomial variation, and a chi-square statistic should be used to test the null hypothesis that there are no differences in the "true" ISPMR indexes. The CHISQ statistic given above had a computed value of 1,625 for the sample of 504 hospitals. Therefore, the null hypothesis must be rejected ($p < .0001$), and it must be concluded that a significant proportion of the observed 8-fold difference in the empirical effectiveness indexes is attributable to actual differentials in the quality of perinatal medical care in California hospitals.

An estimate of the variance of the "true" effectiveness indexes can be obtained by taking the difference between the sample variance for the measured ISPMR indexes and the mean variance attributable to the Bernoulli process. The variance estimate is than

$$\text{var}[I(i)] = \text{SmplVar}[\text{ISPMR}(i)] - 1/N \sum_i \text{var}[\text{ISPMR}(i)]$$

$$\text{var}[I(i)] = 0.0642 - (12.9/504) = 0.0642 - 0.0256 \times 0.0386$$

where the $I(i)$ are the true ISPMR indexes. Here we see that about 40 percent (.0256/.0642) of the observed variance in the measured ISPMR's can be attributed to sampling error. Taking the square root of $\text{var}[I(i)]$ above yields a standard deviation in the true ISPMR's of about 0.2. We therefore conclude that approximately 68 percent of the sample hospitals have ISPMR indexes that lie inside the 0.8 to 1.2 interval, i.e., plus or minus one standard deviation. Alternatively, about 95 percent have ISPMR indexes within the 0.6 to 1.4 range, i.e., plus or minus 2 standard deviations. Thus, the 8-fold range in the observed ISPMR's for all the sample hospitals reduces to slightly over a two-fold (1.4/.6 = 2.33) range for the true ISPMR's in 95 percent of the sample hospitals. As another alternative measure, a Bayesian procedure,[19] designed to adjust the observed ISPMR indexes for their relative reliability, was applied. The resultant index ranged from .77 to 1.42, again an approximate factor of two.

Multiple Regression Models

Generalized least squares regression techniques were applied to the data to isolate the independent effects of the intercorrelated hospital characteristic variables listed in Table 18.3. A stepwise procedure[5] selected those variables which contributed most in explaining the variation in the ISPMR index. Only those variables meeting the prespecified "significance level of entry" of $p<.05$ were included in the models.

The main sample of 504 hospitals was used to construct the first regression model using ISPMR as the dependent variable. In addition to the independent variables described in Table 18.3, the group of variables used in the stepwise procedure included BIRTH—SQ, defined as the square of the annual number of births (BIRTHS). This variable was used to test for the presence of nonlinear scale effects. From the results in Table 18.4 the effectiveness of perinatal care was found to be higher in larger hospitals and in hospitals performing relatively more cesaren sections. Conversely, the effectiveness index was lower in hospitals serving larger proportions of Spanish-surnamed mothers, and in private proprietary hospitals. Significant nonlinear scale effects were observed with a "U-shaped" curve reaching a minimum at 2,850 annual births. That is, the risk-adjusted perinatal mortality rate decreased with the size of delivery service until 2,850 births, then increased thereafter. This estimate is in good agreement with various recommendations for the regional development of perinatal care,[8,15] which call for 2,000 annual deliveries in community perinatal care facilities (Level II), and for 2,000 + births in regional perinatal care centers (Level III).

The regression results for the smaller but more descriptive ACOG sample are reported in Table 18.5. The model is consistent with that derived from the main sample in that hospital size, percentage Spanish surnames, percentage cesarean sections, and for-profit ownership again have statistically significant partial correlations with the effectiveness index. Additionally, the risk-adjusted mortality rates are lower in urban hospitals, in hospitals having larger specialist-to-generalist ratios, and in hospitals routinely recording Apgar scores in 1968. Not only does the model seem quite plausible, but it also reveals some unforeseen factors of importance related to the effectiveness of perinatal care. For example, while it is not surprising that the effectiveness of care is higher in large hospitals and in those routinely recording Apgar scores, the magnitude of the effect of the cesarean section rate is unexpected. Similarly, the higher risk-adjusted mortality rates, holding other factors constant, in proprietary hospitals and in hospitals serving larger proportions of Spanish-surnamed mothers are notable policy-related results.

Table 18.4: Stepwise GLS Regressions Using 1960, 1965–1973 California Vital Record Data: Dependent Variable Is ISPMR = Indirectly Standardized Perinatal Mortality Ratio (N = 504)

Step	Variable	(Expected Sign)	B Value	Std. Error	F	Prob>F	R-Square
0	CONSTANT	...	1.12426	0.01874	3597.58	0.0001	...
1	BIRTHS	(−)	−0.08844	0.01693	27.28	0.0001	0.4515
2	SPANISH	(+)	+0.00193	0.00026	51.33	0.0001	0.5038
3	CSECTION	(−)	−0.01332	0.00211	39.58	0.0001	0.5442
4	BIRTH SQ	(+)	+0.01548	0.00435	12.67	0.0004	0.5581
5	PROFIT	(+)	+0.02597	0.01291	4.05	0.0448	0.5606

Table 18.5:   Stepwise GLS Regressions Using 1960, 1965–1973 Vital Record Data Linked with 1968 ACOG Data: Dependent Variable Is ISPMR = Indirectly Standardized Perinatal Mortality Ratio (N = 312)

Step	Variable	(Expected Sign)	B Value	Std. Error	F	Prob>F	R-Square
0	CONSTANT	...	1.11729	0.02276	2409.61	0.0001	...
1	BIRTHS	(−)	−0.02005	0.00578	12.03	0.0006	0.3220
2	SPANISH	(+)	+0.00198	0.00030	41.32	0.0001	0.4119
3	CSECTION	(−)	−0.01083	0.00277	15.18	0.0001	0.4620
4	APGAR	(−)	−0.02675	0.01332	4.03	0.0456	0.4720
5	SPECIAL	(−)	−0.05524	0.02414	5.24	0.0228	0.4782
6	URBAN	(−)	−0.04645	0.01801	6.65	0.0104	0.4849
7	PROFIT	(+)	+0.03904	0.01591	6.02	0.0147	0.4932

We observe that the BIRTH—SQ term did not enter into the stepwise model derived from the ACOG sample. This, coupled with the significant negative sign for BIRTHS in Table 18.5, indicates that there is an increasing effectiveness of perinatal care throughout the measurable range of scale. In order to test the scale effects more completely with the ACOG sample, both BIRTHS and BIRTH—SQ were "forced" into the regression equation before the stepwise procedure began. The results were virtually identical to those in Table 18.5 except that large correlations between BIRTHS, BIRTH—SQ, and other independent variables gave rise to multicollinearity so that the standard errors for the two scale terms were inflated. Nonetheless, the values of the estimated coefficients were reasonable and the maximum effectiveness was computed to lie in the vicinity of 5,000 annual births. This value is considerably beyond the range of the largest hospital in the sample which had 3,800 births. These and other results suggest that as the model becomes more completely specified, the scale effect becomes more linear and of lesser importance. That is, as more of the specialized input factors associated with large hospitals are identified and added to the model, the effect of scale alone diminishes in its relative importance.

Because the regression models were successful in explaining more than one-half the GLS variance in the effectiveness index, it is of interest to separate the ISPMR index into its two components: the observed (OBPMR) and the expected (EXPMR) perinatal mortality rates. The regression equation may then be respecified to take the observed rate as the dependent variable with the expected rate as a predictor. Under this specification the sample variance for the dependent variable becomes

$$\text{var}[OBPMR(i)] \ = \ \text{var}[PDTH(i)]/BRTH(i)^2$$

When the GLS stepwise procedure was applied to both the main and the ACOG samples using OBPMR as the dependent variable, regression models identical to those described earlier were selected. The results for the ACOG sample are shown in Table 18.6. Here we see that 82 percent of the (GLS) variance in the observed perinatal mortality rates can be explained using the regression model.* Not surprisingly, the expected perinatal mortality rate is the dominant variable, accounting by itself for 72 percent of the weighted variance. Moreover, the estimated regression coefficient for EXPMR does not differ significantly from unity, thus revealing a one-to-one correspondence between the expected and observed rates. That is, holding other things constant, a one percent increase in the expected rate is, on the average, associated with a one percent increase in the observed rate.

The results in Table 18.6 also suggest that, again holding all else constant, urban hospitals have a perinatal mortality rate that is on the average about one per 1,000 lower than their nonurban equivalents; that proprietary hospitals have mortality rates that are almost one per 1,000 higher compared with other types of ownership; and that hospitals routinely recording Apgar scores in (1968) have mortality rates about one-half per 1,000 less than those that did not. The mean sample value for the cesarean section rate was 6 percent, so that the average effect of the CSECTION variable was to lower the observed rate by about 1.3 deaths per 1,000. It would be incorrect, however, to attribute this effect solely to the efficacy of the cesarean procedure, since hospitals having larger proportions of cesarean deliveries are also likely to be characterized by specialized forms of personnel and equipment which might not be captured by the regression model.

Because the average California hospital had about 20 percent Spanish-surname births, the mean effect of the SPANISH variable was to increase the observed rate by about 0.9 deaths per 1,000. Also, the average hospital in

Table 18.6: Stepwise GLS Regressions Using 1960, 1965–1973 Vital Record Data Linked with 1968 ACOG Data: Dependent Variable Is OBPMR = Observed Perinatal Mortality Ratio (N = 312)

Step	Variable	(Expected Sign)	B Value	Std. Error	F	Prob>F	R-Square
0	CONSTANT	...	1.29044	0.87500	2.17	0.1413	...
1	EXPMR	(+)	+1.05462	0.03173	1104.09	0.0001	0.7230
2	BIRTHS	(−)	−0.49328	0.14659	11.32	0.0009	0.7631
3	SPANISH	(+)	+0.04296	0.00768	31.24	0.0001	0.7911
4	CSECTION	(−)	−0.22084	0.06650	11.03	0.0010	0.8061
5	SPECIAL	(−)	−0.05520	0.01870	8.71	0.0034	0.8100
6	URBAN	(−)	−1.07307	0.41941	6.55	0.0110	0.8131
7	PROFIT	(+)	+0.91420	0.37995	5.79	0.0167	0.8164
8	APGAR	(−)	−0.60833	0.31185	3.81	0.0520	0.8181

*The reader should be aware that this value is computed according to the GLS goodness of fit criterion (R-square) given by Buse.[7] When ordinary least squares (OLS) is applied the model explains at least 60 percent of the variance. This finding is consistent with the estimate reported above wherein 40 percent of the observed variance in the ISPMR's can be attributed to sampling error.

California has almost 800 births per year; thus the mean scale effect amounts to about 0.4 deaths per 1,000. It is interesting to note, however, that more than one-half of California maternity hospitals have fewer than 500 annual births. The regression estimates suggest that an increased perinatal mortality rate of about 0.8 per 1,000 can be attributed to size alone for this group compared with an institution having 2,000 + annual deliveries. Of course larger values for such variables as APGAR, CSECTION, and SPECIAL would increase the estimated difference in mean rates between small and large hospitals. The specialist-generalist ratio appears to have an impact on perinatal mortality which is statistically significant, but rather small in magnitude. However, its observed range was 0–55 with a mean of about unity and a standard deviation of about 4. If we take 0 to 10 as a reasonable range, the impact of that variable on the observed rate is about 0.5 per 1,000.

In summary, with the exception of EXPMR, the variables selected by the stepwise regression procedure have independent effects on observed perinatal mortality rates in the order of 0.5 to 1.5 per 1,000 births. These magnitudes are in basic agreement with a recent study[13] which suggests that electronic fetal monitoring has a benefit of about 1 to 2 lives per 1,000. The absolute effect of the expected perinatal mortality rate is much higher. For the main sample the mean for EXPMR was about 24 per 1,000; hence with the observed regression coefficient near unity, the average contribution of EXPMR was about 24 per 1,000. Further, since the range in EXPMR varied from 12 to 67 per 1,000, impact of the expected rate on the observed rate far outweighs the individual effects of the hospital-related factors.

DISCUSSION

The extent to which hospital characteristics influence perinatal mortality rates has not been adequately studied in the past. Early studies concentrated on international differences in infant mortality with diverse, sometimes paradoxical findings. Comparative studies using individual hospitals have attempted to evaluate specific programs and have rarely produced results that are applicable to large populations of hospitals and patients. In general, there is an increasing degree of skepticism regarding the relationship between medical care services and patient outcomes. For example, a recent study[14] making comparisons between an inner-city and a suburban hospital concluded that health care services are "peripheral" to the health of the community, and that socioeconomic differences form the central aspect of levels of health status.

Such views are reinforced by studies which report statistically weak linkages between outcomes and more traditional process and structural measures of the quality of medical care.[12] The lack of correlations have been reported not only for adults but for newborn patients as well. Ashford et al.[4] analyzed 161 geographic units in Great Britain using perinatal mortality rates adjusted for birth weights less than 2,501 g. Only about one-third of the variance in the adjusted rates could be accounted for with 88 "descriptive" variables, and those variables directly related to maternity services had little explanatory power. Tokuhata et al.,[22] also using linked vital record data, observed positive correlations between adjusted perinatal mortality rates and such traditional indicators of quality as medical residency and internship programs, medical school, and a blood bank. Birth weight, income, ethnicity, and other factors were adjusted for using the Mantel-Haenzel technique, yet a number of the observed correlations were opposite from expectations.

With one minor exception, the observed first-order correlations between the ISPMR index and the structural and process measures of medical care were statistically significant and had the anticipated algebraic signs (Table 18.3). The relative success reported here can be attributed to three principal attributes of the study. First, because there is a large variation in perinatal mortality as a function of birth weight, it is essential that birth weight be classified into more than the two traditional categories of "normal" ($>2,500$ g) and "premature" ($<2,501$g). In this study 250 g intervals were used, and other newborn factors were accounted for as well. Second, attention was devoted to the statistical methodology with an emphasis on accounting for the sampling error in the observed indexes. And lastly, a very large population was chosen so as to minimize the magnitude of the sampling errors.

While this study has demonstrated that the expected perinatal mortality rate, which is determined largely by factors outside the direct control of hospitals, has by far the largest impact on observed perinatal death rates, it has also shown that a number of hospital characteristics, which may be subject to control by regulatory agencies, have significant marginal impacts on risk-adjusted outcomes. That is, in spite of strong link between perinatal mortality and numerous intervening factors such as nutrition, genetics, and environment, it *is* possible to measure the marginal effectiveness of perinatal medical care.

CONCLUSIONS

After accounting for newborn risk differentials between hospitals as well as variations resulting from sampling error, we conclude that there remains a variation in the efficacy of perinatal medical care that spans an approximate range of two. That is, the medical care delivered to mothers and newborns appears to be as much as twice as effective in lowering perinatal mortality for the highest versus lowest ranked hospitals, even after accounting for a variety of factors beyond their direct control. That disparity, though not extreme, is nonetheless one which should not be dismissed, especially in view of the patterns of variation which were revealed by the multiple regression analysis. Of particular importance was the higher mortality rates, holding other factors constant, in hospitals with a larger fraction of Spanish-surnamed deliveries. Also, it is likely that improvements in the organization of perinatal health services in California could be made in view of the large number of urban hospitals having small delivery services.

Since the size of delivery service has been shown to be correlated positively with the effectiveness of perinatal care, programs emphasizing the development of regionalized perinatal care could make significant contributions toward lowering perinatal mortality rates.

Although this study has demonstrated that it is possible to measure the effectiveness of perinatal care using a large aggregate of births for many hospitals, the practical value of the technique lies in similar evaluations over shorter time intervals. The next logical step should therefore be to study individual hospitals and other units of observation using more recent data. That issue was not addressed here since it was desirable to minimize the amount of binomial variation in order to analyze the observed-expected index under optimal conditions; hence large numbers of births were called for. Because the sampling error associated with small hospitals for a single year is likely to be excessive, it may be necessary to aggregate across geographic regions for purposes of contemporary policy-relevant inferences. Also, in order to minimize the error in computing the expected rates, additional maternal and newborn factors such as maternal age and length of gestation should probably be accounted for.

Since it is unrealistic to expect all hospitals to perform equally well regardless of their many diverse characteristics, future work might also continue the development of the regression model to predict observed perinatal mortality rates based on expected rates as well as such intrinsic hospital characteristics as size, location, and the presence of specialized equipment and personnel. A quantitative model could then be used to identify those hospitals or regions which are significantly better or worse than the norm, after adjusting not only for patient risk, but also for hospital characteristics. Finally, because of the increasing emphasis on comprehensive and preventive care, birth weight must ultimately be considered to be a factor which is influenced by the medical care system. Therefore, in order to implement improved evaluation strategies we need a more thorough understanding of the social, economic, environmental, biological and medical determinants of birth weight.

ACKNOWLEDGMENTS

The author wishes to acknowledge the participation in the research project of George C. Cunningham, M.D., Steve Edison, B.A., Warren E. Hawes, M.D., Carol Madore, M.A., Frank Norris, M.A., and Michiko Tashiro, M.S. of the California Department of Health. The author is also indebted to Robert H. Brook, M.D., Alfred C. Hexter, Ph.D., Joel C. Kleinman, Ph.D., Lawrence L. Levin, Ph.D., Charles M. Wylie, M.D., and two anonymous reviewers for their constructive comments.

REFERENCES

1. Abernathy, J. R., Greenberg, B. G., and Donnelly, J. R.: Application of discriminant functions in perinatal death and survival. Am. J. Obstet. Gynecol. 95: 860, 1967.
2. Aitken, A. C.: On least squares and linear combinations of observations. Proc. Roy. Soc. Edinb. 55: 42, 1934.

3. American College of Obstetricians and Gynecologists: Committee on Maternal Health: National Study of Maternity Care Survey of Obstetric Practice and Associated Services in Hospitals in the U.S., 1970.
4. Ashford, J. R., Read, K. L. Q., and Riley, V. C.: An analysis of variations in perinatal mortality amongst local authorities in England and Wales. Int. J. Epidemiol. 2: 31, 1973.
5. Barr, A. J., Goodnight, J. H., Sall, J. P., and Helwig, J. T.: A User's Guide to SAS76. Raleigh, SAS Institute, 1976, p. 251.
6. Brook, R. H., et al.: Assessing the quality of medical care using outcome measures: An overview of the method. Med. Care 15 (Suppl): 1, 1977.
7. Buse, A.: Goodness of fit in generalized least squares estimation. Am. Stat. 27: 106, 1973.
8. Committee on Perinatal Health: Toward Improving The Outcome of Pregnancy. White Plains, N.Y., The National Foundation—March of Dimes, 1976.
9. Gruenwald, P.: Fetal growth as an indicator of socioeconomic change. Public Health Rep. 83: 867, 1968.
10. Kessner, D. M., Kalk, C. E., Singer, J., and Schlesinger, E. R.: Infant Death: An Analysis by Maternal Risk and Health Care. Washington, D.C., Institute of Medicine, 1973.
11. Lane, D. S. and Kelman, H. R.: Assessment of maternal care quality: Conceptual and methodologic issues. Med. Care 13: 791, 1975.
12. Nobrega, F. T., Morrow, G. W., Smoldt, R. K., and Offord, K. P.: Quality assessment in hypertension: Analysis of process and outcome methods. N. Engl. J. Med. 296: 145, 1977.
13. Paul, R. H. and Hon, E. H.: Clinical fetal monitoring. V. Effect on perinatal outcome. Am. J. Obstet. Gynecol. 118: 529, 1974.
14. Reeves, B. D., McCue, S., Wagner, A., and McElin, T. W.: A perspective of peripheral care. Ill. Med. J. 145: 34, 1974.
15. Ryan, G. M., Jr.: Toward improving the outcome of pregnancy. J. Obstet. Gynecol. 46: 375, 1975.
16. Scott, W. R., Forrest, W. H., and Brown, B. W.: Hospital structure and postoperative mortality and morbidity: Preliminary findings from a survey of 17 hospitals. Inquiry 13 (Suppl): 72, 1976.
17. Shah, F. K. and Abbey, W.: Effects of some factors on neonatal and postneonatal mortality. Milbank Mem. Fund Q. 49: 33, 1971.
18. Shapiro, S.: Influence of birthweight, sex, and plurality on neonatal loss in the United States. Am. J. Public Health 44: 1142, 1954.
19. Stanford Center For Health Care Research: Study of Institutional Differences in Postoperative Mortality, Washington, D.C.: National Academy of Sciences (PB-250-940-LK, Springfield, VA, National Technical Information Service), 1974.
20. Stanford Center For Health Care Research: Comparisons of hospitals with regard to outcomes of surgery. Health Serv. Res. 11: 112, 1976.
21. Susser, M., Marolla, F. A., and Fleiss, J.: Birth weight, fetal age, and perinatal mortality. Am. J. Epidemiol. 96: 197, 1972.
22. Tokuhata, G. K., Colfesh, V. G., Mann, K., and Digon, E.: Hospital and related characteristics associated with perinatal mortality. Am. J. Pub. Health 63: 227, 1973.
23. Williams, R. L.: Outcome-Based Measurements Of Medical Care Output: The Case Of Maternal And Infant Health, unpublished Ph.D. thesis, University of California, Santa Barbara, 1974.
24. ———: Explaining a health care paradox. Policy Sci. 6: 91, 1975.
25. ———: Intrauterine growth curves: Intra- and international comparisons with different ethnic groups in California. Prev. Med. 4: 163, 1975.

Chapter 19

Problems with Small Numbers

The study that follows highlights an important distinction between outcome studies that assess hospital structural characteristics, such as volumes, and outcome studies that attempt to assess individual hospital performance. Because many hospitals have relatively few patients in a particular diagnostic or procedure category, the problem of small numbers coupled with a poor-outcome rate in the range of 0.01 percent to 5 percent may preclude confident identification of either high or low outliers. Luft and Hunt demonstrated this problem using the example of cardiac catheterization, which is generally a low-risk procedure, and which has diffused widely among hospitals. In spite of this, volumes are rather high; only a fifth of hospitals offering the procedure had 200 or fewer cardiac catheterization patients.

Luft and Hunt first demonstrated that there was a significant correlation between the log of volume and inpatient mortality. This relationship could also be observed in the distributions of hospital outcomes within volume categories. Four hospitals with very low volumes had outcomes that were significantly worse than expected and none had outcomes that were better than expected, although less than one of each would be expected by chance. In contrast, with somewhat fewer hospitals in the group with very high volumes, five had significantly better than expected outcomes and three were significantly worse.

Although low-volume hospitals are correlated with poorer outcomes, it is difficult to identify any one hospital as having significantly better or worse outcomes. In fact, it is statistically impossible for a low-volume hospital to perform significantly better than average, because a perfect outcome rate—that is, no deaths—is well within the usual statistical confidence limits when the expected number of deaths is low, as is usually the case with low-volume hospitals. In high-volume settings, however, the confidence intervals become much more narrow, making it easier to detect hospitals with results that may differ from the expected. In a similar fashion, Williams (1979) explored the variability among hospitals and found that the variance in the indirectly standardized mortality rate is approximately equal to the inverse of the number of expected deaths.[1]

There are two basic approaches to monitoring individual hospital outcomes using routinely available data. The first is to group large numbers of patients across widely varying procedures and diagnoses, including enough risk factors to account for differences in case mix. Statistical problems arising from small numbers are avoided, but identifying a hospital as an outlier gives no clue as to the types of patients or services in which the "poor results" are concentrated. The second approach is to focus on a specific group of patients within a narrowly defined procedure or diagnosis and then accept the reality that confidence intervals will be much wider. This method has the political problem of allowing very widely divergent mortality rates to be considered "acceptable" because they are not outside the statistical confidence intervals.

With both approaches, it is important to remember that chance variability will often account for apparently poor results, and it is impossible to determine from the available data whether an outlier hospital is a true or chance outlier. One must examine more detailed medical records data to determine whether the hospital actually provided poor-quality care (DuBois, Brook, and Rogers 1987). When volume-outcome studies are done, however, the focus of attention is on the patterns of outcomes, not the detection of individual hospitals, so the task is much easier.

NOTE

1. The study by Williams (1979) is reprinted in Chapter 18 of this volume.

Evaluating Individual Hospital Quality through Outcome Statistics

Harold S. Luft
Sandra S. Hunt

The quality of care in hospitals has traditionally been evaluated through the review of individual cases. While such an approach allows for the consideration of the clinical complexity presented by each patient, case review is time-consuming and expensive and does not allow a broad overview of the patterns of care across a large number of patients. The development of computerized case abstract files makes it possible to examine selected information for not only all patients in a particular hospital, but also from large numbers of hospitals. Several abstracting services, such as the Commission on Professional and Hospital Activities (CPHA) and McAuto, collect data from over 1,000 hospitals; the peer review organizations (PROs) will be collecting data on all Medicare patients; and some states, such as California, New York, Massachusetts, and Maryland, have mandatory collection of data on all discharges.

Routinely collected case abstract data have proved invaluable for certain types of research that focus on patterns of performance across hospitals. For example, a growing body of research indicates that patient outcomes are better, using both measures of morbidity and mortality, in hospitals having higher volumes of patients with the particular procedure or diagnosis.[1-7] This observation has led to the suggestion that policies be developed to encourage patients to be treated in hospitals with high volumes. Not all high-volume hospitals have good outcomes, however, so it will be necessary to identify particular hospitals with better than average performance. Preferred provider organizations and Medicaid programs such as California's have already established contracts with selected hospitals and channel their enrollees toward those hospitals.[8] To date, these contracts have not focused on patient outcomes, but quality has been at least a secondary consideration. Even without active efforts to encourage regionalization, case abstract data can be used to provide consumers with uniform data on hospital outcomes. The Department of Health and Human Services has announced that the PRO data on hospital-specific outcomes for Medicare patients must be made publicly available (*New York Times*, April 16, 1985, sect II, p 20). There have already been controversial instances in which similar data have been

Journal of the American Medical Association 255, no. 20 (1986): 2780–84. Copyright 1986, American Medical Association. Reprinted with permission.

used in public settings to criticize specific hospitals and physicians for allegedly poor outcomes[9,10] (*Washington Post*, Aug 13, 1982, p. 1; *Los Angeles Times*, March 12, 1982, p 1).

While case abstract data may be adequate for research on outcomes across a large number of hospitals, and highly significant statistical relationships can be recognized, such data are often inadequate for the identification of individual hospitals as having particularly good or poor outcomes. One reason is the inherent variability in outcomes across patients even with similar diagnoses and treatments, coupled with the relatively low rate of adverse outcomes and small numbers of patients with a particular diagnosis or procedure seen in any one hospital. When hundreds of hospitals and thousands of patients can be included in the study, much of the random variation can be ignored as unexplained "noise." When the focus is just on outcomes in hospital A, however, much of what is seen is probably random variation. To illustrate this problem, this article utilizes case abstract data for patients undergoing cardiac catheterization in 1982 in 151 hospitals. The in-hospital death rate for these patients is about 1%, a figure about in the middle of the range for procedures and diagnoses. The number of patients undergoing catheterization in particular hospitals is relatively high, reducing the problem of statistical variation and making our presentation of the problems somewhat conservative. It will be shown that, while a strong inverse relation exists between mortality and volume for these patients, the identification of hospitals with significantly better or worse than average outcomes is quite difficult. The last part of the article discusses the application of the approach to categories of patients with varying volumes and rates of adverse outcomes.

METHODS

The data for this study were derived from the Professional Activity Studies of the CPHA of Ann Arbor, Mich. All 757 hospitals that subscribed to the system for the entire year of 1982 and that were also respondents to a national Survey of Specialized Clinical Services (SSCS)were included. Only 151 of the 757 hospitals in our sample reported having a cardiac catheterization laboratory, and we excluded hospitals reporting catheterizations without having a laboratory. (The 1982 SSCS was sent to all US community hospitals and had a response rate of 66%. While small hospitals were somewhat less likely to respond to the SSCS, there were no other significant response biases.)

Patient records were excluded at the outset if data were missing on age, sex, discharge status, or length of stay. All data were aggregated to the hospital level, and identifiers were removed by the CPHA. DIfferences in case mix across hospitals were measured by developing a risk-factor matrix based on characteristics known to be associated with differential mortality rates. There were 12 cells (age 35 to 49, 50 to 64, and more than 64 years, dysrhythmia [*International Classification of Diseases, Ninth Revision (ICD-9)* 427], heart failure [*ICD-9*

428], any other single diagnosis [such as renal failure], and any multiple diagnoses). Patients were allocated to the appropriate cells, and cell-specific death rates were calculated. An expected death rate for each hospital was derived by summing over all cells the national cell-specific death rate times the proportion of patients in the hospital falling into each cell. This indirectly standardized mortality rate, or expected death rate, is what would be anticipated if the hospital achieved outcomes equivalent to the national average within each cell, adjusting for differences in case mix at the hospital level. Expected death rates were calculated for groups of hospitals in an analogous way.

Hospitals were grouped into volume categories according to the number of patients seen in a year within a procedure category. The cutoff levels for each category were determined after examining the distribution of hospitals by volume. Groups were formed with attention to having a reasonable number of patients in each category, and break points were designed to reflect natural patterns in the distribution. Outcome differences were not considered in the formation of groups. The volume categories were one to 200, 201 to 400, 401 to 500, 501 to 750, and more than 750 patients per year.

Analysis of the relation between volume and outcome used regression for the evaluation of trends. The binomial distribution was used for the examination of individual hospital outcomes.

RESULTS

There was a highly significant inverse relation between the in-hospital mortality rate, adjusting for case mix, and the number of patients undergoing catheterization in a hospital. The regression of the difference between actual and expected death rates on the log of volume of patients undergoing catheterization yielded a coefficient of $-.013$, with a P value of .0014. The log form captured the curvilinear relation, with substantially higher mortality rates observed at very low values. An inverse relation between volume and outcome for coronary arteriography was first reported by Adams et al in 1973.[11] While the causal relationship is still in dispute—that is, does higher volume lead to better outcomes or do better outcomes attract higher volumes—this does not affect the issue at hand.[1,2,5,12-15] The question posed in this article is whether such data can be used to identify particular hospitals as having significantly better or worse than average outcomes.

The binomial distribution was used to determine the likelihood that the number of observed deaths came from a distribution with a mean death rate equal to the expected rate in that hospital. For individual hospitals, the combination of low probabilities of death and low volumes means that one often expects to observe zero deaths. It is really the case that we have no useful information about how well the hospital is performing. In Table 19.1, only two hospitals met this criteria and were excluded. They had one and two patients, but the observance of no deaths conveys almost no information. (Both these hospitals reported having catheterization laboratories, although it is possible they began operation only at the end of the year.) The next two lowest-volume hospitals had 13 and 52 patients, with seven and three deaths, respectively, which was significantly worse than would be expected by chance.

Not surprisingly, there was substantial variability of performance within volume categories, but most hospitals were found in the center of the table, with probability values between .10 and .90, indicating that it would be inappropriate to identify them as being better or worse than average based solely on these outcome data. On the other hand, more hospitals appeared in the extreme categories than would be expected purely by chance, suggesting that some hospitals, in fact, have significantly better or worse outcomes. Among the 31 very-low-volume hospitals, four had death rates greater than what would be expected 97.5% of the time.

In contrast, none of the very-low-volume hospitals exhibited better than expected performance at usual levels of statistical significance. However, before one assumes that low-volume catheterization units cannot have better than average outcomes, one must recognize that the nature of the binomial distribution makes it an impossibility for such hospitals to record performances significantly better than expected. With a death rate of 1%, and with the maximum number of patients for this category (200), there would be only 2.0 deaths per year if the hospital's performance was just average, and we would expect to observe zero deaths about 14% of the time just due to random variation. Since fewer than zero deaths cannot be observed, it is impossible without more data to reliably identify low-volume hospitals as having better than average performance for patients with a low mortality rate.

In the intermediate-volume categories for cardiac catheterization, an occasional hospital was identified as having a better than expected outcome, but it is important to recall that some such observations occur by chance. On the other hand, five of the 25 very-high-volume hospitals had much better than expected performance. (The probability value of .025 means that fewer than one hospital $[25 \times .025 = .625]$ will, on average, present such good results merely by chance.) Yet, the fact that three very-high-volume hospitals had substantially worse than expected performance suggests that volume does not guarantee success.

The use of hospital-specific probabilities means that we can narrow our focus from all 151 hospitals to the 23 with results outside the .025 to .975 range or the 34 outside the .05 to .95 range. This does not mean that all hospitals with outcomes within the confidence interval are truly average performers, but that if one had to choose just a few hospitals for detailed review, it is the outliers that might best be put at the top of the list. Thus, one should view the finding of significantly "better" or "worse" than expected performance not as a final classification, but as a yellow flag that warrants investigation. As an example, Table 19.2 presents some characteristics of illustrative hospitals with significantly

Table 19.1: Distribution of Hospitals by Results for Patients Undergoing Cardiac Catheterization

Probability That Observed Outcomes Are What Would Be Expected Given Case Mix*	Volume (Patients/Year)					
	Very Low (1–200)	Low (201–400)	Medium (401–500)	High (501–750)	Very High (>750)	Total
Outcomes much better than expected						
<.025	0	1	1	1	5	8
.025–.050	0	1	1	0	3	5
.051–.100	1	3	1	2	2	9
.101–.500	11	22	9	11	8	61
.501–.900	9	14	2	10	4	39
.901–.950	3	2	1	0	0	6
.951–.975	1	3	0	2	0	6
Outcomes much worse than expected						
>.975	4	3	4	1	3	15
Total	29†	49	19	27	25	149

*For each hospital, the probability is calculated using the binomial distribution that the observed number of deaths would occur given the number of patients and the mortality rate expected based on the age and diagnosis of the patients.
†Two hospitals, with one and two patients each, are excluded.

Table 19.2: Characteristics of Selected Hospitals

Hospital	No. of Patients	No. of Cardiac Catheterization Deaths	Ratio of Observed/ Expected Deaths	Expected Death Rate	Probability	No. of Beds	No. of Neighboring Hospitals	No. With Catheterization Laboratories	Medical School Affiliated
A	70	6	6.261	0.0137	.99995	100	0	0	No
B	161	24	6.179	0.0241	.99999	200	26	12	No
C	423	1	0.163	0.0145	.01493	500	7	6	No
D	474	0	0.000	0.0051	.08877	300	8	2	No
E	1,036	27	1.631	0.0159	.99403	600	29	7	Yes

higher and lower than expected death rates, and some hospitals that might stand out to the casual observer. While in a real situation one would have substantially more data available about each hospital, even this limited information is instructive.

Hospital A has a death rate more than six times what would be expected based on its case mix, which is highly unlikely as a chance occurrence. The hospital has only 100 beds and is not affiliated with a medical school. It has no neighboring hospitals within 15 miles, and there may be few alternatives available within any reasonable distance. In contrast, hospital B is within 15 miles of 26 other hospitals, 12 of which have catheterization laboratories, so it is difficult to justify its similarly poor performance on the grounds of access. With 24 deaths among 161 patients, hospital B is likely to be quickly chosen for review, but what about hospital E with 27 deaths among 1,036 patients? This is a large, medical school–affiliated hospital, with many neighboring facilities, yet its death rate is almost two thirds above what would be expected based on its case mix, and given the large number of patients, such outcomes are extremely unlikely by chance. It may be the case, however, that careful review of the patients' charts, such as in a mortality and morbidity conference, will uncover risk factors that account for the deaths and are not included in the risk measure.

Probabilities are also useful in evaluating what may appear to be very favorable death rates. The performance of hospital D, with zero deaths among almost 500 patients, at first glance appears superior to that of hospital C, with one death among about 400 patients. However, hospital D's case mix is at substantially lower risk of death, and its zero death rate is not significantly different than what would be expected by chance.

COMMENT

These data demonstrate that for a procedure such as cardiac catheterization, one can use readily available case abstract data for a large sample of hospitals to discern an inverse relation between the number of patients treated in a hospital and their subsequent mortality. Recognition of such a relationship may suggest to some that patients should be directed away from low-volume institutions and toward high-volume hospitals. However, even if this were an appropriate conclusion for policy purposes, there is much more to consider than just volume. Some low-volume hospitals have quite good outcomes and some high-volume hospitals have outcomes significantly worse than expected for their case mix. In designing policies in response to these findings, it is important to distinguish policies that are appropriately directed toward groups or classes of institutions and those directed toward individual hospitals. The observation of a general relation between volume and outcome suggests that if there is no way to obtain better, more specific data, then volume may be a useful indicator for certain situations. For example, if general advice is to be given to the public about cardiac catheterization, it would not be inappropriate to mention that institutions with higher volumes generally have better outcomes than those with very low volumes of fewer than 200 procedures per year. Third-party payers seeking selective contracts may choose to negotiate only with high-volume centers, both because their outcomes in general are better and because even if low-volume centers have good results, it cannot be proved because of the wide confidence intervals. Similarly, hospital malpractice carriers might want to take volume into account in adjusting their premiums if they find that claims experience is related to volume. In each instance, the recommendations are based on general guidelines that are appropriate for probabilistic situations.

If one needs to refer a specific patient for a procedure, much more information than volume is usually available and should be used. For example, a certain physician or medical center having a particularly good reputation in the area may be recognized as being the place to go for extremely complicated cases. This implies that any strategy designed to influence existing referral patterns must proceed with caution in the identification of the preferred hospitals.

The situation is even more complex if one is undertaking a review of hospital performance to assess quality of care, such as is mandated for PROs. The inherent variability in patient outcomes means that death rates even several times the expected value may not be significantly different from the norm. More importantly, the observation of zero deaths may provide little useful information if the expected death rate is low and the number of patients small.

The data presented in this article refer to in-hospital death rates after cardiac catheterization, but the general observations apply to any outcomes with similar rates of occurrence. Similar analyses have been performed for other procedures and diagnoses. In general, if the rate of adverse outcomes is substantially higher than 1%, such as the 16% death rate for acute myocardial infarction, then it is easier to identify good or poor performance with some degree of statistical confidence. On the other hand, diagnoses and procedures with very high mortality rates often involve extremely ill patients for whom the underlying clinical factors dominate physician or hospital performance, and few hospitals have enough such patients to identify significantly better or worse results. However, one need not be limited to the analysis of mortality. Rates of postoperative complications, infections, or readmissions are similar to the range explored herein of about 1% to 15%.

It is inherently more difficult to identify better or worse than expected performance in hospitals with low volumes because the confidence intervals are so wide. This does not mean, however, that it is fruitless to monitor low-volume hospitals. For example, by pooling several years of data, one can accumulate enough patient observations to reduce confidence intervals to a useful range. Similarly, one may be able to pool patients undergoing related procedures while including controls for the risks of each procedure to increase the sample size.

Once the limitations of small numbers of patients and infrequent occurrences are recognized, there are still roles for routinely collected data in evaluating hospital outcomes. Third-party payers might choose to selectively contract only with hospitals providing outcome measures and to reject those with significantly poor results. Routinely collected data can also be used as an indicator of where more detailed case review is likely to uncover real problems. If abstracts are to be used as indicators, then it is appropriate to cast a wider rather than a narrower net, or, in statistical terms, it is preferable to have many false-positives at the first stage to minimize the number of false-negatives. Thus, Tables 19.3 and 19.4 identify for various combinations of volumes and probabilities the 80% confidence intervals instead of the more conventional 90% or 95% intervals. These are designed to be somewhat conservative, and therefore they identify the points that are above what would be expected by chance 10% of the time and below what would be expected by chance 10% of the time.

Table 19.3 shows the minimum number of deaths that would have to be

Table 19.3:   Number of Deaths Consistent with a Statistically Significant Poor Outcome (at .10 Significance Level)

Expected Death Rate	No. of Patients						
	5	10	20	50	100	200	500
0.001	1*	1*	1*	1*	1*	2	2
0.005	1*	1*	1*	2	2	3	6
0.01	1*	1*	2	2	3	5	9
0.05	2	2	3	6	9	15	32
0.10	2	3	5	9	15	27	60
0.15	3	4	6	12	21	38	86
0.20	3	5	7	15	26	48	113

*Zero deaths are expected to be observed more than 90% of the time with these combinations of death rates and patients. The observation of one death is highly unlikely by chance.

Table 19.4:   Maximum Number of Deaths Consistent with Statistically Significant Good Outcomes (at .10 Significance Level)

Expected Death Rate	No. of Patients						
	5	10	20	50	100	200	500
0.001	NP*	NP	NP	NP	NP	NP	NP
0.005	NP	NP	NP	NP	NP	NP	0
0.01	NP	NP	NP	NP	NP	NP	1
0.05	NP	NP	NP	0	1	5	18
0.10	NP	NP	NP	1	5	14	40
0.15	NP	NP	0	3	10	23	64
0.20	NP	NP	1	5	14	32	88

*NP indicates not possible to show statistically significant good outcomes for this combination of expected death rate and volume level.

observed to reject, with a 10% significance level, the null hypothesis that the outcome in a given hospital is not different from the expected rate. For example, if there is an expected death rate of 15%, such as for abdominal aortic aneurysm, at least six deaths would have to be observed among 20 patients to indicate significantly poor results at the .10 level. If only five deaths are observed, even though the calculated death rate of 25% is substantially above the expected rate of 15%, it is not statistically significant.

Table 19.4 shows the maximum number of deaths consistent with significantly good outcomes, again at the 10% level. For example, the observation of no deaths among 20 patients with a 15% expected death rate is likely to occur less than 10% of the time. The large number of cells labeled not possible indicates how difficult it is to identify a hospital or physician as performing significantly better than average even if no deaths are observed. For example, even a zero death rate is not significant for a hospital with 200 patients whose expected death rate is .01.

Even if a hospital is identified as having significantly better or worse than expected performance, one is not justified in either ordering champagne or demanding closure, because such results do occur by chance. Statistically significant results are not definitive, but should be interpreted as warning flags that require further investigation. Hospitals with significantly worse than expected performance should be selected for intensive chart audit or other appropriate quality review activities. Such a process or routine monitoring with feedback of results for institution-specific examination and review offers the potential for important improvements in quality.[16] Similarly, before policies are designed to channel patients toward specific hospitals with apparently better than expected outcomes, or before they are even publicly identified as good performers, it is important that other types of evaluations support the designation.

If precautions are not taken before acting on outcome statistics, average performers will occasionally be mistakenly identified as being either worse or better than they truly are. In the first instance, they will be incorrectly labeled as having worse than expected outcomes, and libel suits might ensue. In the second instance, patients may be inappropriately redirected toward hospitals with performance not truly better than average, and there may be some liability in this case for worse outcomes than would have occurred had the shift not taken place.

In spite of these statistical caveats, it is quite reasonable to use large data sets to examine general patterns of performance such as the relation between volume and outcome. Such results might be useful to malpractice carriers in rate setting or to third-party payers seeking to limit their negotiations to high-quality institutions. Furthermore, much of the problem identified in this article arises from the low death rate associated with most hospitalizations. If complications are considered, then it is possible to examine interhospital differences with smaller samples.

As the focus of attention shifts to the evaluation of individual hospital or even physician performance, much more attention needs to be paid to the unmeasured aspects of the cases, and less reliance should be placed on general patterns.

Hebel et al[10] have demonstrated how case abstract data can be used as the starting point in examining why a hospital appears to have a higher death rate than its neighbors. They begin with overall mortality, adjust for case mix and other factors, then narrow their focus to specific diagnostic categories. However, the shift from the general to the specific means that the number of patients quickly becomes very small. The inherent variability in patient outcomes, especially if one focuses on rare events such as death, means that statistical confidence becomes increasingly difficult to attain. It would help if attention were to shift to complication rates, both during hospitalization through charts and more detailed abstract review and after hospitalization through the analysis of insurance claims. Thus, while readily available data are a powerful and inexpensive guide they can only be used to begin the process of evaluating performance of hospitals and physicians.

This research was supported in part by grant HS-04329 from the National Center for Health Services Research. We are grateful for comments from Warren Browner, MD, John Bunker, MD, Stephen McPhee, MD, Nancy Ramsay, MA, and Susan Sacks, PhD.

REFERENCES

1. Flood AB, Scott WR, Ewy W: Does practice make perfect: I. The relation between hospital volume and outcomes for selected diagnostic categories. *Med Care* 1984; 22:98–114.
2. Flood AB, Scott WR, Ewy W: Does practice make perfect: II. The relation between volume and outcomes and other hospital characteristics. *Med Care* 1984;22:115–125.
3. Shortell S, LoGerfo J: Hospital medical staff organization and quality of care: Results for myocardial infarction and appendectomy. *Med Care* 1981;19:1041–1055.
4. Luft HS, Bunker J, Enthoven A: Should operations be regionalized? The empirical relation between surgical volume and mortality. *N Engl J Med* 1979;301:1364–1369.
5. Luft HS: The relation between surgical volume and mortality: An exploration of causal factors and alternative models. *Med Care* 1980;18:940–959.
6. Riley G, Lubitz J: Outcomes of surgery in the Medicare aged population: Mortality after surgery. *Health Care Financing Rev* 1985;6:103–115.
7. Farber B, Kaiser D, Wenzel R: Relation between surgical volume and incidence of postoperative wound infection. *N Engl J Med* 1981;305:200–203.
8. Iglehart JK: Cutting costs of health care for the poor in California: A two-year follow-up. *N Engl J Med* 1981;311:745–748.
9. Bargmann E, Grove C: *Surgery in Maryland Hospitals, 1979 and 1980, Charges and Deaths*. Washington, DC, Public Citizen Health Research Group, 1982.
10. Hebel JR, Kessler I, Mabuchi K, et al: Assessment of hospital performance by use of death rates. *JAMA* 1982;248:3131–3135.
11. Adams DF, Fraser DB, Abrams HL: The complications of coronary arteriography. *Circulation* 1973;48:609–618.
12. Dranove D: A comment on "Does practice make perfect?" *Med Care* 1984;22:967.

13. Flood AB, Scott WR, Ewy W: Letter in reply. *Med Care* 1984;22:967–969.
14. Luft HS, Hunt SS, Maerki SC: *The Volume-Outcome Relationship: Practice Makes Perfect or Selective Referral Patterns?* San Francisco, Institute for Health Policy Studies, 1985.
15. Maerki SC, Luft HS, Hunt SS: Selecting categories of patients for regionalization: Implications of the relationship between volume and outcome. *Med Care* 1986;24:148–158.
16. Moses LE, Mosteller F: Institutional differences in postoperative death rates. *JAMA* 1968;203:492–494.

References

Adams, D. F.; Fraser, D. B.; and Abrams, H. L. (1973). "The Complications of Coronary Arteriography." *Circulation* 48 (3): 609–18.

Aronow, D. B. (1988). "Severity-of-Illness Measurement: Applications in Quality Assurance and Utilization Review." *Medical Care Review* 45 (2): 339-66.

Asher, H. (1956). *Cost-Quantity Relationships in the Airframe Industry.* Santa Monica, CA: The Rand Corporation.

Blumberg, M. S. (1986). "Risk Adjusting Health Care Outcomes: A Methodologic Review." *Medical Care Review* 43 (2): 351–93.

——— (1987). "Comments on HCSF Hospital Death Rate Statistical Outliers." *Health Services Research* 21 (6): 715–40.

Center for the Study of Services (1987). "Hospitals." *Consumer Checkbook* 6 (3): 13–26.

Chassin, M. R.; Kosecoff, J.; Park, R. E.; Winslow, C. M.; Kahn, K. L.; Merrick, N. J.; Keesey, J.; Fink, A.; Solomon, D. H; and Brook, R. H. (1987). "Does Inappropriate Use Explain Geographic Variations in the Use of Health Care Services?" *Journal of the American Medical Association* 258 (18): 2533–37.

Davies, A. R.; and Ware, J. E.; Jr. (1988). "Involving Consumers in Quality of Care Assessment." *Health Affairs* 7 (1): 33–48.

DesHarnais, S. I.; Chesney, J. D.; Wroblewski, R. T.; Fleming, S. T.; and McMahon, L. F.; Jr. (1988). "The Risk-Adjusted Mortality Index: A New Measure of Hospital Performance." *Medical Care* 26 (12): 1129–48.

Dranove, D. (1984). "A Comment on 'Does Practice Make Perfect?'" *Medical Care* 22 (10): 967.

DuBois, R. W.; Brook, R. H.; and Rogers, W. H. (1987). "Adjusted Hospital Death Rates: A Potential Screen for Quality of Medical Care." *American Journal of Public Health* 77 (9): 1162–66.

Farber, B. F.; Kaiser, D. L.; and Wenzel, R. P. (1981). "Relation between Surgical Volume and Incidence of Postoperative Wound Infection." *New England Journal of Medicine* 305 (4): 200–204. [This study is reprinted in Chapter 9 of this volume.]

Fleiss, J. L. (1981). *Statistical Methods for Rates and Proportions.* New York: Wiley.

Flood, A. B.; Ewy, W.; Scott, W. R.; Forrest, W. H., Jr.; and Brown, B.W., Jr. (1979). "The Relationship between Intensity and Duration of Medical Services and Outcomes for Hospitalized Patients." *Medical Care* 17 (11): 1088–1102.

Flood, A. B.; and Scott, W. R. (1987). *Hospital Structure and Performance.* Baltimore: The Johns Hopkins University Press.

Flood, A. B.; Scott, W. R.; and Ewy, W. (1984a). "Does Practice Make Perfect? Part I: The Relation between Volume and Outcomes for Selected Diagnostic Categories. Part II: The

Relation between Volume and Outcomes and Other Hospital Characteristics". *Medical Care* 22 (2): 98–114, 115–25. [Part I is reprinted in Chapter 14 of this volume.]

——— (1984b). "Reply to Dranove." *Medical Care* 22 (10): 967–69.

Fowles, J.; Bunker, J. P.; and Schurman, D. J. (1987). "Hip Surgery Data Yield Quality Indicators." *Business and Health* 4 (8): 44–46.

Garnick, D.; Luft, H.; McPhee, S.; and Mark, D. (1989). "Surgeon Volume vs Hospital Volume: Which Matters More?" *Journal of the American Medical Association* 262 (4): 547.

Glass, G. (1976). "Primary, Secondary, and Meta Analysis of Research." *Educational Researcher* 5: 3–8.

Gonnella, J. S.; Hornbrook, M. C.; and Louis, D. Z. (1984). "Staging of Disease: A Case-Mix Measurement." *Journal of the American Medical Association* 251 (5): 637–44.

Hannan, E. L.; O'Donnell, J. F.; Kilburn, H., Jr.; Bernard, H. R.; and Yazici, A. (1989). "Investigation of the Relationship between Volume and Mortality for Surgical Procedures Performed in New York State Hospitals." *Journal of the American Medical Association* 262 (4): 503–10.

Hertzer, N. R.; Avellone, J. C.; Farrell, C. J.; Plecha, F. R.; Rhodes, R. S.; Sharp, W. V.; and Wright, G. F. (1984). "The Risk of Vascular Surgery in a Metropolitan Community." *Journal of Vascular Surgery* 1 (1): 13–21.

Hsia, D. C.; Krushat, W. M.; Fagan, A. B.; Tebbut, J. A.; and Kusserow, R. P. (1988). "Accuracy of Diagnostic Coding for Medicare Patients under the Prospective Payment System." *New England Journal of Medicine* 318 (6): 352–55.

Hughes, R. G.; Garnick, D. W.; Luft, H. S.; McPhee, S. J.; and Hunt, S. S. (1988). "Hospital Volume and Patient Outcomes: The Case of Hip Fracture Patients." *Medical Care* 26 (11): 1057–67.

Hughes, R. G.; Hunt, S. S.; and Luft, H. S. (1987). "Effects of Surgeon Volume and Hospital Volume on Quality of Care in Hospitals." *Medical Care* 25 (6): 489–503. [This study is reprinted in Chapter 17 of this volume.]

Hughes, R. G.; and Lee, D. E. (1990). "Public Information on Private Practice: The Availability of Physician Inpatient Data." *Hospital & Health Services Administration* 35 (1): 55–69.

Iglehart, J. K. (1984). "Cutting Costs of Health Care for the Poor in California: A Two-Year Follow-Up." *New England Journal of Medicine* 311 (11): 745–48.

Institute of Medicine (1980). "Reliability of National Hospital Discharge Survey Data." Washington, DC: National Academy of Sciences.

Jencks, S. F.; Williams, D. K,; and Kay, T. L. (1988). "Assessing Hospital-Associated Deaths from Discharge Data." *Journal of the American Medical Association* 206 (15): 2240–46.

Kelly, J. V. (1988). "Deaths in Teaching and Nonteaching Hospitals: Quality of Care and Severity of Illness Differences." National Center for Health Services Research Working Paper.

Kelly, J. V.; and Hellinger, F. J. (1986). "Physician and Hospital Factors Associated with Mortality of Surgical Patients." *Medical Care* 24 (9): 785–800.

——— (1987). "Heart Disease and Hospital Deaths: An Empirical Study." *Health Services Research* 22 (3): 369–95. [This study is reprinted in Chapter 10 of this volume.]

Kempczinski, R. F.; Brott, T. G.; and Labutta, R. J. (1986). "The Influence of Surgical Specialty and Caseload on the Results of Carotid Endarterectomy." *Journal of Vascular Surgery* 3 (6): 911–16.

Light, R. J,; and Pillemer, D. B. (1984). *Summing Up: The Science of Reviewing Research.* Cambridge, MA: Harvard University Press.

Luft, H. S. (1978). "Why Do HMOs Seem to Provide More Health Maintenance Services?" *Milbank Memorial Fund Quarterly/Health and Society* 56 (2): 140–68.

———— (1980). "The Relation between Surgical Volume and Mortality: An Exploration of Causal Factors and Alternative Models." *Medical Care* 18 (9): 940–59. [This study is reprinted in Chapter 16 of this volume.]

Luft, H. S.; Bunker, J. P.; and Enthoven, A. C. (1979). "Should Operations Be Regionalized: The Empirical Relation between Surgical Volume and Mortality." *New England Journal of Medicine* 301 (25): 1364–69. [This study is reprinted in Chapter 12 of this volume.]

Luft, H. S.; Garnick, D. W.; Mark, D. H.; Peltzman, D. J.; Phibbs, C. S.; Lichtenberg, E.; and McPhee, S. J. (1990) "Does Quality Influence Choice of Hospital?" *Journal of the American Medical Association*. In press.

Luft, H. S.; and Hunt, S. S. (1986). "Evaluating Individual Hospital Quality through Outcome Statistics." *Journal of the American Medical Association* 255 (20): 2780–84. [This study is reprinted in Chapter 19 of this volume.]

Luft, H. S.; Hunt, S. S.; and Maerki, S. C. (1987). "The Volume- Outcome Relationship: Practice Makes Perfect or Selective Referral Patterns?" *Health Services Research* 22 (2): 157–82.

Maerki, S. C.; Luft, H. S.; and Hunt, S. S. (1986). "Selecting Categories of Patients for Regionalization: Implications of the Relationship between Volume and Outcome." *Medical Care* 24 (2): 148–58.

Manning, W., Jr.; Liebowitz, A.; and Goldberg, G. A. (1984). "A Controlled Trial of the Effect of a Prepaid Group Practice on Use of Services." *New England Journal of Medicine* 310 (23): 1505–10.

Neutra, R. (1977). "Indications for the Surgical Treatment of Suspected Acute Appendicitis: A Cost-Effectiveness Approach." In *Costs, Risks and Benefits of Surgery,* edited by J. P. Bunker, B. Barnes, and F. Mosteller, 277–307. London: Oxford University Press.

Paul-Shaheen, P.; Clark, J. E.; and Williams, D. (1987). "Small Area Analysis, A Review of the North American Literature." *Journal of Health Politics, Policy and Law* 12 (4): 741–809.

Pilcher, D. B.; Davis, J. H.; Ashikaga, T.; Bookwalter, J.; Butsch, D. W.; Chase, C. R.; Ellman, B. R.; Vacek, P. M.; and Lord, F. C. (1980). "Treatment of Abdominal Aortic Aneurysm in an Entire State over 7½ Years." *American Journal of Surgery* 139 (4): 487–94.

Riley, G. and Lubitz, J. (1985). "Outcomes of Surgery among the Medicare Aged: Surgical Volume and Mortality." *Health Care Financing Review* 7 (1): 37–47. [This study is reprinted in Chapter 15 of this volume.]

Roos, L. L.; Cageorge, S. M.; Roos, N. P.; and Danzinger, R. (1986). "Centralization, Certification, and Monitoring: Readmissions and Complications after Surgery." *Medical Care* 24 (11): 1044–66. [This study is reprinted in Chapter 8 of this volume.]

Roos, L. L., and Roos, N. P. (1983). "Assessing Existing Technologies: The Manitoba Study of Common Surgical Procedures." *Medical Care* 21 (4): 454–62.

Roos, L. L.; Roos, N. P.; and Sharp, S. M. (1987). "Monitoring Adverse Outcomes of Surgery Using Administrative Data." *Health Care Financing Review* (Annual Supplement) 5–16.

Roos, N. P. (1984). "Hysterectomy: Variations in Rates Across Small Areas and Across Physicians' Practices." *American Journal of Public Health* 74 (4): 327–35.

Rosenblatt, R. A.; Reinken, J.; and Shoemack, P. (1985). "Is Obstetrics Safe in Small Hospitals? Evidence from New Zealand's Regionalised Perinatal System." *Lancet* 2 (8452): 429–32.

Rosenthal, R. (1979). "The 'File Drawer Problem' and Tolerance for Null Results." *Psychological Bulletin* 86: 638–41.

———— (1984). *Meta Analytic Procedures for Analytic Research.* Beverly Hills, CA: Sage Publications.

Rosenthal, R., and Rubin, D. B. (1988). "Comment: Assumptions and Procedures in the File Drawer Problem." *Statistical Science* 3 (1): 120–26.

Shortell, S. M.; and LoGerfo, J. P. (1981). "Hospital Medical Staff Organization and Quality of Care: Results for Myocardial Infarction and Appendectomy." *Medical Care* 19 (10): 1041–53.

Showstack, J. A.; Rosenfeld, K. E.; Garnick, D. W.; Luft, H. S.; Schaffarzick, R. E.; and Fowles, J. (1987). "Association of Volume with Outcome of Coronary Artery Bypass Graft Surgery." *Journal of the American Medical Association* 257 (6): 785–89. [This study is reprinted in Chapter 11 of this volume.]

Sloan, F. A.; Perrin, J. M.; and Valvona, F. (1986). "In-Hospital Mortality of Surgical Patients: Is There an Empiric Basis for Standard Setting?" *Surgery* 99 (4): 446–53. [This study is reprinted in Chapter 13 of this volume.]

Steinbrook, R. (1988). "Hospital Quality in California." *Health Affairs* 7 (3): 235–36.

Trauner, J. B. (1983). "Preferred Provider Organizations: The California Experiment." San Francisco: Institute for Health Policy Studies. University of California, San Francisco. Working paper.

U. S. Congress (1988). Office of Technology Assessment. *The Quality of Medical Care: Information for Consumers*. Washington, DC: U.S. Government Printing Office.

U. S. Department of Health and Human Services (1987). "Medicare Hospital Mortality Information 1986." Health Care Financing Administration.

——— (1988). "Medicare Hospital Mortality Information 1987." Health Care Financing Administration. HCFA Pub. No. 01–002.

Wennberg, J. E.; Blowers, L.; Parker, R.; Gittelsohn, A. M. (1977). "Changes in Tonsillectomy Rates Associated with Feedback and Review." *Pediatrics* 59 (6): 821–26.

Wennberg, J. E.; and Gittelsohn, A. M. (1973). "Small Area Variations in Health Care Delivery." *Science* 182 (4117): 1102–8.

——— (1975). "Health Care Delivery in Maine I: Patterns of Use of Common Surgical Procedures." *Journal of the Maine Medical Association* 66 (May): 123–30, 149.

Wennberg, J. E.; Roos, N. P.; Sola, L.; Schori, A.; and Jaffe, R. (1987). "Use of Claims Data Systems to Evaluate Health Care Outcomes: Mortality and Reoperation Following Prostatectomy." *Journal of the American Medical Association* 257 (7): 933–36.

Whiting-O'Keefe, Q. E.; Henke, C,; and Simborg, D. W. (1984). "Choosing the Correct Unit of Analysis in Medical Care Experiments." *Medical Care* 22 (12): 1101–14.

Williams, R. L. (1979). "Measuring the Effectiveness of Perinatal Medical Care." *Medical Care* 17 (2): 95–109. [This study is reprinted in Chapter 18 of this volume.]

Index

Abdominal aortic aneurysm, 40, 41, 44,
98, 110-12; and hospital volume, 110;
and mortality, 110; and physician volume, 110; and volume-outcome
relationship, 102, 106
Abdominal hysterectomy, 39, 181
Abrams, Herbert L., 31
Acute myocardial infarction, 39-40,
126-28, 173, 190, 191, 202, 206-8,
338, 390; case selection, 215; and coronary care units, 208, 209; and
hospital volume, 126, 127; and mortality, 45, 388; and physician volume,
126, 127, 207, 340; and types of
patients, 126, 127; and volume-outcome relationship, 208, 209
Adams, Douglass F., 31
Age, volume-outcome relationship and,
11, 302
American College of Obstetricians and
Gynecologists, 369
American College of Surgeons, 216, 217,
225, 341
American Hospital Association, 196, 263,
342
American Journal of Surgery, 38
American Medical Association, 193
American Peer Review Organization, 163
American Society of Anesthesiologists,
237
Amputation of lower limb: and mortality,
273, 274; and patient risk level, 274
Angina pectoris, 202

Angiography, 117, 202
Angioplasty, 117
Aorto-femoral reconstruction, 40
Apgar scores, 369, 370, 373, 375
Appendectomy, 39, 40, 115-17, 181, 338;
and hospital volume, 115-16; infection
rates, 182, 185; and mortality, 115; and
physician volume, 116, 340
Area Resource File, 342
Arteriography, 205
Asher, H., 11
Ashikaga, Takamuru, 38
Association of American Medical Col-
leges, 194
"Association of Volume with Outcome of
Coronary Artery Bypass Graft Sur-
gery" (Showstack et al.), 47-48, 216
Avellone, Joseph C., 40

Biliary tract surgery, 113-15; and hospital
volume, 115; and physician volume,
115; and volume-outcome relationship,
101, 104, 114, 237
Births (California), selected charac-
teristics, 368
Bookwalter, John, 38
Bowel operations, and mortality, 276
Brook, R. H., 21
Brott, Thomas G., 43
Bunker, John P., 5, 33, 45, 146
Business and Health, 45
Butsch, David W., 38

About the Authors

Harold S. Luft is Professor of Health Economics and Associate Director of the Institute for Health Policy Studies at the University of California, San Francisco. He received his undergraduate and graduate training at Harvard University, majoring in economics with a specialization in health economics. Prior to joining the University of California, San Francisco in 1978, Dr. Luft was Assistant Professor in the Health Services Research Program at Stanford University. He is a member of the Institute of Medicine of the National Academy of Sciences. His research has covered a wide range of areas, including applications of benefit-cost analysis, studies of medical care utilization, the relationship between hospital volume and patient outcomes, regionalization of hospital services, adverse selection in multiple-option health insurance settings, competition in the medical care market, and health maintenance organizations. In addition to numerous articles in scientific journals, he is the author of *Poverty and Health: Economic Causes and Consequences of Health Problems* and *Health Maintenance Organizations: Dimensions of Performance*.

Deborah W. Garnick joined the Department of Health Policy and Management, Program on Health Care Financing and Insurance, at Harvard University's School of Public Health in 1989. Previously, she was a Senior Research Associate for five years at the University of California, San Francisco. Since completing her doctoral training at the Johns Hopkins University School of Hygiene and Public Health, her research interests have included hospital competition, managed care, the relationship between hospital volume and patient outcomes, and the quality of care.

David H. Mark, M.D., is Director of Research in the Department of Family Medicine, Medical College of Wisconsin. He received his degree in medicine from Harvard Medical School and trained in surgery at Virginia Mason Hospital in Seattle, Washington, and preventive medicine at the University of California in San Francisco and Berkeley. He was a Pew Postdoctoral Fellow at the Institute for

Health Policy Studies at the University of California, San Francisco. Dr. Mark's research interests include quality assurance in medical care and the assessment of various surgical procedures.

Stephen J. McPhee, M.D., is Associate Professor of Medicine in the Division of General Internal Medicine and a faculty member in the Institute for Health Policy Studies, both at the University of California, San Francisco. He received his degree in medicine from the Johns Hopkins University School of Medicine and completed his internal medicine training at the Johns Hopkins Hospital in Baltimore, Maryland. Dr. McPhee has a background in health services research, obtained as a Henry J. Kaiser Family Foundation Fellow in General Internal Medicine at the Johns Hopkins University School of Medicine prior to his appointment to the faculty at the University of California, San Francisco. He has research experience in and has published articles on several areas of health services research, including disease prevention and health promotion, methods of changing physicians' behavior, graduate medical education, health care cost containment, medical technology assessment, and quality assurance. He is coeditor of the annually updated textbook *Current Medical Diagnosis and Treatment*.